BASIC METHODS IN

Antibody Production
and
Characterization

BASIC METHODS IN
Antibody Production
and
Characterization

Edited by

Gary C. Howard
Castro Valley, CA

Delia R. Bethell
BioSeparations, Inc.
Tucson, AZ

CRC Press
Boca Raton   London   New York   Washington, D.C.

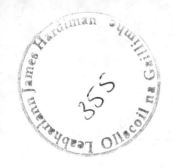

Library of Congress Cataloging-in-Publication Data

Basic methods in antibody production and characterization / edited by Gary C. Howard
and Delia R. Bethell
      p. cm.
Includes bibliographical references and index.
ISBN 0-8493-9445-7 (alk. paper)
1. Immunoglobulins—Laboratory manuals. I. Howard, Gary C. II. Bethell, Delia R.

QR186.7 .B37 2000
616.07′98—dc21
                                      00-033729
                                          CIP

Visit the CRC Press Web site at www.crcpress.com

Preface

Antibodies have become indispensable tools for biomedical research. Their extraordinary specificity of binding is matched by their ease of use and adaptability to many experimental and now even some therapeutic applications.

Basic Methods in Antibody Production and Characterization is a cookbook of methods for the production and use of antibodies. We have attempted to cover all aspects of polyclonal and monoclonal antibodies. Many of the procedures are well established. Others (e.g., phage display) are quite new. Although we have sought to present this material in a simple step-by-step manner, no methods book can cover every experimental protocol. Each contributor has provided introductory material to give a basic understanding of the methods and references to other applications of his or her chapter's particular technology.

The methods presented are more or less in chronological order. The most important element in making antibodies is the ultimate purpose of the experiments. Time, experience, expense, and the scientific questions to be answered will direct the choice of methods for antibody production.

We want to thank each of the contributors to this volume. Without their professional knowledge and enthusiastic efforts, the book would not have been possible. We also thank Yale Altman for his encouragement, guidance, and unflagging support throughout the project.

The Editors

Gary C. Howard, Ph.D., received a B.A. in zoology in 1971 and an M.S. in biology from West Virginia University, Morgantown, and a Ph.D. in biological sciences from Carnegie Mellon University, Pittsburgh, PA. After fellowships at Harvard and Johns Hopkins, Dr. Howard spent 10 years with biotech companies. He edited *Methods in Nonradioactive Detection* (Appleton & Lange, 1993) and, with W. E. Brown, is currently preparing a volume on the practical aspects of advanced methods in protein chemistry for CRC Press. Dr. Howard is a freelance editor and writer and a senior scientific editor for the J. David Gladstone Institutes, a private biomedical research institution affiliated with the University of California, San Francisco.

Delia R. Bethell, Ph.D., received a B.S. in biology from Newcomb College, Tulane University, New Orleans, LA, in 1968, an M.S. in biology from University of Denver, Denver, CO, and a Ph.D. in physiology at Hershey Medical Center, Pennsylvania State University. Dr. Bethell has worked with the production of monoclonal antibodies and their use in the area of *in vitro* diagnostics for a number of years. She has served on the Executive Board of the Society for In Vitro Biology for the past 10 years, holding the office of President from 1998 to 2000. Dr. Bethell is currently director of research with BioSeparations, Inc., in Tuscon, AZ.

Contributors

Peter Amersdorfer, Ph.D.
Phylos
300 Putnam Avenue
Cambridge, MA 02139
pamersdorfer@phylos.com

Jory R. Baldridge, Ph.D.
Ribi ImmunoChem Research, Inc.
553 Old Corvallis Road
Hamilton, MT 59840

Eric S. Bean, Ph.D.
HTI Bio-Products
P.O. Box 1319
Ramona, CA 92065
esbean@home.com

Lee Bendickson
Department of Biochemistry,
  Biophysics and Molecular Biology
Iowa State University
Ames, IA 50011

Delia R. Bethell, Ph.D.
BioSeparations, Inc.
245 South Plumer Avenue, Suite 28
Tuscon, AZ 85719
dbethell@bioseparations.com

Kathryn Elwell
Genzyme Diagnostics, Inc.
1531 Industrial Road
San Carlos, CA 94070
kjelwell@webtv.net

Michael J. Gramer
Cellex Biosciences
8500 Evergreen Boulevard
Minneapolis, MN 55433

Nicholas R. Griffin, M.D.
Consultant Histopathologist
Histopathology Department
Airedale General Hospital
Skipton Road near Keighley
Yorkshire BD20 6TD
England

Neil M. Hand
Chief Medical Laboratory
  Scientific Officer
Histopathology Department
  University Hospital
Queen's Medical Centre
Nottingham NG7 2UH
England
mpznhand@unix.ccc.nottingham.ac.uk

Kristi R. Harkins, Ph.D.
Iowa State University
1104 Molecular Biology Building
Ames, IA 50011
kharkins@iastate.edu

Mark D. Hirschel, Ph.D.
Cellex Biosciences
8500 Evergreen Boulevard
Coon Rapids, MN

Gary C. Howard, Ph.D.
17015 High Pine Way
Castro Valley, CA 94546
gsrahoward@aol.com

Michael J. Lacy
Ribi ImmunoChem Research, Inc.
553 Old Corvallis Road
Hamilton, MT 59840

Warren Ladiges, Ph.D.
Associate Professor
Department of Comparative Medicine
T-140 Health Science Building
School of Medicine
University of Washington
Seattle, WA 98195
wladiges@u.washington.edu

Donald H. Lewis, Ph.D.
Professor
Department of Veterinary Pathobiology
College of Veterinary Medicine
Texas A&M University
College Station, TX 77843
dlewis@ cvm.tamu.edu

James D. Marks, M.D.
Professor
Department of Anesthesia, 3C38
University of California, San Francisco
San Francisco General Hospital
San Francisco, CA 94110
marksj@anesthesia.ucsf.edu

Kendrick J. Morrell
Immunocytochemistry Laboratory
   Manager
Histopathology Department
University Hospital
Queen's Medical Centre
Nottingham NG7 2UH
England

Marit Nilsen-Hamilton, Ph.D.
Professor
Department of Biochemistry,
   Biophysics and Molecular Biology
Iowa State University
3206 Molecular Biology Building
Ames, IA 50011
marit@iastate.edu

Beverly J. Norris
Cellex Biosciences
8500 Evergreen Boulevard
Minneapolis, MN 55433
bnorris@bilbo.intexp.com

Gamal E. Osman, Ph.D.
Senior Research Manager
Antigenics Inc.
34 Commerce Way
Woburn, MA 01801
gosman@antigenics.com

Sigmund T. Rich, D.V.M.
1574 Holt Avenue
Los Altos, CA 94024

Sandy J. Stewart, Ph.D.
Paradigm Genetics
P.O. Box 12257
Research Triangle Park, NC 27709
sstewart@paragen.com

Contents

1 Starting Out

Delia R. Bethell and Gary C. Howard

CONTENTS

1.1 MONOCLONALS VS. POLYCLONAL ANTIBODIES

Antibodies are extraordinarily useful molecules. Their highly specific binding to a wide range of molecules, including peptides, carbohydrates, and nucleic acids, and their ability to identify specific antigenic determinants in these molecules make them extremely valuable — perhaps even irreplaceable — adjuncts to biomedical research.

Antibodies can be obtained from a number of sources. The original antibodies were obtained from the sera of immunized animals. These polyclonal antibodies were a mixture of different immunoglobulin types binding to multiple sites on the antigen used for immunization. In 1975, Georges Kohler and Cesar Milstein developed the process for creating monoclonal antibodies, of a single immunoglobulin type binding to a single specific site on the antigen used for immunization. They fused antibody-producing mouse B cells, cells with a finite life span, with "immortalized" cells of a mouse myeloma, and selected for the immortalized, antibody producing cells. Each cell, or clone, was capable of producing large amounts of a single type of antibody, that antibody bound to a single epitope. For this work, they shared the Nobel Prize. More recently, the DNA coding for specific antibodies and fragments of antibodies has been introduced into bacteria, yeast, and mammalian cell lines by recombinant molecular genetics techniques. This allows even greater yields of antibodies from cultured cells.

As the name indicates, polyclonal antibodies from antisera bind to a number of epitopes. Polyclonal antibodies are isolated from the serum of an immunized animal. There are typically thousands of different antibodies reacting with numerous epitopes. Polyclonal antisera usually contain most of the immunoglobulin types and a large range of affinities for the different epitopes. For many applications, such as electron microscopy, polyclonal antibodies offer some important advantages over monoclonal antibodies. For example, when searching for an antigen with multiple epitopes, one polyclonal antibody can reach many binding sites, increasing the detection sensitivity.

In contrast to polyclonal antibodies, monoclonal antibodies are highly selective and unlimited amounts of equal quality can be produced in *in vitro* culture or in animals. They have powerful applications in biomedical research, diagnosis, and therapy due to this ability to reproduce exactly the same binding characteristics. Monoclonal antibodies have been generated against a seemingly endless array of compounds, including toxins, drugs, blood proteins, cancer cells, viruses, hormones, environmental pollutants, food products, metals, and plant materials. Monoclonal antibodies are routinely used to create sensitive tests for detecting small amounts of substances in a highly reproducible fashion. Scores of monoclonal antibody-based tests are used in human and animal clinical diagnostic tests. Monoclonal antibodies can be used to isolate and purify specific compounds from complex mixtures (i.e., immunoaffinity chromatography). Great strides have been made in adapting mono-clonal antibodies for the treatment of diseases such as cancer. Another novel spin-off of monoclonal antibody technology has been the creation of catalytic antibodies, or abzymes, produced by immunizing mice with enzyme transition-state analogs. Abzymes represent a whole new approach to the study of enzyme mechanisms and the creation of useful biological catalysts.

Production of recombinant antibodies by linking DNA sequences which code for antibody binding regions onto generic immunoglobulin molecules and transfer-ring the DNA into bacteria has introduced another set of advantages. Although a more complicated procedure, it eliminates many of the problems of traditional methods, such as allergic reactions in humans when exposed to a mouse monoclonal antibody. Recombinant antibodies also give researchers additional control of the final product.

Whatever their source, antibodies are extraordinarily useful. They are often stable for years in solution, lyophilized, or frozen. They can be easily modified with other combining groups or markers.

The choice of a polyclonal or monoclonal antibody for a specific experiment or assay requires careful consideration. Often a pool of well-defined monoclonal anti-bodies can accomplish many of the same things as a polyclonal reagent.

> *Sensitivity:* Monoclonal antibodies can play a role in identifying antigens present in minute quantities — such as those that may be present on cancer cells — that are often missed by heterogeneous, polyclonal, antibody prep-arations such as those made in normal immune responses.
>
> *Supply:* Monoclonal antibodies, in theory, can supply a virtually unlimited amount of antibody indefinitely. In practice, the clones can be overgrown with nonproducer strains, requiring costly and time-consuming re-cloning. Animals yielding polyclonal antiserum can likewise provide very large amounts of serum and antibody. However, every new immunization has some potential to modify the mixture of epitopes recognized, and every animal has a limited life span.
>
> *Time:* This usually relates to availability of a commercial monoclonal or polyclonal antibody. To develop either antibody takes a considerable

investment of time with no certain guarantee of success in a given application. However, many monoclonal and polyclonal antibodies are available from commercial houses or academic laboratories.

Cost: New developments in the use of bioreactors for the growth of hybridoma cell lines producing monoclonal cells have greatly reduced the cost of producing large quantities of antibodies while also reducing the requirement for the use of large numbers of animals. The cost and yield of bioreactor-grown mammalian cells is further reduced by the use of bioreactor-produced bacterial products. Yet there are still specific roles and limitations for antibodies of each category.

Ethics: Today strict regulations govern the use of animals. Although it is still usually necessary to use animals for the initial immunizations, monoclonal and recombinant procedures can greatly reduce the requirement for animals. Phage display work has the potential of totally eliminating the use of animals.

Patents: For some specific applications, there may be legal issues to consider. For example, a patent covers tests using monoclonal antibodies as capture-and-detection antibodies in ELISA and other formats. In addition, there may be limitations on the use of antibodies obtained from academic institutions. Although patents exist, many are available through license opportunities.

1.2   USING THIS MANUAL

This volume describes basic methods in the production and use of antibodies. Many of the procedures are well known and have been in use for some time. Others (e.g., phage display) are quite new. Our goal is to present this material in a simple step-by-step manner. However, no methods book covers all experimental protocols. Therefore, we have asked each contributor to include enough theoretical material to give a basic understanding of the method and references to other applications of that particular technology. Several have also included hints for troubleshooting problems.

The book follows the making of antibodies in a somewhat chronological order. The early chapters describe the various preparations for making antibodies. First, it is clearly important to think through the experiments that will ultimately use the antibodies. That will dictate the type of antibodies needed (monoclonal, polyclonal, or recombinant produced by bacteria). An overview of the legal and ethical issues surrounding the use of laboratory animals follows. Guidance concerning specific regulations should be sought before any use of animals. Antigens and adjuvants are key to the successful production of antibodies of any kind.

Chapters 5 through 10 describe the procedures for making polyclonal and monoclonal antibodies. Methods for screening monoclonal antibodies and for producing and growing them in bioreactors or as ascites in mice are covered. A final chapter reviews the phage display, a technique for producing antibodies and other protein molecules in bacteria.

Chapters 11 through 14 review methods for dealing with antibodies after they are made. These chapters provide methods for the purification, characterization, and storage of antibodies. One chapter details methods for labeling antibodies with fluorescent, biotin, or other probes to prepare them for specific applications. Later chapters describe the uses of antibodies in immunohistochemistry and western blot analysis, two widely used applications for antibodies.

1.3 LABORATORY SAFETY

The procedures described in this book involve the use of laboratory animals, radioactive labels, toxic chemicals, and other biohazards. All of these require significant levels of training and the appropriately protective clothing and methods. We encourage the researcher to ensure that proper training is provided to all persons working in the laboratory.

1.3.1 LABORATORY ANIMALS

Laboratory animals are a significant part of the production and use of antibodies. Their care and treatment are matters of law and regulation. Institutions and companies are required to have policies and procedures to ensure the health and humane treatment of animals. Appropriate care must also be exercised in the safe handling of the animals and any biological waste.

1.3.2 RADIOACTIVE MATERIALS

Low-level radioactive materials are often used as tracers and labels. The use of radioactive materials is subject to strict regulations governing use and disposal. Only trained laboratory personnel should handle radioactive materials.

1.3.3 TOXIC CHEMICALS

Many chemicals are extremely toxic. Fume hoods, gloves, proper disposal, and good technique are needed for their safe use. MSDS (Material Safety Data Sheets) are provided by all manufacturers and should be readily available in the laboratory. Disposal must be in accordance with the applicable laws and regulations.

1.3.4 GENERAL LABORATORY SAFETY

Safety is always a concern in laboratories. Solvents, biohazards, electrical hazards, and equipment safety all require specific and constant attention. Eating, drinking, and smoking have no place in laboratories. Manufacturers' instructions are also excellent sources of information for the safe use of equipment.

2 Animal Welfare and Regulatory Issues

Sigmund T. Rich

CONTENTS

2.1 INTRODUCTION

The welfare, humane care, and use of animals are governed by a number of guidelines, principles, laws, rules, and regulations. These are issued by the federal, state, and local governments and by academic and scientific societies, industrial organizations, and, most important, the institutions themselves.

Institutional Animal Care and Use Committees (IACUCs) are the most common and effective means of complying with all activities involved in the use of animals in the various biomedical fields, including research, development, teaching, training, testing, and production.

2.2 LEGAL ASPECTS

There are two major national laws governing the care and use of animals. The Animal Welfare Act (AWA) is implemented by the regulations published in the Code of Federal Regulations (9 CFR1–3) and administered by the U.S. Department of Agriculture (USDA). The Health Research Extension Act is implemented by the Public Health Service Policy on Humane Care and Use of Laboratory Animals (PHS Policy) and administered by the National Institutes of Health (NIH) Office of Laboratroy Animal Welfare (OLAW). The PHS Policy requires compliance with the AWA and that institutions use the *Guide for the Care and Use of Laboratory Animals* (Institute of Laboratory Animal Resources [ILAR], Commission on Life Sciences, National Research Council [NRC]).

2.3 COMPLIANCE PROBLEMS

Although well intentioned, these two laws result in different regulations and requirements at different times by a variety of proponents with different agendas. In addition, the National Academy of Sciences, a quasi-governmental agency that serves as an independent adviser to the federal government, produces its own standards. It should be no surprise that compliance with all the provisions of both statutes can be challenging.

Different standards apply for different species. Under the AWA, an animal is defined as "any live or dead dog, cat, nonhuman primate, guinea pig, hamster, rabbit, or any other warm-blooded animal, which is being used, or is intended for use for research, teaching, testing, experimentation, or exhibition purposes, or as a pet." However, according to the AWA regulations, "rats of the genus *Rattus* and mice of the genus *Mus* bred for use in research" are excluded from the term *animal*, and therefore are not animals under the regulatory authority of the USDA.

In contrast, under the PHS policy, the definition of *animal* is "any live vertebrate animal used or intended for use in research, research training, experimentation, biological testing, or related purposes."

Different standards are also applied according to the nature of the work and intended purposes. For example, if rabbits, sheep, or goats are used for the production of antibodies that are to be used in the diagnosis, treatment, or prevention of animal diseases, a USDA license is required. Furthermore, the entire process of production (methods, records, quality control, testing, labeling, and packaging) falls under the purview and inspection of the USDA's Animal and Plant Health Inspection Service (APHIS). If the antibodies are to be used in the treatment or prevention of human diseases, or for biomedical research, the APHIS has the same responsibility for oversight and inspection.

However, if the animals under experimentation are used "for the purposes of improving animal nutrition, breeding, management, or production efficiency, or improving the quality of food or fiber," a USDA animal welfare license is not required. Instead, different sets of standards and oversight are involved. *A Guide for the Care and Use of Agricultural Animals in Animal Research and Teaching* has been developed and is used by institutions that use agricultural animals in their programs (see Resource 10).

Depending on funding and various other factors, animal experimentation activities may be subject to federal, state, and local laws, and additional standards adopted by scientific societies and industrial organizations. The above examples are not intended to intimidate or confuse the reader. They are just a few examples to demonstrate that compliance is complicated and challenging.

The information required to comply with nearly all the various guidelines, standards, laws, and regulations is contained in a relatively few publications.

2.4 COMPLIANCE SOLUTIONS

The most effective solution to the problem of rapidly changing standards and laws is through the IACUC. The USDA requires a minimum of three members, the PHS a minimum of five. The committee is charged with being knowledgeable in the regulations and to provide oversight of animal activities, as well as information and advice to top management of corporations and scientific staffs of research institutions.

Hundreds of IACUCs perform effectively in a variety of institutions, from multicampus universities and international pharmaceutical firms to small start-up biotechnology companies with two rooms of mice or a family farm enterprise with a small herd of goats, some chickens, and rabbits. Careful selection of an IACUC and the provision of an appropriate mandate, support, and authority will solve most animal care regulatory problems.

2.5 SYNOPSIS OF THE ANIMAL WELFARE ACT

The Animal Welfare Act of 1966 and its amendments regulate the transportation, purchase, sale, housing, care, handling, and treatment of animals used in research, for exhibitions, and sold as pets. The act specifically includes dogs, cats, nonhuman primates, guinea pigs, hamsters, rabbits, wild animal species, and any other warm-blooded animals that the Secretary of Agriculture determines are used, or are intended for use, in research, testing, experimentation, for exhibition purposes, or as pets.

The act has been amended in major areas three times (in 1970, 1976, and 1985) and is likely to be amended in the future. New rules and regulations, and interpretations of existing requirements of the act are issued frequently.

The amendments of 1985 affected animal research conducted intramurally by government agencies as well as grants and contracts funded by the federal government and resulted in an amended Public Health Service Policy on the Humane Care and Use of Laboratory Animals.

Other amendments addressed such issues as exercise for dogs; care of nonhuman primates (to ensure their psychological well being); the composition and duties of the Institutional Animal Care and Use Committee, adequate veterinary care; and responsibilities of the attending veterinarian, including record keeping and the training of all personnel using laboratory animals in humane methods of animal maintenance and experimentation.

Another recent amendment to the act resulted in the establishment of the Animal Welfare Information Center located in the National Agriculture Library. This center, in cooperation with the National Library of Medicine, provides reference material and services that cover many aspects of animal welfare and comparative medicine, resources that can be very helpful to research staffs and veterinarians.

All federal research facilities must comply with regulations and standards, but responsibility for enforcement is left to each agency. Most government agencies have indicated that they will abide by all provisions of the Animal Welfare Act as amended, as well as the PHS Policy on Humane Care and Use of Laboratory Animals.

Many areas of the act will not be addressed in this synopsis, i.e., registration, record keeping, reports, identification of animals, definitions of terms, space requirements, husbandry, transportation of designated species, facilities standards, operating standards, penalties, dealers, and exhibitors. These areas are important for people involved with logistic support and compliance.

Sections of the act that are addressed in this volume are limited to the bare essentials that will be of interest to this specific audience.

The research facility is responsible to ensure that personnel are qualified to perform their duties. The facility administrator must periodically review personnel qualifications of the staff; provide training in the humane care and use of animals; ensure that the needs of each species is met; and see to their proper handling, care, pre- and post-operative care, and aseptic surgical methods. The facility is responsible for covering the concept, availability, and use of research and/or testing methods that limit the use or minimize the distress of animals. This includes the proper use of anesthetic, analgesic, and tranquilizing drugs as well as providing information on alternatives to the use of live animals and the prevention of unnecessary duplicative research.

An Institutional Animal Care and Use Committee, appointed by the chief executive officer of the facility, must include a minimum of three members with the experience and expertise to assess animal programs, facilities, and procedures. The Committee must also have a veterinarian with training and experience in laboratory animal medicine who can direct or delegate responsibility for animal "activities" and an "outside" member who is not affiliated in any way with the facility to represent the general community interests in the care and use of animals.

The Committee reviews the program for humane care and use of animals, inspects animal facilities and animal study areas at least every 6 months, and prepares written and signed reports of its activities.The reports must describe the nature and extent of compliance with regulations and standards, and especially identify departures.

The act also provides for a review of individual research protocols including the rationale for using animals, and the appropriateness of the species and numbers; measures to ameliorate pain and distress; and the method of euthanasia. It further must provide assurance of the availability of professionally trained surgeons and qualified medical care for the animals. The institution must have a formal arrangement (a contract) with an attending veterinarian and must provide adequate facilities and authority for the veterinarian to work effectively.

RESOURCES

1. *Guide for the Care and Use of Laboratory Animals*, Institute of Laboratory Animal Resources (ILAR), National Research Council, National Academy of Sciences, National Academy Press, Washington, D.C. (This is the "bible" for personnel in the biomedical sciences.)
2. *ILAR Journal* (formerly *ILAR News*). ILAR, 2101 Constitution Avenue, NW, NAS 347, Washington, D.C. 20418 A quarterly publication for biomedical investigators, laboratory animal scientists, institution officials, and members of animal care and use committees.
3. *Public Health Service Policy on Humane Care and Use of Laboratory Animals*. U.S. Department of Health, Office for Protection from Research Risks, 6100 Executive Blvd., MSC 7507, Rockville, MD 20892.

4. *Code of Federal Regulations* (9 CFR1–3). The Animal Welfare Act, U.S. Department of Agriculture, Animal and Plant Health Inspection Service, Regulatory Enforcement and Animal Care, 4700 River Road, Unit 84, Riverdale, MD 20737.

5. Animal Welfare Information Center, National Agricultural Library, 5th Floor, Beltsville, MD 20705. (Established by the 1985 amendments to the Animal Welfare Act, AWIC provides information on employee training, improved methods of experimentation [including alternatives], and animal care and animal use topics through the production of bibliographies, workshops, resource guides, and the *Animal Welfare Information Center Newsletter*. AWIC services are geared for those who must comply with the Animal Welfare Act, such as researchers, veterinarians, exhibitors, and dealers.)

6. *Contemporary Topics in Laboratory Animal Science*, 70 Timber Creek Drive, Cordova, TN 38018. A bimonthly publication, this journal serves as the official communication vehicle for the American Association of Laboratory Animal Science and includes a section of refereed articles and book reviews, editorials, committee reports, philosophical topics, and association news.

7. *Lab Animal*, 345 Park Avenue South, New York, NY 10017. Published 11 times a year by Nature Publishing Co. This peer-reviewed journal for professionals in animal research emphasizes proper management and care.

8. Scientists Center for Animal Welfare, 7833 Walker Drive, Suite 340, Greenbelt, MD 20770. This independent organization, supported by individuals and institutions involved in research with animals, is concerned about maintaining the highest standards of humane care. SCAW organizes conferences, publishes resource materials, and supports a wide variety of educational activities.

9. National Association for Biomedical Research, 818 Connecticut Avenue, NW, Suite 303, Washington, DC 20006. NABR is a nonprofit organization comprised of 350 institutional members from academia and industry whose mission is to advocate public policy that recognizes the vital role of laboratory animals in research, education, and safety testing. NABR is a source of information for existing and proposed animal welfare legislation and regulations at the national, state, and local level.

10. Guide for the Care and Use of Agricultural Animals in Agricultural Research and Teaching, January 1999. Federation of Animal Science Societies, 1111 N. Dunlap Ave., Savoy, IL 61874.

3 Antigens

Donald H. Lewis

CONTENTS

3.1 INTRODUCTION

The selection of an antigen represents one of the very first steps in the preparation of antibodies. Antigens are critical to the process. While some methods of making antibodies offer forgiveness (monoclonal antibodies), the purity and effectiveness of the antigen bear a direct relationship to the purity and specificity of the resulting antibodies. A few definitions will be useful.

First, complete antigens are substances capable of both inducing a specific immune response and reacting specifically with the products of that response. Certain substances sometimes referred to as incomplete or partial antigens (also called haptens) are capable of forming immune complexes in serologic reactions, but are unable to stimulate an immune response unless coupled to another (usually larger) reactive substance. Hence, the terms *immunogenicity* and *antigenicity* are related, but distinct terms. All immunogens are antigens, but not all antigens are immunogens. Immunogenicity is the ability of a component to induce a humoral and/or cell mediated immune response, whereas antigenicity is the ability to combine specifically with products of that response.

3.1.1 CONSIDERATIONS FOR SELECTING ANTIGENS

At least four factors determine the effectiveness of a particular component's antigenic characteristics (i.e., molecular size and structural relationships, foreignness, structural stability, and degradability). In addition, the nature of immune cell–cell interaction is a fundamental consideration for immunogenic activity.

3.1.1.1 Molecular Size and Structural Relationships

Large molecules in general stimulate a better immune response than do small molecules. In addition, the immune system recognizes some macromolecules better than others. Proteins and polysaccharides are some of the most potent immunogens, whereas lipids and nucleic acids are usually poor immunogens unless coupled to proteins or polysaccharides. Furthermore, the immune system does not recognize the entire immunogenic molecule. Discrete macromolecular sites called *epitopes*, or antigenic determinants, interact with the specific antigen-binding site in the variable region of the immunoglobulin molecule known as a *paratope*. An individual immunogenic molecule usually possesses several different epitopes capable of interacting with immunoglobulin, usually 5 to 6 amino acid or polysaccharide residues, and the most intense immune responses are directed against epitopes that are the most "foreign." As a result, some epitopes are much more immunogenic than others. Thus rabbits immunized with the enzyme lysozyme of human origin, for example, preferentially respond to a single favored epitope, and the remainder of the molecule is essentially nonimmunogenic. Those epitopes are referred to as *immunodominant*. In general, the number of epitopes possessed by an immunogenic molecule is directly related to molecular size. Immunogenic molecules usually possess about one epitope per 5 to 10 kDa of molecular mass.[1]

The fit and subsequent binding between epitope and paratope is based on their three-dimensional interaction and noncovalent union. As a result, the orientation of the determinant may influence the nature of the epitope–paratope interaction. A *conformational determinant* depends upon three-dimensional relationships of the immunogenic molecule and is composed of noncontiguous residues brought into close proximity to each other by folding of the molecule. The immunogenicity of these determinants is destroyed by denaturation procedures. A second group of determinants, *linear determinants*, are characterized by possessing adjacent amino acid residues in the covalent sequence of the molecule. Molecules containing linear determinants are not inactivated by usual denaturation procedures and, in fact, linear determinants present in the folded states of native proteins are not usually available for immunogenic activity until the molecules have been denatured to reveal those reactive sites. A third group of determinants referred to as *neoantigenic determinants* require proteolysis of the immunogen molecule so as to reveal epitopes for immunogenic activity.

3.1.1.2 Foreignness

Cells involved in immunogenic interaction are selected by the host's system early in life in such a way as to not respond to self-antigens — a situation referred to as tolerance. Those cells will respond to other, non-self, foreign molecules that differ even in minor respects from the self-antigens, and that response is the fundamental basis for immune function. However, certain self-tissue components are isolated from that early selecive process (e.g., lens proteins, sperm cells). If the tissue barriers are compromised by trauma or infection, an immune response to those tissues will develop as if they were foreign. Foreign molecules differ in their *immunogenicity* or their ability to stimulate an immune response. The immunogenicity of a molecule largely depends on its degree of foreignness. The greater the difference between a foreign antigen and self-antigens, the greater will be the intensity of the immune response.

3.1.1.3 Structural Stability

Recognition of an immunogen involves both the shape of the molecule and the peptide or polysaccharide sequence. Highly flexible molecules (e.g., gelatin, a protein known for its structural instability) are poorly immunogenic. For this same reason, proteins are better immunogens than large, repeating polymers such as lipids, carbohydrates, and nucleic acids.

3.1.1.4 Degradability

Immune cells recognize only small molecular components of the immunogen molecule. If the molecule cannot be broken up or solubilized, it cannot function as an immunogen. Plastic joints and stainless steel pins commonly used in medical applications do not trigger immune responses in patients. Starch and other simple repetitive polysaccharides are poor immunogens both because they are relatively easily degraded, and because they do not assume a stable configuration. Polymers of D-amino acids are nonimmunogenic because they do not occur naturally in vertebrates and vertebrate enzymes cannot degrade them. In contrast, L-amino acids in most proteins can be degraded into fragments that can be recognized by the immune system.

3.1.2 REQUIREMENT FOR CELL-TO-CELL INTERACTION AND LYMPHOCYTE ACTIVATION

Immune cells are not autonomous in the sense that they recognize their antigen in toto and are activated to realize their full functional potential without the involvement of other cells. Instead, the immune system is designed so that cooperative interaction between major groups of cells occurs to provide the diversity for recognizing the infinite number of structures a pathogen might evolve, and to regulate the response of the system to "self" components.

Cooperative cell-to-cell interactions are mediated by receptors. Those receptors are carried by specialized cells of the immune system, the lymphocytes. These cells are of two forms, the B and T lymphocytes. Both originate from multipotential cells, which are continuously self-renewing and present in the bone marrow. During differentiation, each B or T lymphocyte develops a particular type of receptor specialized for one particular binding unit or *ligand*. The receptors are designated the B-cell antigen receptor (*BcR*) and the T-cell antigen receptor (*TcR*). B lymphocytes continue to originate from the bone marrow, whereas T lymphocytes are generated in the thymus from precursors immigrating from the bone marrow.

Because the system must be prepared for an infinite variety of ligands, a large number of different lymphocytes, each with specificity for one particular antigenic determinant, must be available. After contact with the immunogen and complex interactions between lymphocytes and the accessory cells, the lymphocytes become activated, multiply, and transform into *effector* cells.

B cells and T cells differ in fundamental ways concerning the immunogens with which they can interact and the components they are able to recognize. B-cell receptors can interact with immunogenic molecules, which may be either cell-bound or soluble. The antigens recognized can be portions of proteins, glycoproteins, lipids, or DNA, or even small chemical compounds such as steroid hormones. T cells, on the other hand, do not recognize antigenic determinants per se. Their receptors are specialized to recognize immunogenic components complexed with particular molecules expressed on the cell surfaces of the host in which the immune response occurs. These cell-surface molecules are the products of the major histocompatibility complex (MHC). Immunogenic peptides from proteins derived from an infectious agent, for example, associate with the glycoproteins encoded by the MHC, and immunogenic fragments along with MHC molecules are displayed on cell surfaces of the host. Because protein–protein interactions are involved in MHC expression of the immunogenic fragment, only proteins can serve as donors of T-cell antigenic determinants. MHC molecules may also be expressed with peptides originating from altered self molecules (e.g., tumor components or viral peptides). Such alteration of the MHC molecules alerts the T cells with receptors for the altered self molecules to become activated and destroy cells possessing the altered MHC-associated peptides.[3]

The TcR only recognizes antigenic epitopes presented together with MHC. One may conclude that two types of MHC molecules (i.e., MHC class I and MHC class II) are expressed on cell surfaces and that those MHC molecules interact with two subpopulations of T cells. T cells that recognize antigenic peptides associated with MHC I (e.g., tumor or virus-associated peptides) express a co-receptor, *CD8*, which interacts with the nonpolymorphic regions of the MHC molecule, strengthening the TcR-MHC/antigen interaction. Referred to as "cytotoxic T cells, " CD 8+ T cells develop lytic systems that enable them to kill virus-infected or tumor cells bearing the immunogen plus MHC. The second type of T cells (CD 4+ T cells) recognizes antigen together with MHC class II and uses the CD4 glycoprotein as co-receptor, strengthens T-cell–MHC II interactions, and elaborates a number of regulatory proteins. Since many of the regulatory proteins are required in B-cell functioning and serve as precursors of cytotoxic T cells, these T cells are called helper T cells.

B-cell activation proceeds by two different routes, depending on the nature of the antigen.[4] One such route is dependent upon direct contact with helper T cells and involves thymus-dependent (TD) antigens. Antigens that can activate B cells in the absence of direct contact by helper T cells are known as thymus-independent (TI) antigens. Two types of TI antigens, type 1 and type 2, are recognized and activate B cells by different mechanisms. Examples of type 1 TI antigens (TI-1) include some bacterial lipopolysaccharides and other bacterial cell wall components. Type 2 TI (TI-2) antigens are highly repetitious molecules, such as polymeric proteins (e.g., bacterial flagellin) or bacterial cell polysaccharides with repeating polysaccharide units. TI-1 antigens are polyclonal B-cell activators (mitogens). When exposed to low levels of these antigens, only those B cells specific for epitopes of the antigen will be activated. At higher concentrations, TI-1 antigens will stimulate B-cell proliferation and antibody production by a large number of those cells. TI-2 antigens activate by cross-linking of the BcR, but differ from TI-1 antigens by their inability to function as B-cell mitogens.

The nature of antibody response to TI antigens differs from that associated with TD antigens. The response to TI antigens does not result in the production of memory cells. It results in the predominance of one class of immunoglobulin (IgM) and is generally weaker than that associated with TD antigens. For a variety of polysaccharide antigens, it may be the only response to microbial invaders observed initially and may serve as the critical first immune defensive strategy to those agents. TD antigens provide a characteristic biphasic response. Typified initially by the emergence of IgM, they later form relatively long-lived plasma cells that produce high-affinity and high-titer, predominantly non-IgM (mostly IgG or IgA) antibody and memory B cells capable of differentiation into similar plasma cells in subsequent exposures to antigen. The presence of previously primed memory B cells accounts for the characteristic rapid emergence of high-affinity antibody in secondary or later immunizations that serves to prevent reinfection with many microbial agents.

3.2 HAPTENS, IMMUNOSPECIFICITY, AND IMMUNOGEN–ANTIBODY INTERACTIONS

Haptens do not, alone, elicit an immune response. They usually bear only one epitope to which antibodies can only be elicited by complexing them to a larger, carrier molecule before immunization. Hapten-carrier molecule conjugates require both T and B cells. The carrier portion of the conjugate activates T cells, whereas antibodies to both hapten and carrier are elicited by B cells. The carrier is immunogenic in its own right and immunization with the hapten-carrier conjugate elicits antibody to both carrier and hapten. Landsteiner and Van der Scheer[5] pioneered these techniques for elucidating the specificity of antibodies for antigenic determinants using diazotization techniques. This method involves introducing a diazo group ($-N^+ \equiv N^-$) into a molecule by first reacting an aromatic amine with nitrous acid generated through the combination of sodium nitrite with hydrochloric acid. The diazonium salt is then combined with the protein at a slightly alkaline pH. Reaction products include monosubstituted tyrosine and disubstituted histidine and lysine residues. A number of coupling procedures for attaching haptens to protein carriers have been reviewed elsewhere.[6]

Once the method for raising antibodies to small chemically defined haptens was developed, it became possible to relate variations in chemical structure of a hapten to binding to a particular immunoglobulin. Thus, testing antibodies raised to meta-aminobenzosulfonate reveals that aminobenzene sulfonate synthesized with the sulfonate group in the ortho position combines poorly with that antibody, whereas haptens with the sulfonate group in the para position do not combine with the antibody.

Antibodies to a specific hapten can be studied with pure hapten (without carrier) in equilibrium dialysis, hapten coupled to a different (non-cross-reacting) carrier, or inhibition of precipitation with free hapten. Equilibrium dialysis involves placing a mixture of the hapten and its specific antibody inside a dialysis bag and measuring the rate and extent to which hapten diffuses into the surrounding fluid until equilibrium is established between free hapten and hapten-antibody complex. If the exterior fluid is continually renewed, all hapten will eventually be removed, indicating the reversible nature of the antibody-hapten complex. The strength of the binding between the antibody and the hapten reflects the affinity of the immunoglobulin for that epitope. Low-affinity antibodies bind immunogens weakly and tend to dissociate readily, whereas high-affinity antibodies bind immunogens more tightly and remain bound longer.

The affinity at one binding site does not always reflect the strength of the antigen–antibody interaction. When complex antigens containing multiple epitopes are mixed with antibodies containing multiple binding sites, the interaction between the antibody molecule with the antigen molecule at one site will increase the probability of reaction between those two components at a second site. The strength of such multiple interactions between a multivalent antibody and antigen is referred to as *avidity*. The multivalency of most immunogens of infectious agents provides an enhanced effect. The binding of immunogen to immunoglobulin by multiple links is much greater than might be expected by individual bonds. High avidity is advantageous for a variety of functions *in vivo* (e.g., immune elimination of agent, virus neutralization).

3.3   SPECIFICITY AND CROSS-REACTIVITY

Immune specificity is defined by the ability of antibody to discriminate between the immunogen against which it was made (homologous antigen) and other antigenic components. Karush[7] defined selectivity as the ability of an antibody to discriminate, in an all-or-none fashion, between two related ligands. Thus, selectivity depends not only on the relative affinity of the antibody for the two ligands, but on the experimental lower limit for detection of reactivity. Cross-reactivity may be defined as the ability of antibody to react with ligands other than the immunogen. In most cases, cross-reactive ligands possess lower affinity than the immunogen for a particular antibody.

Often in practical situations, cross-reactivity is ascertained by methods such as agarose gel immunoprecipitation procedures or similar methods which do not distinguish between differences in concentration. Coupled with the heterogeneity of immune antisera, this factor has led to ambiguities in specificity and cross-reactivity. Berzkofsky and Schechter[8] have defined two forms of cross-reactivity. Type 1 cross-reactivity, or true cross-reactivity, is affinity-related and defined as the ability of two ligands to react with the same site on the same antibody molecule but with different affinities. Type 2 cross-reactivity, or shared reactivity, occurs when the ligand reacts with all or only a subpopulation of the antibodies in a heterogenous population of antibody molecules. In reality, both phenomena are displayed simultaneously in most antibody preparations.

3.4   PEPTIDES AS IMMUNOGENS

The use of peptides as immunogens has emerged as DNA sequence information became available in the last 20 or so years and the potential application of polypeptides construction to vaccine development, became known. Much of the current interest in this subject can be traced back to the report in 1980 by Walter et al.[9] of the production of antibody probes to SV40 large T antigen using small peptide immunogens. Concurrently, Sutcliffe et al.[10] demonstrated that this technique could be used to identify previously unrecognized gene products of the Moloney leukaemia virus genome. Demonstrations of the power of using short peptide immunogens to produce antibody probes for complete proteins have stimulated research in a number of areas including the potential use of completely synthetic vaccines, avoiding the problems of using biological products as immunogens; the development of anti-tumor reagents, the development of molecular probes to specific sites on antigens; the development of antibodies to sites on proteins which will not normally act as epitopes; and identification of as yet uncharacterized gene products.

The principal considerations for producing peptide immunogens relate to (a) the sequence of the peptide, (b) the length of the peptide to be produced, (c) whether or not to link the peptide to a carrier protein and the type of carrier to be used, (d) the type of assay to be used to assess the immune response, and (e) the immunization protocol.

The sequence of suitable peptide immunogen can be estimated by one of the programs described by Stern.[11] Peptides as short as 6 amino acids have been shown to produce antiserum, but increasing peptide length to 12 amino acids enhances immunogenicity.[12] Longer peptides may be able to produce a secondary structure which mimics that in complete proteins and enhances the probability that an immune response to peptide will be similar to that produced by natural protein.[13]

Initial efforts to develop antiserum to short peptides involved the use of free peptides.[14] It is now recognized that such peptides elicit a weak immune response, and that better response can be achieved by linking the peptides to carrier protein. A number of carrier proteins have been successfully used. Bacterial toxoids, for example, have been regarded as suitable, in part because they are immunogenic, and because most recipients will have been preimmunized to them and secondary T-cell response could be expected. Other carrier proteins include keyhole limpet hemocyanin, bovine serum albumin, ovalbumin, and thyroglobulin. Although it is possible that any of these carriers may be useful, the choice of carrier may be critical in some instances. It may be necessary, for example, to link the peptide to one carrier for immunization purposes and to a second for assay purposes, since some peptides may not easily bind to the microtiter plates usually used in screening.

3.5   POTENTIAL PITFALLS

The standard approach for use of peptides as immunogens has been to attach multiple copies of a B-cell epitope (usually a single sequence) to a carrier protein, the latter of which serves as a source of T-cell determinants, and many of the pitfalls are related to these considerations. Often in the case of substituting polypeptides for viral immunogens, not only are important B-cell epitopes discontinuous, but adjacent molecules contribute to native immunogenicity, and in these instances, there is no general way to synthesize corresponding B-cell epitopes. Even when the B-cell epitope is linear, single mutations outside the sequence can affect the antigenic specificity of the epitope by altering molecular configuration of the native immunogenic molecule. The need to include several B- and T-cell determinants could make this approach impracticable.

REFERENCES

1. Sela, M., Ed., 1973, *The Antigens*, Academic Press, New York.
2. Cruse, J.M. and Lewis, R.E., 1999, *Atlas of Immunology*, CRC Press, Boca Raton, FL.
3. Schimpl, A., 1993, *Methods of Immunological Analysis,* 1, 24–43, Masseyeff, R.F., Ed., VCH Publishers, New York.
4. Paul, W.E., 1999, *Fundamental Immunology*, 4th ed., Raven Press, New York.
5. Landsteiner, K. and Van der Scheer, K., 1934, *J. Exp. Med.,* 59, 751–768.
6. Hosada, H. and Ishikawa, E., 1993, *Methods of Immunological Analysis,* 2, 431–445, Masseyeff, R.F., Ed., VCH Publishers, New York.
7. Karush, F., 1978, *Comprehensive Immunology,* 5, 85–116, Litman, G.W. and Good, R.A., Eds., Plenum Books, New York.
8. Berzofsky, J.A. and Schechter, A.N., 1981, *Mol. Immunology,* 18, 751–763.
9. Walter, G., Scheidtmann, K.H., Carbone, A., Laudano, A.P., and Doolittle, R.F., 1980, *Proc. Natl. Acad. Sci. U.S.A.*, 71, 5197–2000.
10. Sutcliffe, J.G., Shinnick, T.M., Green, N., Lin, F.T., Niman, H.L., and Lerner, R.A., 1980, *Nature,* 287, 801–805.
11. Stern, P.S., 1991, *Trends Biotechnol.*, 9, 163–169.
12. Janin, J., 1979, *Nature,* 277, 491–492.
13. Rhodes, G., Houghten, R., Taulane, J.P., Carson, D., and Vaughan, J., 1984, *Mol. Immunol.*, 21, 1047–1054.
14. Atassi, M.Z., Lee, C.L., 1978, *Biochem. J.,* 171, 429–434.

4 Adjuvants

Jory R. Baldridge and Michael J. Lacy

CONTENTS

4.1 INTRODUCTION

Immunological adjuvants nonspecifically enhance or modify the immune response to coadministered antigens. Thus, antibody production is more vigorous than if antigen is administered alone. A variety of mechanisms contribute to this adjuvant-induced amplification including (1) the formation of a depot of immunogen resulting in the slow release and presentation of antigen to the immune system over an extended period of time, (2) optimizing the immune stimulus by focusing a general immunostimulant and antigen in the same microenvironment where they can interact with antigen-presenting cells and lymphocytes simultaneously, and (3) nonspecific activation of the cells of the immune system thus facilitating those interactions that favor the production of antibody. This chapter will deal primarily with commercially available adjuvants designed for the production of antisera in the research setting (see Table 4.1).

The most widely recognized and utilized adjuvants are the water-in-oil emulsions initially developed by Freund.[1,2] These emulsions are generated by mixing an aqueous solution of soluble antigen with an equal volume of oil through a process known as emulsification. During this procedure the antigen-containing water droplets become entrapped in the oil, forming particulates in a very viscous emulsion. For adjuvant activity, it is critical that these thick emulsions remain stable and that the components do not separate after mixing. Upon administration into the host's tissue, this viscous mixture acts as a depot of antigen. The potency of water-in-oil emulsions can be increased by incorporating immunostimulants. The classic example is complete Freund's adjuvant (CFA), which consists of the aqueous antigen solution,

TABLE 4.1
Sources for Adjuvants

Adjuvant	Manufacturer/Address	Phone
AdjuPrime	Pierce Chemical Co.	1-800-874-3723
	P.O. Box 117	
	Rockford, IL 61105	
Adjuvax	Alpha-Beta Technologies, Inc.	1-800-833-0503
	373 Plantation Street	
	Worcester, MA 01605	
Alum	Several sources	
Complete Freund's Adjuvant	Several sources	
Gerbu Adjuvant	C-C Biotech Corporation	1-888-379-6534
	16766 Espola Road	
	Poway, CA 92064	
Incomplete Freund's Adjuvant	Several sources	
Quil A	Accurate Chemical and Scientific	1-516-333-2211
	Corporation	
	300 Shanes Drive	
	Westbury, NY 11590	
Ribi Adjuvants	Ribi ImmunoChem Research Inc.	1-800-548-7424
	553 Old Corvallis Road	
	Hamilton, MT 59840	
TiterMax	CytRx Corporation	1-800-345-2987
	154 Technology Parkway	
	Norcross, GA 30092	

mineral oil, an emulsifying agent, and heat-killed *Mycobacterium tuberculosis*, a very potent immunomodifier. Incomplete Freund's adjuvant (IFA) is identical to CFA except that the M. tuberculosis is omitted. Freund's adjuvants have been used and continue to be used extensively with antigens to stimulate the production of high concentrations of good quality antibodies. There are, however, complicating factors that need to be considered. The emulsions are rather tedious to generate and can contribute to the degradation of protein antigens.[3] Freund's adjuvants are known to be inherently toxic, frequently resulting in granulomas, sterile abscesses, and ulcerations following administration.[4,5] To reduce the extent of these complications, most protocols recommend using CFA for the primary immunization only and then using IFA for all subsequent vaccinations. Furthermore, due to increasing concerns for research animals, many animal care facilities have banned or restricted the use of CFA, while encouraging the use of other adjuvants. Several alternatives are now available which are generally as effective as CFA/IFA for enhancing antibody production and have greatly reduced toxicity.[6,7,8]

TiterMax® is a water-in-oil emulsion developed specifically for the production of antibodies in research animals. TiterMax has three primary ingredients: (1) a block copolymer, CRL 89-41; (2) squalene, a metabolizable oil; and (3) a microparticulate silica. The nonionic block copolymer is a synthetic immunomodifier which acts in part by adhesion of protein antigens to oil, thereby enhancing delivery of high concentrations of antigen-to-antigen presenting cells. By utilizing squalene instead of mineral oil, TiterMax emulsions result in greatly reduced toxicity compared with Freund's.[8] The emulsification of TiterMax with antigen is easier to prepare and more stable than Freund's emulsions.[8]

Another product is the Ribi adjuvant system (RAS), which was developed as an alternative to Freund's for producing antibodies in research animals. To reduce the toxicity found in Freund's water-in-oil emulsions, the RAS emulsions were designed as oil-in-water emulsions with a final concentration of only 2% metabolizable squalene oil.[9] These emulsions include one or more of the following bacterial-derived immunostimulators: (1) synthetic trehalose dimycolate (TDM), (2) monophosphoryl lipid A (MPL®*), and (3) cell wall skeleton from *Mycobacterium phlei* (CWS). The immunostimulants nonspecifically induce immune activation resulting in the production of inflammatory cytokines which facilitate antibody production. The RAS emulsions are thin fluids that are easy to use, compared to the thick, viscous Freund's water-in-oil emulsions. Three variations of RAS are available for use, depending upon the antigen and the animal to be immunized.

4.2 GENERAL GUIDELINES AND PRECAUTIONS FOR WORKING WITH ADJUVANTS

1. Adjuvants designed for the production of antisera are very strong immunostimulants which will induce intense inflammatory reactions upon introduction into tissues. Protective eyewear and gloves should be worn when working with these materials.
2. Adjuvants are sold as sterile reagents and should be handled aseptically. Any introduction of contaminants during vaccine preparation can adversely affect the desired antisera. The contaminants can be more immunogenic than the antigen, resulting in the production of antisera specific for the contaminant rather than the antigen. If the adjuvant becomes contaminated, it should be discarded.
3. Excessive amounts of adjuvant can be immunosuppressive, resulting in low yields of antibody. Adjuvants, therefore, should be used at or near doses recommended by the manufacturer.
4. For peptides or other poorly immunogenic antigens, it can be beneficial to covalently couple them to a helper protein before using them with adjuvants. Several protocols for attaching helper proteins to antigens can be found in *Current Protocols in Immunology*.[10]
5. Higher titers of antibody are normally generated by immunizing multiple times with small amounts of antigen, rather than by immunizing one time with a large dose of antigen. This may be a consideration when antigen is scarce.
6. Some adjuvants, including RAS and TiterMax, can increase the generation of antibodies of the IgG2a subclass in mice.[9,11,12]

---

* Registered Trademark of Ribi ImmunoChem Research, Inc., Hamilton, MT.

4.3   PROTOCOLS FOR USING FREUND'S ADJUVANTS

- *Some research institutions have restricted the use of CFA. Check with the appropriate animal care and use committee at your institution before using CFA.*
- *CFA should be used for primary vaccinations only. Subsequent immunizations with CFA will lead to severe lesions at the site of injection. Therefore, IFA or another adjuvant should be used for all subsequent boosts.*

4.3.1   Low-Tech Emulsifications for Injection of 1 to 5 Mice

Materials:

CFA (or IFA)	Antigen in PBS
Sterile round bottom cryovial, 2.0 ml	High-speed drill or stirrer
Adjustable clamp	Ring stand and clamp
Safety eyewear	Syringe for injection
Latex gloves	

Autoclaved paper clip for stirring rod (see Figure 4.1)

Procedure for 1.0 ml of vaccine.

1. Securely fasten a small (1/4 in.) high-speed electric drill in a vertical position, or use a commercial high-speed motorized stirrer.
2. Form a large metal paper clip into the shape shown in Figure 4.1. Autoclave it in foil or paper and store until needed. Insert the paper clip stirring rod into the chuck of the drill or stirrer, leaving the loop end covered and sterile.
3. Calculate the amount of antigen required and the volume desired per injection. Allow 10 to 100 µg of antigen per mouse, in a volume of 200 µl per mouse for IM or SC injections. For IP injections, allow 200 to 500 µl volume per mouse. *Detergents will weaken the emulsion and should be avoided.*
4. Place the capped cryovial into an adjustable clamp. Align it directly below the stirring rod allowing space to remove the vial's cap.
5. Warm CFA to 37°C prior to use and vortex vigorously for 1 to 2 min to resuspend the *M. tuberculosis.*
6. Remove the cap from the cryovial and add 500 µl of CFA (or IFA). Uncover the stirring rod and move the cryovial up until the stirring-rod loop is emersed in the adjuvant. Begin stirring at low speed and increase to high speed (>1000 RPM). Add 250 µl of aqueous antigen (reserve the remaining 250 µl until the next step) to the CFA (or IFA). Stir for an additional 30 s.

   Note: Exercise caution with the high-speed stirrer. The round bottom vial should be clamped firmly so that the tube does not change position during

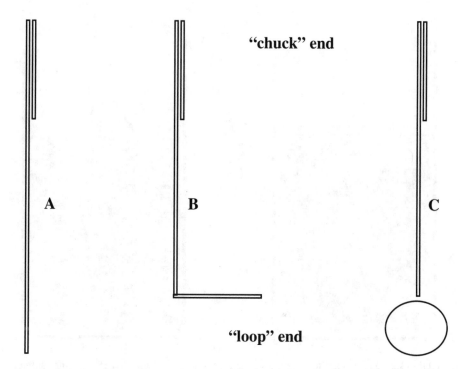

FIGURE 4.1 A large metal paper clip can be formed into a stirring rod to be used for small volume emulsifications. The entire rod should be about 3-in. long with a small loop at one end and a doubled thickness of metal at the "chuck" end. (A) Using a needle-nosed plier, bend a paper clip, as shown, so that the chuck end has a double thickness. (B) At the opposite end to the chuck end, bend a 1/2-in. length at 90 degrees to the shaft section. Then, grasp the end of the 90-degree-angled section, as shown, and begin to roll the wire into a loop (C) Form a loop whose diameter is no greater than 1/4 in.

the emulsifying process and cause the stirring rod to rub. The stirring rod should be firmly secured within the stirrer chuck.

7. Using a sterile pipet tip, add the remaining 250 µl of antigen and continue stirring at high speed for 1 to 2 min.
8. To determine if the emulsion is ready, use a sterile pipet tip to drop 10 to 50 µl of emulsion onto the surface of tap water in a beaker. The emulsion should form a stable "bead" on the water's surface (see Figure 4.2). If the emulsion does not form a bead, or the bead dissipates after 10 s, stir again at high speed for 2 to 3 min, and retest it as above. If no bead forms, add an additional 50 µl of CFA (or IFA) to the emulsion and stir at high speed for 2 to 3 min. Repeat as necessary.
9. When a stable emulsion has been formed, draw the emulsion into a syringe using a needle with a wide bore (16 to 18 gauge). It should be noted that it is possible to emulsify the mixture to the extent that the resulting emulsion will be too stiff to be forced through a hypodermic needle.

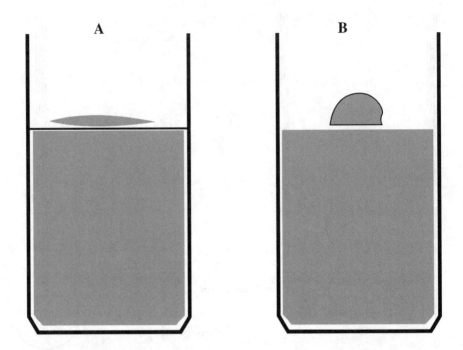

FIGURE 4.2 Diagram to illustrate the testing for a stable emulsion. (A) This mixture did not form a single, large bead when dropped upon water. Instead the oily mixture partially or completely dispersed across the surface of the water. The mixture is not a stable emulsion adequate for injection. Do not inject. Continue with the emulsification procedure. (B) The emulsion formed a bead when dropped upon water. This is a stable emulsion that is suitable for injection.

4.3.2   EMULSIFICATION USING SYRINGES

CFA (or IFA) can be emulsified aseptically using two syringes, subsequently requiring only the addition of the hypodermic needle.

Materials:

CFA (or IFA)   Antigen in PBS
Safety eyewear   Latex gloves
Two identical glass syringes, 1, 3, or 5 ml
Double-hub Luer-lock syringe needle (connector)

Procedure:

1. Calculate the amount of antigen required and the volume desired per injection. Allow 10 to 100 µg of antigen per mouse in a volume of 200 µl per mouse for IM or SC injections. For IP injections, allow 200 to 500 µl volume per mouse. *Detergents will weaken the emulsion and should be avoided.*

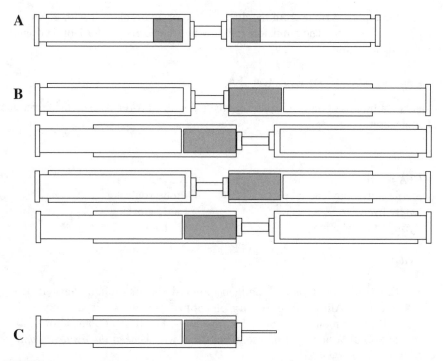

FIGURE 4.3 Emulsification of aqueous antigen and adjuvants using a dual-syringe method. (A) Attach the syringes securely to a Luer-lock double-hulled connector. (B) First, push the aqueous antigen solution into the oil, then continue to force the mixture through the connector in an alternating pattern. (C) After a stable emulsion has formed, remove the connector and add a needle for injection or transfer the emulsion to a 1 ml syringe for injection.

2. Select syringe size according to total volume of materials to be added. Warm CFA to 37°C prior to use and vortex vigorously for 1 to 2 min to resuspend the *M. tuberculosis*. Aspirate the required volume of CFA (or IFA) into a syringe. Connect the syringe to a double-hub needle with Luer lock and expel any air.
3. Aspirate the aqueous antigen into the second syringe and expel any air.
4. Attach the antigen-containing syringe to the free end of the double-hub needle. Make certain both syringes are securely fastened to the double-hub needle via the Luer locks.
5. Firmly depress the plunger forcing all of the antigen solution through the double-hub needle and into the CFA (or IFA). In an alternating pattern continue to force the mixture from one syringe to the other (see Figure 4.3).
6. Continue to emulsify as in the preceding step, until a stable emulsion is formed. This may take several minutes. Test for a stable emulsion by expelling a small drop onto the surface of some water in a beaker. The droplet should form a stable bead (see Figure 4.2).
7. Force the entire volume of emulsion into one syringe. Remove the double-hub needle and add a needle for injections. Alternatively, remove

the empty syringe from the dual-connector and replace it with a sterile 1-ml syringe. The emulsion can now be transferred to the 1-ml syringe for injection.

4.3.3 Sonication of CFA (or IFA)

Aqueous solutions of antigen can be emulsified with CFA (or IFA) by the technique of sonication.

Materials:

CFA (or IFA)   Antigen in PBS
Sterile polypropylene tube   Probe sonicator
Safety eyewear   Latex gloves
Syringe for injection   Ice bath

Procedure:

1. Calculate the amount of antigen required and the volume desired per injection. Allow 10 to 100 μg of antigen per mouse, in a volume of 200 μl per mouse for IM or SC injections. For IP injections, allow 200 to 500 μl volume per mouse. *Detergents will weaken the emulsion and should be avoided.*
2. Warm CFA to 37°C prior to use and vortex vigorously for 1 to 2 min to resuspend the *M. tuberculosis*. Into a sterile polypropylene tube, add CFA (or IFA) and an equal volume of aqueous antigen.
3. Sonication can generate a great deal of heat, which may lead to denaturation of protein antigens. To avoid overheating the mixture, place the tube on ice during sonication or between pulses. Begin emulsifying the mixture by pulsing for 5 to 10 s at a time with the probe sonicator.
4. Invert tube slowly in order to determine the thickness of the emulsion. Continue sonicating with 10-s pulses until a stable emulsion is formed. The process is complete when the emulsion remains immobile in the inverted tube or when a drop forms a stable bead on the surface of tap water (see Figure 4.2).
5. Transfer to a 1 ml syringe for injection by aspirating the emulsion into the syringe. Alternatively, the transfer technique of Spack and Toavs[13] can be used. Obtain a sterile plunger from a syringe whose barrel diameter is the same as the tube in which the emulsification was performed. Swab the bottom of the emulsification tube with alcohol to sterilize, then pierce a hole in the bottom of the tube using a sterile 18-gauge needle. Hold the top of a sterile 1 ml syringe (without its plunger) directly beneath the hole in the emulsification tube. Insert a snug-fitting syringe plunger into the emulsification tube and push the emulsion into the 1-ml syringe.

4.4 PROTOCOL FOR USING TITERMAX®

Materials:

TiterMax®	Antigen in PBS
Safety eyewear	Latex gloves
Syringe for injection	One 3-way stopcock
	or double-hub needle

Two 2.5 ml all-plastic syringes (rubber plungers will stick to the syringe barrels) or siliconized all-glass Luer-lock syringes.

Procedure:

1. Warm TiterMax to room temperature and vortex for 30 s or longer, in order to ensure that TiterMax is a homogeneous suspension.
2. For 1.0 ml of emulsion, load one syringe with 0.5 ml of TiterMax. Load second syringe with 0.25 ml of aqueous antigen. *Detergents will weaken the emulsion and should be avoided.* Retain 0.25 ml of aqueous antigen for further use.
3. Connect the two syringes to the 3-way stopcock. It is important to begin the emulsification process by forcing the aqueous antigen into the Titer-Max. Force the materials back and forth through the stopcock for about 2 min (see Figure 4.3).
4. Force all of the emulsion into one syringe and disconnect the empty syringe. Load the empty syringe with the remaining 0.25 ml of antigen that was previously withheld.
5. Reconnect the syringes. Push the aqueous antigen into the emulsion first, then repeat the emulsification process for an additional 60 s.
6. Push all the emulsion into one syringe, and disconnect the empty syringe.
7. Test for a stable emulsion by expelling a small drop of the mixture onto the surface of some water in a beaker. The droplet should form a stable bead (see Figure 4.2). If the droplet flattens or dissipates upon the surface of the water, reconnect the syringes to the 3-way stopcock and continue the emulsification process until a stable emulsion is formed, which may take several minutes.

4.5 USE OF RIBI ADJUVANT SYSTEM

Materials:

Ribi adjuvant	Antigen in saline
Syringe for injection	Vortex mixer
Safety eyewear	Latex gloves

Procedure:

1. For use with Ribi Adjuvant System (RAS) it is recommended that the antigen be solubilized at a concentration of 50 to 500 µg/ml in saline (or PBS). Some antigens require detergents to ensure solubility. In these cases, try to make the final detergent concentration 0.2% or less.
2. RAS is supplied in vials as an oil concentrate containing 500 µg of each immunostimulant. Each vial is intended for reconstitution to a final volume of 2 ml with an antigen-containing saline solution. Prior to use, warm the vial for approximately 10 min at 37 to 45°C in a water bath or incubator. This will facilitate in the mixing of the oil into the antigen solution during the next step.
3. Inject 2 ml of antigen solution directly into the stoppered vial (leave the cap seal in place). Vortex vigorously for 2 to 3 min. MPL, TDM, and CWS immunostimulants will be at a final concentration of 250 µg/ml in the antigen–adjuvant emulsion.

OR

Alternatively, if all the adjuvant will not be used initially, reconstitute the vial with 1 ml of PBS or saline alone (without antigen) and vortex vigorously. Using a sterile syringe and 25-gauge needle, withdraw the required volume of adjuvant and mix with an equal volume of antigen-containing saline, then vortex vigorously. Any unused portion of adjuvant will be stable for several months when stored at 4°C (warm to 37°C before use).

Note: The antigen-adjuvant emulsions formed with RAS are not thick, viscous emulsions like those formed using Freund's or TiterMax. They will readily disperse if applied to water.

4. Withdraw the emulsion into a sterile 1 ml syringe for injection and remove any air bubbles.
5. Vaccinate the animals by injecting the antigen-adjuvant emulsion accordingly:
   a. Mice — a total dose of 0.2 ml administered at 2 sites SC (0.1 ml/site) or the entire 0.2 ml IP
   b. Rats or guinea pigs — a total dose of 0.5 ml administered at 2 sites SC (0.2 ml/site) and 0.1 ml IP
   c. Rabbits — a total dose of 1 ml administered as 0.3 ml IM in each thigh, 0.1 ml SC at the back of the neck and the remaining 0.3 ml ID at several sites
   d. Goats — a total dose of 1 ml administered in each hind leg IM (0.5 ml/site)
6. It is recommended that the animals be given vaccine boosts at monthly intervals until the desired titers are obtained.

ACKNOWLEDGMENTS

We would like to thank Y. Hudson, L. Ito, V. Brookshire, and Dr. T. Ulrich for their critical reviews of this chapter. We also thank V. Archer for assistance in the preparation of this chapter.

REFERENCES

1. Freund, J., Casals, J., and Hosmer, E. P., Sensitization and antibody formation after injection of tubercle bacilli and paraffin oil, *Proc. Soc. Exp. Biol. Med.*, 37, 509, 1937.
2. Freund, J., The effect of paraffin oil and mycobacteria on antibody formation and sensitization, *Am. J. Clin. Pathol.*, 21, 645, 1951.
3. Kenney, J. S., Hughes, B. W., Masada, M. P., and Allison, A. C., Influence of adjuvants on the quantity, affinity, isotype and epitope specificity of murine antibodies, *J. Immunol. Methods*, 121, 157, 1989.
4. Broderson, J. R., A retrospective review of lesions associated with the use of Freund's adjuvant, *Lab. Anim. Sci.*, 39, 400, 1989.
5. Claassen, E., de Leeuw, W., de Greeve, P., Hendriksen, C., and Boersma, W., Freund's complete adjuvant: an effective but disagreeable formula, *Res. Immunol.*, 143, 478, 1992.
6. Mallon, F. M., Graichen, M. E., Conway, B. R., Landi, M. S., and Hughes, H. C., Comparison of antibody response by use of synthetic adjuvant system and Freund complete adjuvant in rabbits, *Am. J. Vet. Res.*, 52, 1503, 1991.
7. Lipman, N. S., Trudel, L. J., Murphy, J. C., and Sahali, Y., Comparison of immune response potentiation and *in vivo* inflammatory effects of Freund's and Ribi adjuvants in mice, *Lab. Anim.. Sci.*, 42, 193, 1992.
8. Hunter, R. L., Olsen, M. R., and Bennett, B., Copolymer adjuvants and TiterMax, in *The Theory and Practical Applications of Adjuvants*, Stewart-Tull, D. E. S., Ed., Wiley, New York, 1995, 51.
9. Rudbach, J. A., Cantrell, J. L., and Ulrich, J. T., Methods of immunization to enhance the immune response to specific antigens *in vivo* in preparation for fusions yielding monoclonal antibodies, *Methods Mol. Biol.*, 45, 1, 1995.
10. Maloy, W. L., Coligan, J. E., and Paterson, Y., Production of antipeptide antisera, in *Current Protocols in Immunology*, Vol. 1, Coligan, J. E., Kruisbeek, A. D., Margulies, D. H., Shevach, E. M., and Strober, W., Eds., John Wiley & Sons, New York, 1994, chap. 9.4.
11. van de Wijgert, J. H., Verheul, A. F., Snippe, H., Check, I. J., and Hunter, R. L., Immunogenicity of *Streptococcus pneumoniae* type 14 capsular polysaccharide: influence of carriers and adjuvants on isotype distribution, *Infect. Immunol.*, 59, 2750, 1991.
12. Glenn, G. M., Rao, M., Richards, R. L., Matyas, G. R., and Alving, C. R., Murine IgG subclass antibodies to antigens incorporated in liposomes containing lipid A, *Immunol. Lett.*, 47, 73, 1995.
13. Spack, E. G. and Toavs, D., Transfer techniques for minimizing waste of sonified adjuvant emulsions, *Biotechniques*, 20, 28, 1996.

5 Polyclonal Antibodies

Eric S. Bean

CONTENTS

5.1 INTRODUCTION

This chapter is meant to provide the reader with a general guide to the generation and use of polyclonal antibodies. The protocols and methods that follow are those used in our laboratories and are by no means the only approaches used for these purposes. Instead they represent one set of cohesive practices that result in the consistent generation of high-quality reagents that have proved useful in many different applications.

Polyclonal antibodies have been important research tools for decades. Used in virtually all disciplines of the sciences to identify and quantitate individual molecular species and to dissect the interactions of ligands with their specific binding partners, the speed and ease with which polyclonal antibodies can be generated makes them invaluable reagents for the research community.

When Kohler and Milstein published their hallmark paper on monoclonal antibodies,[1] many thought that polyclonal antibodies were relics of the past. However, there are limitations to the uses of monoclonal antibodies, and recent developments in solid phase synthesis of peptides extend the application of polyclonal antibodies into areas previously thought to be exclusive to monoclonal antibodies. It is now relatively straightforward to produce monospecific polyclonal antibodies via affinity purification using short peptide antigens that represent a single epitope. These same peptides can be used to generate very specific immune responses in host animals and provide the basis for many new diagnostic reagents.

5.2   SELECTION OF HOST

Polyclonal antibodies have been raised in numerous species including mice, rats, hamsters, guinea pigs, rabbits, goats, chickens, horses, donkeys, cattle, sheep, and even emus. The choice of host is predicated on several factors, the most important of which is the intended use of the resulting antibody. If a large volume diagnostic product is the objective, or if extensive research utilizing the resultant antiserum is required, immunizing mice is not a viable approach because of the extremely small volume of serum that is produced. On the other hand, if the antiserum is to be used for the analysis of a dozen western blots, it doesn't make much sense to immunize a horse or a cow, which can provide several liters of antiserum from a single bleeding. For most routine work where small volumes of antiserum are required (i.e., <100 ml), the rabbit is the most common species for polyclonal production, while goats and sheep are the species of choice for large-scale antiserum production. Table 5.1 lists the expected yields of antiserum from various species.

Beyond the question of volume are issues related to the source of the antigen and the expected immunogenicity in a particular host species. Most proteins with molecular weights greater than 6,000 daltons are immunogenic to some degree, and small haptenic molecules can be rendered immunogenic for most species by conjugation to an appropriate carrier molecule, such as bovine serum albumin (BSA), keyhole limpet hemocyanin (KLH), or ovalbumin (OVA). These carrier proteins

TABLE 5.1
Expected Antiserum Yields

Species	Volume (maximum ml per bleed)	Volume (ml per month)
Mouse	0.1–0.2	0.2–0.4
Guinea pig	1–2	3–5
Rabbit	25	50–70
Goat	800	2,000–2,500
Horse	3,000	6,000–8,000
Cow	4,000	8,000–10,000

provide the T-cell epitopes necessary for a successful immune response. Size is not the only consideration, and even large molecules isolated from the immunized species may not provide an immunogenic stimulus because of self-tolerance. Animals avoid the generation of antibodies against self-antigens by elimination of B and/or T cells that recognize host molecules.

Although well-conserved mammalian proteins can be difficult to raise antibodies against, limited success has been achieved with chickens. Phylogenetically divergent from mammals, chickens can respond to many antigens that are otherwise not immunogenic in the more commonly used species, such as rabbits or guinea pigs.[2,3] Some well-conserved proteins prove to be very immunogenic because they are not seen by the immune system under normal circumstances and, when presented in the context of an adjuvant, stimulate a vigorous response. Unfortunately, it is not possible to determine *a priori* if a given protein will be immunogenic or not. The investigator must rely on empirical data for that determination, and success or failure in one species does not provide significant predictive information relative to another species.

One other consideration regarding the host is the number of animals required for immunization. For humane reasons, it is always important to reduce the number to the minimum anticipated to produce a successful project. Understanding that even with genetically identical animals different immune responses will be obtained from a single immunogen preparation, several animals should be used for any immunization program and the animals should be assessed separately to identify those that provide the desired antibodies. With outbred species such as goats or rabbits, the differences between animals are more pronounced, and a minimum of two animals should be used, with three to four preferred where antigen availability is not a great concern. For mice and rats, groups of five are commonly used.

5.3 INJECTION PROTOCOLS

A myriad of injection protocols have been used successfully to generate antibodies to a variety of antigens. Some of the variables include the dose of antigen, route of immunization, frequency of injection, and choice of adjuvant. Many of these reported protocols share common features: (1) a primary immunization, (2) a suitable rest period to allow the primary immune response to subside and memory cells to form, (3) one or more booster injections, and (4) serum collection 10 to 14 days following the last booster.

For the generation of antibodies to be used in routine analytical work, where extremely low concentrations of analyte are not anticipated, a relatively brief immunization protocol can be used:

Day 0: Primary injection (25 to 300 µg antigen), complete Freund's adjuvant (CFA)
Day 21: Booster injection (25 to 300 µg antigen), incomplete Freund's adjuvant (IFA)
Day 42: Booster injection (25 to 300 µg antigen), IFA
Day 56: Serum collection

This generic protocol can be used for most host species and will allow the generation of an effective immune response to a wide variety of antigens. If it is expected or known that the antigen is weakly immunogenic, it is advisable to use CFA for the first booster injection in addition to the primary injection. Subsequent booster immunizations and serum collections can be made at regular intervals to increase the serum yield.

It should be noted that the characteristics of the immune response are changing during this early phase. The primary immunoglobulin response can be detected by typical serological reactions within 5 to 7 days following the initial exposure to the antigen. The antibody titer gradually increases for several days to 2 weeks and afterward begins to drop. The general shape of the primary response is a bell-shaped curve with an extended decay phase, but the exact shape of the response is influenced by many of the same variables mentioned previously.

When booster injections are given, the immune response is characterized by a rise in antibody titer for a period of 10 to 14 days to levels much higher than the primary response. The decay phase is extended because more cells are involved in antibody production and the predominant class of antibodies produced during the secondary immune response is longer lived. Figure 5.1 shows the typical shapes of the primary and secondary immunoglobulin formation curves.

The primary immune response is characterized by relatively high levels of IgM antibody, which has a half-life of 8 to 10 days. The IgG class of antibodies makes up the major proportion of the secondary response, and this class has a half-life of

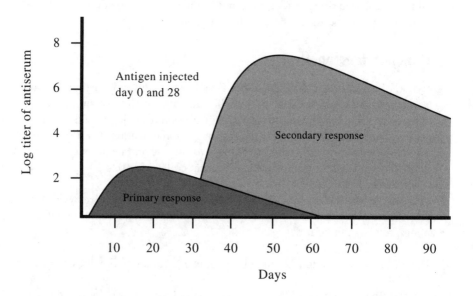

FIGURE 5.1 Primary and secondary immunoglobulin formation. Antibody first becomes detectable in the serum at about day 5 following the primary immunization. The secondary, or anamnestic, response following the second injection at day 28 achieves a very high titer compared to the primary response.

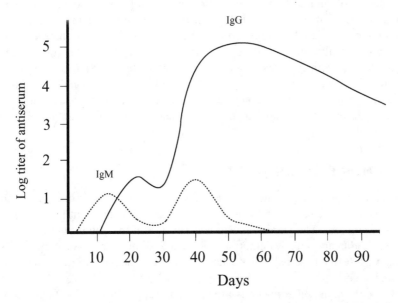

FIGURE 5.2 The IgM response to a typical antigen is about the same magnitude during the primary and secondary responses. The IgG response to the booster injection eclipses the IgM response and is sustained for a much longer period of time. Subsequent injections will result in diminished IgM and heightened IgG responses, respectively, for most antigens.

25 to 35 days. Figure 5.2 shows the relative contribution of IgG and IgM to the primary and secondary antibody responses.

Here too, the nature of the antigen plays an important role in determining the best strategy for generating a good immune response. For most analytical work, IgM antibodies are undesirable because they tend to produce more nonspecific binding than IgG antibodies. For this reason, it is advisable to utilize a protocol with at least three or four booster injections to maximize the IgG response. One note of caution should be mentioned: minor impurities in the antigen will begin to exert their influence on the immune response after multiple immunizations. Unless the immunogen is highly purified, you run the risk of inducing unwanted antibody responses during a prolonged immunization protocol. These undesirable responses can be eliminated by several methods that follow, but in some instances, these remedies are not practical. Keep in mind the fact that a polyclonal immune response is always changing, and that careful evaluation of the quantitative and qualitative aspects of the resulting antibodies is crucial to the generation of an optimal antiserum.

5.4 DOSE OF ANTIGEN

The dose of immunogen required to elicit a good antibody response depends on a number of factors, but it is likely that the amount of antigen that reaches the appropriate antigen-processing cells of the immune system is a major determinant. Thus, the route of administration and the choice of adjuvant will greatly affect the presentation of immunogen and the subsequent antibody response. The intrinsic immunogenicity of the antigen is, by far, the most important factor, and because this is not possible to determine *a priori*, the practical consideration of immunogen availability usually determines the dose. For rabbits and goats, if antigen is abundant, 250 to 500 µg per injection is reasonable, but 100 µg per injection is more common. With rodents, doses from 10 to 100 µg per injection are recommended. It should be noted that many successful immunization schemes have utilized doses as low as a few micrograms per injection, particularly when intra-splenic immunizations have been utilized.[4,5]

5.5   CHOICE OF ADJUVANT

Generation of a strong immune response with immunogens, particularly hapten-carrier conjugates, can be difficult unless a good adjuvant is utilized during the injection protocol. The word *adjuvant* is derived from the Latin *adjuvare*, meaning "to help." Adjuvants are, by definition, nonspecific stimulators of the immune system and serve to extend the half-life of the injected immunogen and to recruit antigen-processing cells.

The most common adjuvant is Freund's adjuvant,[6] a water-in-oil emulsion that provides a depot of immunogen that is slowly released into the surrounding tissues. Freund's complete adjuvant (FCA) contains killed *Mycobacterium tuberculosis* cells while Freund's incomplete adjuvant (IFA) is a simple mixture of paraffin oil and a nonionic surface-active emulsifier. The *Mycobacterium* cells in FCA serve to recruit macrophages to the injection site along with the T cells and B cells necessary for eliciting a good antibody response. Many immunization protocols utilize FCA for the primary injection and IFA for the subsequent booster immunizations because they tend to produce stronger, longer-lasting immune responses compared to other adjuvants. The major drawback to using Freund's adjuvant is the frequent generation of injection-site granulomas. As a result, many institutions have disallowed the use of these adjuvants for protocols conducted under their jurisdiction. Be sure to consult with the appropriate regulatory agency prior to initiating any immunization protocols.

Another commonly used adjuvant is alum, or precipitated aluminum hydroxide. Alum is used with many human vaccines because it is well tolerated and does not produce the injection site reactions associated with Freund's adjuvants. Commercially available preparations provide a convenient method for immunogen formulation that require only the simple mixing of the antigen solution with the alum prior to injection.

Other adjuvants have been developed to provide a potent stimulus to the immune system while reducing the undesirable side effects mentioned above. Hunter's Titer-Max produces stable water-in-oil emulsions using a squalene-based formulation while the Ribi Adjuvant System utilizes bacterial cell-wall components in a stable oil-in-water emulsion to elicit the antibody response. Another new system, GERBU adjuvant, utilizes GMDP, a subunit of the mycobacterial cell wall as the active component. These adjuvant systems provide viable alternatives to the use of Freund's adjuvant, but with some sacrifice in performance for some antigens.

5.6 ROUTE OF IMMUNIZATION

The choice of injection route is dependent on the form and amount of antigen under most circumstances. However, in some cases, a particular route is chosen to facilitate targeting the antigen to a specific set of antigen processing cells, thereby directing the immune system to respond appropriately (e.g., oral immunization to produce gut-associated antibodies, or inhalation immunization to stimulate secretory IgA production). For most soluble antigens prepared with adjuvant, the subcutaneous route is preferred in rabbits and goats, while the intraperitoneal route is more practical for mice and other rodents. Antigens delivered via the intravenous route are metabolized very quickly, while intradermal and intramuscular immunizations slow the presentation of immunogen to the immune system.

The use of animals in the production of polyclonal antiserum is not difficult, but the proper care and handling of animals require experience and patience. Appropriately trained individuals should be consulted prior to the initiation of any antiserum program to ensure the humane treatment of the animals throughout the project.

5.6.1 SUBCUTANEOUS INJECTIONS

Subcutaneous (SC) injections are the most common routes of administration for all animals except mice, and are suitable for all types of immunogens. Typical volumes for rabbits are 0.5 to 1.0 ml total volume delivered to 4 to 6 injection sites. The use of multiple sites provides for an enhanced interaction of the immunogen with the immune system because more lymph nodes are exposed to the preparation. For goats, a total volume of 2 to 3 ml distributed to 6 to 8 sites works well. For immunogens prepared with Freund's adjuvant, sites along the back of the neck, and down both sides of the spine, provide good drainage into the local lymphatic tissues. Mice are typically injected subcutaneously on the back of the neck.

The actual technique for subcutaneous injections is quite simple. Use a 20-gauge needle for immunogen with adjuvant (thick emulsion) and a 22-gauge needle for immunogen without adjuvant:

1. Wipe the appropriate area with an alcohol swab and pinch the skin between the thumb, index, and forefinger. Pull the skin slightly up and away from the body, forming a small skin "tent."
2. Insert the needle through the entire thickness of the skin into the tent, under the area between the fingers, and move it slightly side to side to confirm that the needle has not penetrated muscle or the body wall. Pull back on the plunger to aspirate the syringe. If blood is present, this indicates that the needle is in a vein or small artery. Redirect the needle if blood is present.
3. Inject the required volume of immunogen and wait several seconds prior to removing the needle to prevent any loss of antigen from the site of injection. For rabbits, do not inject more than 0.25 ml per site; for goats, do not exceed 1.0 ml per site; and for mice, 50 to 100 µl per site is recommended.
4. Repeat steps 1 through 3 until all of the immunogen has been injected.

5.6.2   INTRAMUSCULAR INJECTIONS

Intramuscular (IM) injections provide for a slower release of the antigen to the immune system when oil-based adjuvants are used. While goats and rabbits can tolerate injection volumes of 0.3 to 0.5 ml per site, it is not recommended to use this route for mice unless volumes less than 50 µl per site are anticipated. The injection of material into the muscle causes some tissue damage and can be somewhat painful. It may be easier to anesthetize the animal before performing this operation.

If anesthesia is not used, it is best if the muscle is relaxed for these injections, so the use of appropriate restraint devices, or help from an assistant, is required:

1. The semimembranosus/semitendinosus muscles (hindquarter, back leg) are commonly used for intramuscular injections of goats, while the gluteal muscles are preferred for rabbits and mice.
2. Wipe the site with an alcohol swab and insert the needle (22- to 25-gauge for rabbits and goats) with a quick thrust, inserting approximately two thirds of the needle into the muscle. Aspirate the syringe. You should not see any blood in the syringe barrel. If blood is seen, the needle is in a vein or artery and should be repositioned before proceeding.
3. Slowly depress the plunger to administer the immunogen. After withdrawal of the needle, gently massage the injection site to help disperse the inoculum.
4. Repeat steps 2 and 3 until all of the inoculum has been administered.

5.6.3   INTRAVENOUS INJECTIONS

Intravenous (IV) injections are particularly useful for particulate antigens (e.g., whole bacteria) but carry the additional risk of anaphylactic shock when immunizing sensitized animals. This route of injection delivers the inoculum directly to the reticuloendothelial system and results in very rapid metabolism of the immunogen. Virtually all species can be immunized this way, but practice is necessary to accurately deliver the inoculum into the lateral tail vein of a mouse or rat. For rabbits, the marginal ear vein is the preferred site, and with larger species, the jugular vein is appropriate. Oil-based adjuvants should not be injected via the i.v. route.

1. Shave and then clean the area with an alcohol swab.
2. a. For rats and mice, the needle placement should be no closer to the body than half the length of the tail. With the tail under tension, insert the needle approximately parallel with the vein. Insure proper placement by inserting at least 3 mm into lumen of vein and aspirate syringe to confirm intravenous placement.
   b. For rabbits, hold the ear parallel to the ground and insert the needle into the marginal ear vein at a 20° angle. Insure proper placement by inserting at least 3 mm into lumen of vein and aspirate syringe to confirm intravenous placement.

    c. For goats or other large species, apply digital pressure to the jugular furrow so the vein becomes more prominent. Insert the needle into the jugular vein and aspirate syringe to confirm intravenous placement.

3. Inject the inoculum slowly, then remove needle while applying digital pressure to the injection site to prevent excessive bleeding. Continue to hold until bleeding stops, usually about 30 s.

5.6.4 INTRADERMAL INJECTIONS

Intradermal (ID) injections also provide for the slow release of antigen but are technically more difficult to administer. The idea is to deliver the inoculum between the layers of the skin. This is most easily accomplished while the animal is anesthetized, and with mice and rats, anesthesia is absolutely necessary.

1. Clip the hair at the injection site and wipe the site with an alcohol swab.
2. Insert the needle (25-gauge or smaller is recommended, but up to 22-gauge can be used) between the layers of skin at a 20° to 30° angle. It is best to insert 7 to 9 mm of the needle to prevent leakage of the inoculum. Aspirate the syringe. Blood or other fluid in the syringe barrel indicates improper placement. If improper placement occurs, reposition needle.
3. Administer the inoculum slowly and do not inject more than 100 µl per site to prevent tissue trauma. Successful injection results in a small, circular skin welt.
4. Withdraw the needle and apply pressure with the end of a finger simultaneously to the entry point of the needle for several seconds after removal to prevent leakage from the puncture site.
5. Repeat steps 2 to 4 until all of the inoculum has been administered. It is common to use up to 30 injection sites for ID immunization.

5.6.5 INTRAPERITONEAL INJECTIONS

Intraperitoneal (IP) injections are utilized primarily for administering inocula to rodents, but all species can be immunized this way. IP injections are particularly useful for injecting mice and rats, and all forms of immunogens can be employed.

1. For species other than mice and rats, clip hair at the injection site. Wipe the area with an alcohol swab.
2. Insert the needle into the lower right quadrant of the abdomen at a 30° angle. Aspirate the syringe. Blood or other fluid in the syringe barrel indicates improper placement. If improper placement occurs, reposition needle.
3. Administer the inoculum in a steady, fluid motion. Volumes of several milliliters can be injected into mice, and very large volumes can be administered to larger animals.

The brief immunization protocol at the beginning of this section is suitable for the generation of medium titer antiserum to a reasonably immunogenic antigen, is frequently used because most researchers are interested in saving time. However, for the generation of high-titer antiserum, it is necessary to invest more time in the immunization scheme. Ideally, the primary immunization is performed with small amounts of antigen so that only the highest affinity clones are stimulated to proliferate. A longer rest period between the primary injection and subsequent boosts also favors the generation of higher titer antiserum. Once primed, most animals will respond vigorously to secondary immunizations for at least 6 to 8 months. The following schedule, while twice as long, will generally produce a higher quality antiserum than the schedule presented earlier:

Day 0: Primary injection (25 to 100 μg antigen), CFA
Day 35: Booster injection (25 to 100 μg antigen), IFA
Day 56: Booster injection (25 to 100 μg antigen), IFA
Day 77: Booster injection (25 to 100 μg antigen), IFA
Day 98: Booster injection (25 to 100 μg antigen), IFA
Day 108: Serum collection

5.7 BLEEDING

To bleed animals requires a little more skill than to immunize them. It is imperative to insert the needle into a vein. With practice, even mice can be bled with ease. Rabbits are usually bled from the central auricular artery, goats and other larger animals from the jugular vein, and mice or rats from the tail vein. For small test bleeds used to assess the progress of the immunization scheme, a syringe can be used for blood collection, but some hemolysis is inevitable with this technique and should not be used for the collection of larger volumes of serum or where hemolysis may interfere with the eventual use of the antibodies.

For some applications it may be suitable to collect into an anticoagulant such as EDTA or sodium citrate for the preparation of plasma, but for serum production, it is best to collect into clean boroslicate glass containers. These allow for very efficient clotting and produce serum with very little hemolysis.

5.7.1 BLEEDING MICE OR RATS

1. Immobilize the mouse in a suitable restraining device so that the animal is comfortable but unable to twist its body. It is desirable to perform this in a warm environment so that blood is freely circulating to the extremities, including the tail.
2. Clean the underside of the tail with alcohol, approximately 1 to 2 in. from the body. Using a sterile scalpel or razor blade, nick the vein (do not cut all the way through) and collect several drops of blood into a test tube or capillary tube. Apply slight pressure to the site for 15 to 20 s to stop the flow of blood.
3. Allow the blood to clot at room temperature for 2 to 4 h, or alternatively incubate at 37°C for 1 h. Dislodge the clot by gently tapping the tube and transfer to 4°C for 2 to 3 h or overnight.

4. Separate the serum from the clot by centrifugation at 10,000 × g for 15 min.

5. If yield is critical, pour off the serum and spin the supernatant again at 10,000 × g for 10 min before collecting the final serum from above the cell pellet. This will provide about 100 to 200 µl of serum. If yield is not important, aspirate enough serum from above the original clot for testing. This will provide about 50 to 100 µl of serum.

6. For most applications, the addition of sodium azide to 0.05% (final concentration) and storage at 4°C for short periods is acceptable. If azide will interfere with the testing, aliquot and store the serum at −20°C until use.

5.7.2   BLEEDING RABBITS

1. Place the rabbit in a restraining device so that the ears are accessible. The rabbit should be warm so that blood flow to the ears is unimpeded.

2. Shave the ear along the central auricular artery and then clean the area with an alcohol swab.

3. Insert a 22-gauge needle into the central auricular artery and hold a test tube under the needle hub to collect the blood.

4. Gently rubbing the ear with a finger above the area just cleaned will promote blood flow and facilitate blood collection. fifty milliliters can safely be obtained in about 6 to 7 min if the rabbit is calm and warm. If the animal becomes startled, or if the temperature is too low, blood flow to the ears is involuntarily slowed and collection can be difficult or impossible.

5. Allow the blood to clot at room temperature for 2 to 4 h, or alternatively incubate at 37°C for 1 h. Dislodge the clot by rimming the tube with a wooden applicator and transfer to 4°C for 2 to 3 h, or overnight, to allow complete clot retraction.

6. Separate the serum from the clot by centrifugation at 10,000 × g for 15 min.

7. If yield is critical, pour off the serum and spin the supernatant again at 10,000 × g for 10 min. before collecting the final serum from above the cell pellet. If yield is not important, aspirate enough serum from above the original clot for testing.

8. For most applications the addition of sodium azide (to 0.05%) and storage at 4°C for short periods is acceptable. If azide will interfere with the testing, aliquot and store the serum at −20°C until use.

5.7.3   BLEEDING GOATS (OR OTHER LARGE ANIMALS)

1. Immobilize the animal in a suitable restraining device so that its head can be held up to expose the jugular vein.

2. Shave or clip the hair around the vein and clean the area with an alcohol swab.

3. Insert an 18-gauge needle into the jugular and collect the blood into an appropriate size glass container. This can be facilitated by the use of a butterfly needle attached to a piece of tubing with a roller clamp. The flow of blood can then be controlled by use of the valve.

4. Remove the needle while applying digital pressure to the injection site to prevent excessive bleeding. Continue to hold until bleeding stops, usually about 30 to 45 s.

5. Allow the blood to clot at room temperature for 2 to 4 h or alternatively incubate at 37°C for 1 h. Dislodge the clot by rimming the container with a wooden applicator and transfer to 4°C for 2 to 3 h or overnight to allow complete clot retraction.

6. Separate the serum from the clot by centrifugation at $10,000 \times g$ for 15 min.

7. If yield is critical, pour off the serum and spin the supernatant again at $10,000 \times g$ for 10 min before collecting the final serum from above the cell pellet. If yield is not important, aspirate enough serum from above the original clot for testing.

8. For most applications the addition of sodium azide (to 0.05%) and storage at 4°C for short periods is acceptable. If azide will interfere with the testing, aliquot and store the serum at −20°C until use.

5.8 TESTING SERUM SAMPLES

Assessing the progress of an immunization program is critical to the successful development of high-quality polyclonal antisera. Because the immune response is constantly undergoing change, it is imperative to monitor both quantitative and qualitative aspects of the antibody response. While many different techniques are available for evaluating antibodies, the method used should reflect the ultimate use of the antibody, because a polyclonal antiserum that is ideal for ELISA assays may not work very well for immunoprecipitation or immunohistochemistry. The ELISA method is, by far, the most widely used for the initial evaluation of potency, or titer.

5.8.1 ENZYME-LINKED IMMUNOSORBENT ASSAY

Materials

Polystyrene microtiter plates
Pipet: adjustable 20 to 200 μl
25 mM Na$_2$CO$_3$ buffer, pH 8.6
Phosphate buffered saline (PBS): 10 mM Na$_2$HPO$_4$/NaH$_2$PO$_4$, 150 mM NaCl, pH 7.2
Bovine serum albumin (BSA), gelatin or casein
Tween 20
Secondary antibody conjugate (e.g., goat anti-rabbit IgG or rabbit anti-goat IgG conjugated to horseradish peroxidase)
Citrate-phosphate buffer: 50 mM Na$_2$HPO$_4$ −50 mM citric acid, pH 5.0

Orthophenylenediamine (OPD)
Hydrogen peroxide (H_2O_2), 30%
Sulfuric acid (H_2SO_4), $4N$
Microtiterplate reader

By far, the easiest method for testing the resulting antiserum is to use an enzyme linked immunosorbent assay (ELISA). Most antigens can be detected when bound directly to the solid phase (typically an 8×12 96-well polystyrene plate). This is a common assay protocol:

1. Antigen is allowed to bind passively to the plate overnight at 4°C (100 µl, 0.1 to 1.0 µg per well in carbonate buffer.
2. Blocking solution containing excess protein (1 to 2% BSA, gelatin, or casein in PBS) and 0.05% Tween 20 is added (150 to 200 µl) to eliminate the remaining protein binding sites. This is allowed to incubate for 1 to 2 h at room temperature.
3. Primary antibody (the serum to be tested) is titrated across the plate (100 µl of a 1:50 dilution is a good starting point) and incubated for 30 to 60 min followed by washing of the plate to remove unbound antibody.
4. Secondary (anti-species) antibody conjugated to horseradish peroxidase (100 µl per well, dilution depends on specific lot, needs to be in excess) is incubated for 30 to 60 min followed by washing of the plate to remove unbound antibody.
5. Enzyme substrate (100 µl of 10 mg/ml OPD in citrate-phosphate buffer containing 0.1% H_2O_2) is added and incubated for 10 to 30 min, after which the reaction is stopped by the addition of sulfuric acid (50 µl). The plate is read in a microtiter plate reader, and the amount of color developed is directly proportional to the amount of primary antibody in the well. Using this technique, the relative titers of the various serums collected can be compared and ranked.

For very small antigens and haptens, it can be difficult to detect antibody with antigen directly adsorbed to the solid phase. In this case, there are several alternatives:

1. The antigen can be conjugated to a different protein than that used for the immunogen. This antigen conjugate is then coated on the solid phase and presents the antigen in manner similar to the immunogen, thereby increasing the potential for antibody–antigen interaction. It is best to use different conjugation chemistries for the solid-phase antigen and immunogen because some linker molecules elicit strong immune responses. If the same chemistry is used, much of the observed reactivity may be directed at the linker and not the hapten.
2. The antigen can be biotinylated and bound to streptavidin-coated plates. This binds the antigen in an oriented fashion so that detection is relatively straightforward.

One of the drawbacks to this ELISA format is that it requires the antigen to be bound to the solid phase. This can result in conformational changes in the antigen that reduce the affinity of the antibody for the antigen. Conjugation of the antigen to an inert carrier protein and immobilization via biotin–avidin, as mentioned above, are two remedies for this. Another remedy is to utilize a "sandwich" assay format. The limitation to this approach is that you must have two antibodies that are directed at different epitopes and the antibodies must be derived from different species if the indirect method is to be used (anti-species conjugate), or one of the antibodies must be purified and labeled if the direct method is used.

5.8.2 RADIAL IMMUNODIFFUSION

Materials

Antigen solutions of various concentrations
Agarose (1.5% in barbital buffer, pH 8.6)
Pipets: 10 ml, adjustable pipets 1 to 10 and 20 to 200 μl
Plastic radial immunodiffusion (RID) plates (various configurations, dimensions determine volume of agarose required)
Hot water bath
Precision hole punch, 2 mm diameter
Jeweler's eyepiece with calibrated scale
Small, disposable mixing cups (15 to 20 ml)

This technique is commonly used to quantitate antisera directed against serum proteins. Because it relies on the formation of immune complex precipitates, it is not particularly useful for antisera raised against haptens. If a source of antigen is available for which the concentration is reliably known, this technique can provide an absolute titer of a polyclonal antiserum (mg antigen consumed per ml antiserum),[7] otherwise a relative ranking of various bleeds can be obtained.

This protocol assumes the use of 8-cm circular RID plates with 4.6-cm center wells. Pouring 8 ml of agarose into this configuration provides a layer 1.0 mm thick. Use of alternative configurations will require a different volume of agarose or a correction factor in the equation below:

1. Heat the agarose to 68°C. At this temperature the agarose is liquid, but not so hot that it will denature the antibody to be subsequently added.
2. Pipet the appropriate volume of antiserum into a small, disposable mixing cup and add enough agarose to bring the total volume to 10 ml. This combination is quickly mixed to produce a homogeneous solution.
3. Pipet 8 ml of the agarose/antibody mixture evenly into the RID plate. The use of a circular rotatory bed facilitates the even distribution of agarose. Allow the agarose to cool and solidify.
4. Punch holes in the agarose to provide wells for the addition of antigen solution. This can be facilitated by attaching a piece of tubing to the punch

and applying a slight vacuum. Be careful not to apply too much vacuum, as distorted holes will result in inaccurate measurements.

5. Pipet 2 μl of each antigen solution into separate wells. A minimum of three different concentrations should be used, and five standards seem to give consistently reliable results. Allow the antibody–antigen reaction to come to equilibrium. For most proteins an incubation period of 24 h is sufficient, but larger molecules, which diffuse more slowly (e.g., IgM), require additional time. The reaction can be monitored by reading the diameters of the precipitin rings at various times and selecting a time after which no further changes take place.

6. Plot the square of the diameter versus the antigen concentration. From the

$$T = \frac{4 \times V_{ag}}{P \times k_1 \times \pi \times h}$$

slope of the resulting line, the antiserum titer (T, mg/ml) can be calculated: where V_{ag} is the volume of antigen, P is the antiserum concentration in the gel (% v/v), k_1 is the slope of the line, and h is the depth or height of the antiserum-containing gel.

ELISA and RID methodologies provide measurements of potency, but that is only half of the equation. If highly purified antigens are utilized in those assays, it is possible to get a good estimate of the specific antibody titer, but the nature of the other antibodies present in the serum cannot be easily determined with those techniques. Instead, methods that employ a separation step for the antigen prior to introduction of the antiserum provide valuable information regarding the specificity of the antibodies.

5.8.3 WESTERN BLOT ANALYSIS

Western blots (covered in more detail in Chapter 15) are performed in a three-stage procedure. Following separation of an antigenic mixture by SDS-PAGE, the proteins are transferred to a nitrocellulose or PVDF membrane in the second stage. At this point, the membrane-bound antigen mixture is treated in much the same way as an ELISA plate. The excess binding sites are blocked with a solution containing an irrelevant protein and some detergent. Primary antibody is diluted into the blocking buffer and incubated with the membrane. Following washing to remove excess antibody, secondary antibody conjugate is incubated with the membrane to allow binding to any primary antibody captured by the immobilized antigens. After another wash cycle, enzyme substrate is added to disclose where conjugate has been localized. The substrates used for Western blots differ from those used in the ELISA protocol because the final colored product is insoluble and binds to the membrane wherever enzyme conjugate is found. This results in a pattern of colored bands indicating what molecular weight species in the antigenic mixture reacts with the primary antibody mixture. A complex pattern of reactivity indicates that either the antiserum contains undesirable antibodies or that the epitopes recognized by the antiserum are present on a heterogeneous mixture of antigens (e.g., degradation fragments). A single band indicates a monospecific antibody relative to the electrophoresed antigen preparation.

5.8.4 IMMUNOELECTROPHORESIS

Immunoelectrophoresis (IEP) is performed as a two-stage procedure. The first stage separates the antigenic material in biological fluids by their differential migration in an electric field (Figure 5.3B). The second stage of this technique is the immunological characterization of the separated proteins by the immunodiffusion procedure (Figure 5.3C). In this process, antibody diffuses into the gel and the antibody–antigen reaction is visualized by staining the resulting immunoprecipitates. This method is commonly utilized to evaluate the specificity of antisera raised against serum proteins.

Materials

  Agarose IEP slides (1.5% low electroendosmosis agarose dissolved in 0.035 M barbital buffer, pH 8.6)
  Barbital buffer (27 mM barbital, 23 mM sodium acetate, 15 mM sodium azide, pH 8.6 ± 0.1)

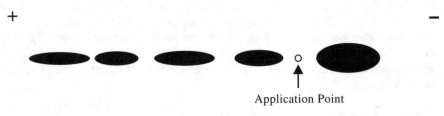

Application Point

FIGURE 5.3B The first stage of immunoelectrophoresis separates the antigenic mixture on the basis of charge.

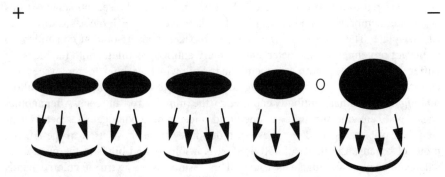

FIGURE 5.3C During the immunodiffusion stage, antibody and antigen migrate and form immuno-precipitates that can be seen best after staining.

Electrophoresis chamber
Constant voltage power supply (up to 200 volts)
Adjustable pipets 1 to 10 and 20 to 200 µl
Bromphenol blue dye, 0.1% (w/v)
Amido black dye, 0.1% (w/v)

1. Pipet 1 to 2 µl of bromphenol blue dye into well #1 and allow this to be adsorbed into the gel. Pipet 4 µl normal serum into well #1, and 4 µl of the appropriate antigens into the other wells (see Figure 5.3A).
2. Fill the electrophoresis chambers with barbital buffer (the same volume on both sides to prevent capillary migration due to hydrostatic pressure).
3. Place the slide into the electrophoresis chamber and make contact with the running buffer.
4. Turn on the power supply and electrophorese the antigens at 170 volts (5 to 7 volts/cm) for 60 to 90 min or until the bromphenol blue tracking dye has migrated 5 to 10 mm from the end of the antiserum trough.
5. Remove the gel from the precut trough if not already done (a small-gauge needle works well).
6. Dispense 90 µl of antiserum into the appropriate troughs and place the slide in a humidified chamber for the immunodiffusion portion of the assay (18 to 24 h at room temperature).
7. Direct analysis of the plate can be performed prior to staining and drying. This is recommended because faint immunoprecipitin lines can be abolished

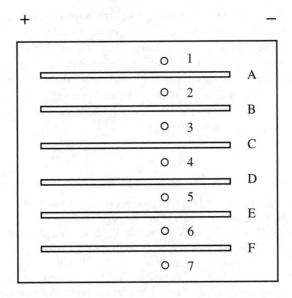

FIGURE 5.3A A typical IEP slide is configured with multiple wells for the placement of the antigenic mixture to be electrophoresed, typically serum (1–7). Adjacent to the antigen wells are troughs that hold the antiserum for the second stage immunodiffusion (A–F).

during the subsequent washing step prior to staining. This is accomplished by viewing the plate against a black background using a point source of light held behind the plate at an angle of approximately 45°.

8. If staining is desired, the plate should be placed in normal saline for 24 to 48 h to leach out soluble, nonprecipitated proteins. A brief soak in distilled or deionized water will remove excess salts prior to staining. Place the slide in the amido black stain for 10 to 15 min and remove excess stain with a brief rinse with distilled water followed by destaining in acetic acid, ethanol (methanol), water (10, 45, 45 by volume). After destaining the gel can be dried and mounted for a permanent record.

9. Interpretation of the resulting immunoprecipitates can be aided by the use of known, specific antisera. A monospecific antiserum results in the generation of a single precipitin line while antiserum containing multiple antigenic specificities will produce multiple arcs. (Figure 5.3c).

5.9   POST PRODUCTION PURIFICATION

Polyclonal antiserum by its very nature contains antibodies that will bind many different antigens. In some assay systems, this is not a problem because the specific antibody titer is high enough that simple dilution eliminates the interference, or the antigens recognized by the nonspecific antibodies are not present in the assay system. When this is not the case, there are approaches for the generation of a monospecific polyclonal antiserum: (1) affinity purification of the specific antibodies, and (2) affinity depletion of the nonspecific antibodies, leaving behind the specific antibodies.

These techniques are covered in more detail in Chapter 11. But the basic method involves the immobilization of the specific antigen on a solid phase (usually activated Sepharose-like beads) for affinity purification or immobilization of the nonspecific antigen(s) on a solid phase for the affinity depletion method. Passing the antiserum over the immobilized antigen(s) results in binding of the appropriate antibodies, which can be recovered following elution (affinity purified antibody) or discarded following elution (depletion methods). These procedures allow the generation of highly specific polyclonal antisera.

REFERENCES

1. Kohler, G. and Milsten, C., 1975, Continuous culture of fused cells secreting antibody of predefined specificity, *Nature*, 256, 495–497.
2. Vieira, J. G. H., Oliveira, M. A. D., Russo, E. M. K., Maciel, R. M. B., and Pereira, A. B., 1984, Egg yolk as a source of antibodies for human parathyroid hormone (hPTH) radioimmunoassay, *J. Immunoassay*, 5, 121–129.
3. Stuart, C. A., Pietrzyk, R. A., Furlanetto, R. W., and Green, A., 1988, High affinity antibody from hen's eggs directed against the human insulin receptor and the human IGF-1 receptor, *Anal. Biochem.*, 173, 142–150.
4. Batova, I. N., Petrov, M. G., Kyurkchiev, S. D., and Kehayov, I. R., 1966, Characterization of a sperm nuclear protein, *Am. J. Reprod. Immunol.*, 36, 49–57.

5. Cardillo, F., Mengel, J., Garcia, S. B., and Cunha, F. Q., 1995, Mouse ear spleen grafts: a model for intra splenic immunization with minute amounts of antigen, *J. Immunol. Methods*, 188, 43–49.
6. Freund, J. and McDermot, K., 1942, Sensitization to horse serum by means of adjuvants, *Proc. Soc. Exp. Biol. N.Y.*, 49, 548.
7. Becker, W., 1969, Determination of antisera titres using the single radial immunodiffusioin method, *Immunochemistry*, 6, 539–546.

6 Monoclonal Antibody Production

Sandy J. Stewart

CONTENTS

6.1 INTRODUCTION

In 1975, Kohler and Milstein[1] began a Nobel Prize-winning revolution in the scientific community. Even then, probably very few individuals could have envisioned the tremendous developments awaiting the future. Monoclonal antibodies have

0-8493-9445-7/00/$0.00+$.50
© 2000 by CRC Press LLC

become powerful tools in virtually every field of biological science and medicine. The discovery of novel applications and their contributions to all fields of research have been limitless. Monoclonal antibodies constitute one of the most important scientific tools for the past two decades. Although research was the first market penetrated, monoclonal antibodies have become a driving force in today's $17 billion medical diagnostics market. Most current home pregnancy and ovulation tests employ monoclonal antibodies and more recently, monoclonal antibodies have moved into the medical therapeutics market with potential products for various cancers and autoimmune diseases.

This chapter deals with the preparation, production, culture, cloning, and freezing of hybridoma cell lines. It assumes that the reader is somewhat versed in the field of mammalian cell culture. Additional aspects are covered in other chapters within this book (see Chapter 1, for example). An enormous number of factors are involved in hybridoma production; the described techniques attempt to present a more conservative, well-accepted protocol for the novice. The following protocol is not the only approach, nor is it always the best, but it will consistently provide good results.

6.1.1   OVERVIEW

Immunization of an animal results in the activation of B lymphocytes and subsequent antibody production recognizing hundreds or thousands of epitopes. The magnitude of the response is dictated by the immunogenicity of the antigen injected. This collection of antibody produced by many different B cells is termed *polyclonal* for the various B cell clones it is derived from. As such, polyclonal serum is comprised of a collection of monoclonal antibodies. Unfortunately, when B-cells are removed from an animal and cultured *in vitro*, they die quickly unless they are somehow transformed and immortalized. A single B cell from the polyclonal mixture which is isolated and immortalized is termed *monoclonal*.

Monoclonal antibodies are those produced by a single B-cell clonal line. Each mammalian B cell contains the capacity to produce an antibody which recognizes a single epitope, generally consisting of 6 to 12 amino acids. Although this single B cell may produce hundreds of antibodies, they will all be identical in the epitope binding region. The conferring of immortality to that single B cell by fusion to a myeloma cell results in a B-cell line (hybridoma) producing a single epitope-binding monoclonal antibody.

6.1.2   SCHEDULE

1. Choose mutant cell line, media, selection method, and antigen source for immunization and screening.
2. Immunize animals.
3. Develop screening method (discussed in detail in Chapter 7).
4. Fusion.
5. Screen supernatants.
6. Clone and cryopreserve.
7. Screen clones and cryopreserve.

6.2 CELL LINES AND MEDIA

The choice of animal is restricted to those with compatible mutant cell lines available for fusion. Since most mutant cell lines are BALB/c mouse derived, mice and rats are most commonly used as donor animals. The BALB/c strain is preferred, unless it responds poorly to a specific immunogen, primarily since there will be no subsequent histocompatibility problems when fused with a typical BALB/c myeloma line. Resultant hybridomas will easily proliferate into tumors when injected intraperitoneally into BALB/c mice and produce high titer ascites. Rat–mouse hybrids appear as stable as mouse–mouse hybrids, but require the use of nude athymic mice for ascites production.[2] However, ascites production from interspecies hybridomas can also be accomplished in artificially immunosuppressed animals.[3] Bifunctional hybrids can be produced by the fusion of two hybridomas and yield antibodies that specifically bind with two antigens.[4] A method of selection must be developed to distinguish such hybrids. Typical mutant cell lines used are SP2/0-Ag 14, P3-X63-Ag8.653, S194/5.XXO, and FO. All of these myeloma cell lines are BALB/c derived, do not secrete immunoglobulin, and have been used extensively for fusions.[5] In many cases the literature will describe which cell line is most appropriate for a specific application. These cell lines must be maintained in a sterile, humidified incubator at 37°C and at 5% CO_2 in air, and should be kept growing in log phase at 3–6×10^5 cells/ml. If the myeloma line is allowed to overgrow to 1×10^6 cells/ml, its hybrid-forming efficiency irreversibly declines. The reason is not well understood and the only recourse is to thaw a new aliquot. The mutant cell line that is to be used should be put into culture at least 2 to 3 weeks before the anticipated fusion.

6.2.1 MEDIA

Three commonly used media are RPMI-1640, DMEM, and IMDM, which can be purchased as powders or ready-to-use sterile liquids (see reference 6 for a detailed list of components). Several components should be added prior to use, specifically glutamine, an antibiotic, and fetal bovine serum (FBS), which are described in Section 6.2.3, Preparation of Media. Glutamine is very labile and decomposes at temperatures above freezing, releasing toxic ammonia into the culture media. Short-term storage at 4°C will minimize this problem. Antibiotics such as penicillin, streptomycin, and gentamycin are often added singularly or in combination to offer broad-spectrum protection against microbes while avoiding the higher toxicity of some other antibiotics. A number of labs currently use a medium commercially sold as serum-free and can be equally effective as serum-supplemented media in certain cases. However, the inclusion of serum is almost always advantageous and well worth the additional investment. Which FBS supplier to use is very subjective, but it is also a very critical factor. If possible, obtain some from a colleague who is using a specific lot which works well for the myeloma cell line and medium which you are planning to use. Heat inactivate the FBS at 56°C for 30 min. The next best approach is to obtain samples (about 100 ml) from at least four lots from a supplier. The supplier will reserve a specific amount of each of these lots while you run your tests. Culture the myeloma cells in each lot and perform a fusion with spleen cells. Then culture the fusion products in each of the four lots. This is obviously very time consuming but is regarded as necessary when setting up to perform a number of fusions. When this task is completed, the fusion efficiency variations between lots of serum will justify the time invested. There are additional media supplements that some investigators add at various times during the fusion, selection, and culturing processes for a variety of reasons, for example, attempting to increase specific antibody production by addition of IL-6.[7] While many of these components may offer some degree of benefit, their omission will not inhibit a successful fusion. Once a level of comfort and success is achieved with the basic protocol, experimentation is always encouraged to optimize specific needs. Finally, all culture media must be filter sterilized and undergo a sterility check for at least 1 week at 37°C without antibiotics or 2 weeks with antibiotics.

6.2.2 SELECTION METHOD

After the fusion process, several cell types are present in the culture; however, all except the hybridomas and unfused mutant cells will die out. There must be a method to select for the hybridomas specifically, since the mutant cells would eventually outgrow the hybrids. The most commonly used method is to use mutant cell lines that are deficient in the enzyme hypoxanthine guanine phosphoribosyl transferase (HGPRT) and culturing the cells in medium supplemented with hypoxanthine, aminopterin, and thymidine (HAT).[8] Aminopterin blocks the biosynthetic pathway for nucleic acids. Normal cells produce HGPRT and can use a salvage pathway if supplied with hypoxanthine and thymidine (HT), whereas the mutant cell lines cannot do. By culturing the fusion products in HAT, eventually the only cells able to survive will be the hybridomas, since they can produce HGPRT (characteristic derived from the normal spleen cell) and they can survive in cell culture (characteristic from the mutant cell line). Figure 6.1 illustrates this selection process. The BALB/c derived SP2/0 myeloma cell lines deficient in HGPRT are commonly used in this scheme. An additional method involves using mutant cell lines deficient in thymidine kinase and following a similar premise.

6.2.3 PREPARATION OF MEDIA

Complete Dulbecco's Modified Eagles Media (DMEM)

900 ml	1× liquid medium, DMEM
10 ml	Penicillin-streptomycin solution (10,000 units/ml)
10 ml	L-glutamine (200 mM)
100 ml	FBS (heat inactivated)

Sterilize through a 0.2-µm filter and store at 4°C for 3 to 4 weeks.

HAT medium: Prepare a 100× stock that is sterilely filtered and stored frozen, protected from light. Aminopterin is light sensitive and can easily degrade to the point of being ineffective.

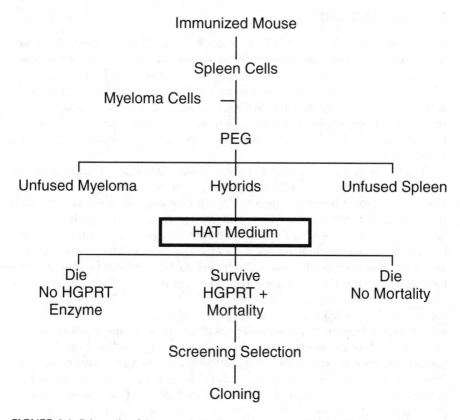

FIGURE 6.1 Schematic of the procedure of producing monoclonal antibodies and the selection process employing HAT.

136 mg	hypoxanthine
1.9 mg	aminopterin (light sensitive)
39 mg	thymidine

It is convenient to mix the hypoxanthine and thymidine together, since this solution can be split for both HAT and HT. Heat the hypoxanthine and thymidine to 45°C to aid in solubilization. Also, a few drops of 1 *N* sodium hydroxide added to the aminopterin-containing solution will aid in solubilization. Sterilize by filtration and store in 1-ml aliquots at –20°C. This can now be diluted 1:100 in complete DMEM for use.

HT medium: Same as above without aminopterin.

Polyethylene glycol (PEG): Make up a 50% solution of PEG 1200 in PBS by heating to 50°C. Autoclave to sterilize and store at 4°C.

6.3   IMMUNIZATION

A significant amount of time and effort can be saved and chances of success increased if one takes time at this stage. Although a major advantage of hybridoma production is the ability to immunize with crude antigen and screen for specificity, it is certainly advantageous, when possible, to immunize with the highest purity of antigen available. This will not only increase the chance of success, but will also significantly reduce screening complexity and time. In some cases, pure antigen will be needed for either the immunization or screening, although generally less amounts are needed for screening.

The immunization schedule employed is very important. Adequate time is required for maturation of affinity and isotype class switch to occur. The first exposure of a naive immune system to a specific immunogen will result primarily in production of IgM antibody. Following the initial response, individual B cells can undergo a class switch of their immunoglobulin isotype. It is thought that a somatic gene recombination occurs within the B-cell heavy chain locus such that the heavy chains of the Ig change from IgM to IgG, but the variable epitope-binding region remains the same.[9] The cytokines IL-4 and IL-5 are thought to direct the switching to specific isotypes. Within 4 to 5 days B-cell affinity maturation and class switch begin.[10] If a rest period of at least 3 weeks follows before a boost immunization, then the products will be primarily antibodies of the IgG and IgA subclasses (see Figure 6.2). This is a very simplified scheme of an only partially understood process. For many antibody uses, such as capture or detection in a sandwich assay, immunoaffinity purification of antigen, etc., IgG antibodies are generally desired due to their stability and physical advantages over the pentameric IgM isotype.

The interval between subsequent immunizations can also greatly affect the affinity of antibody produced. As the interval is increased, antigen levels decrease and only higher affinity B cells remain ready to respond to a subsequent boost such that the response becomes mostly directed against the more immunogenic antigen. Most of this process occurs in germinal centers formed by antigen-activated B cells and follicular dendritic cells. The most likely theory involves somatic hypermutation of the V-D-J regions of the B-cell genome followed by antigen selection of high affinity cells.[1] Hypermutation only seems to occur in activated B cells and is thought to cease with the onset of class switching. Almost all antibodies produced after secondary immunizations show signs of hypermutation.

Consideration must also be given to the expected life span of mice and the possible development of fibroblasts with age. Typically, 6- to 8-week-old mice are initially immunized with the fusion performed within 6 months. A minimum of three injections with a maximum of 200 μl of volume per mouse should be planned. At least three mice should be identically immunized to safeguard against premature death due to a variety of reasons. The primary immunization should be subcutaneous and equally distributed in two to four locations in the abdominal area. The second immunization should be given intraperitoneally. A final boost 3 to 4 days prior to fusion should be administered intravenously through the tail vein to maximize immunogen reaching the spleen and activating B cells.

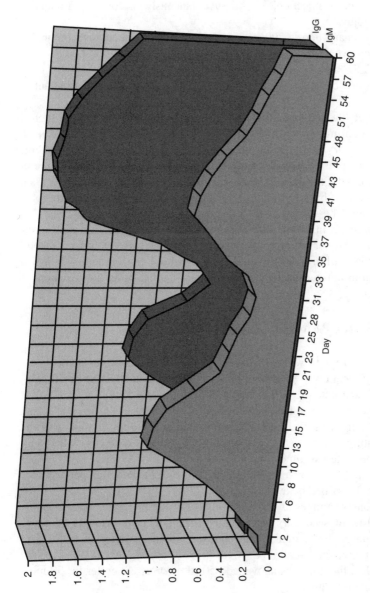

FIGURE 6.2 Demonstration of the anamnestic response due to a challenge immunization administered at day 31 and the comparison of the associated switch in IgG predomination over IgM. Isotype measurements reflect only those levels associated with the specific response against antigen immunized and not the total population.

6.3.1 IMMUNIZATION PROTOCOL

Animal: BALB/c male mouse, 8 weeks old.
Day 0   Take a blood sample to be used as a negative control.
Day 0   Primary injection, 200 μl subcutaneously in complete Freund's
          adjuvant.
Day 28   Primary boost, 200 μl intraperitoneally in incomplete Freund's
          adjuvant.
Day 38   Take blood sample for test screen.
Day 60   Final boost, 50 μl intravenously (tail vein) soluble, no adjuvant.

If the titer of the test screen at day 38 is not deemed satisfactory, then the animal should continue to be immunized at 3- to 4-week intervals, as on day 28, until a satisfactory titer is achieved. The final intravenous boost should entail all the customary precautions of any intravenous injection and cannot include adjuvant. Specifically, the antigen must be soluble in a physiological buffer, such as 0.85% phosphate buffered saline (PBS) pH 7.2 and the concentration of immunogen should be only one fifth of the amount previously injected. This small dose will result in activating only the highest affinity B cells and increase the chance for a higher affinity monoclonal. Utmost care should be taken to avoid air bubbles within the syringe. A single bubble can immediately kill the animal. If soluble antigen is not available, then a final boost intraperitoneally should be given.

6.3.2 TEST SCREEN PROTOCOL

1. Coat a microplate with 50 μl/well of solubilized antigen at maximal coating (generally 5 μg/ml) in borate buffered saline (BBS) or 50 mM sodium carbonate pH 8.5 overnight at 4°C.
2. Wash the plate five times with ELISA wash buffer.
3. Fill the wells with ELISA block buffer and incubate for 30 min at room temperature.
4. Wash the plate five times as above.
5. Add 50 μl of test serum diluted in ELISA diluent buffer per well at dilutions described below.
6. Wash plate five times as above.
7. Add 50 μl of secondary antibody–enzyme conjugate, such as alkaline phosphatase-labeled donkey anti-mouse antibody at 1 μg/ml in ELISA diluent buffer for 1 h at 37°C.
8. Wash plate five times as above, add 50 μl of substrate buffer for 30 min at room temperature.
9. Stop the reaction with 3 N NaOH and read plate.

Pre-immune and test serum dilutions are 1:300, 1,000, 3,000, 10,000, 30,000, 100,000, and 0.

6.3.3   ELISA Reagents

Borate buffered saline (BBS):

   100 mM boric acid
   25 mM sodium borate
   75 mM sodium chloride
   pH 8.5

ELISA wash buffer:

   10 mM Tris
   0.05% Tween-20
   0.03% sodium azide
   pH 8.0

ELISA block and diluent buffers:

   0.05% Tween-20
   1.0% BSA (grade V)
   0.03% sodium azide
   Add to PBS at pH 7.4, no need to adjust pH

ELISA substrate buffer:

   9.6% diethanolamine (v/v)
   1.0 mM magnesium chloride
   Adjust pH to 9.8 with HCl

ELISA substrate:

   15 mg p-nitrophenyl phosphate in 25 ml ELISA substrate buffer
   No need to adjust pH

6.4   HYBRIDIZATION PROTOCOL

The actual hybridization of two cells is simply a physical and/or chemical manipulation forcing cells to adhere and fuse with each other. The resultant hybrid contains the DNA from both cells and is thus tetraploid if all DNA is accounted for. This manipulation is completely random and results in fusion between a variety of cells, not just the desired fusion products. The hybridization chemical is also extremely detrimental to cells and results in considerable stress to surviving cells and also considerable cell death. Therefore, the most widely used hybridization chemical, polyethylene glycol (PEG), is probably the most crucial medium element in the fusion process. PEG actually causes cells to adhere to one another and their membranes fuse such that two cells become one and the resultant cell contains much of the DNA from both cells. The mechanics of this are solely dependent upon the solution of PEG.[12] Molecular weights of PEG are actually only averages, although most researchers use from 1000 to 3000 Da. If possible, obtain a solution of PEG from a colleague who has had success with it. If this is not possible, then you must test your PEG solution in a fusion before use in an actual experiment. If you do not have success, another batch made the same way will probably work. There is no rationale for this. Make up a 50% solution of PEG 1200 in PBS by heating to 50°C. Autoclave to sterilize and store at 4°C. For reasons previously mentioned, a successful PEG solution should be carefully stored for future use.

6.4.1 FEEDER CELLS

Hybridomas, like most lymphoid cell lines, grow poorly at very low densities. The reasons are not well understood but are thought to include requirements for growth factors such as IL-6, trace elements such as selenium, and the neutralization of cellular toxins. Feeder cells are generally thymocytes, macrophages, or fibroblasts, which are co-cultured with the fusion products to aid in their proliferation. They will eventually die out in culture; however, fibroblasts should be irradiated to keep them from dividing and outgrowing the hybrids. The addition of feeders is always advantageous to the culture and is considered essential by many investigators.

Macrophages, for use as feeders, can be harvested through lavage of the murine peritoneal cavity with PBS. One mouse can yield approximately 3×10^6 macrophages, which is generally enough to plate out ten 96-well plates. Using a fire-polished glass Pasteur pipette, suspend the cells to eliminate clumping. Centrifuge for 10 min at $400 \times g$ and resuspend the pellet in culture medium. Perform a cell count, dilute in complete DMEM to 3×10^4 cells/ml, and plate out 50 µl/well 1 to 2 days prior to the fusion. Generally, one spleen will contain approximately 100 million B cells and yield enough cells for 10 to 15 96-well plates. However, this is completely dependent upon how good an immune response was generated and how many cells could be adequately harvested. Make sure you have enough plates for the best scenario (at least 15 to 20) since you do not want to find an enormously swollen spleen and have to discard cells because you did not prepare enough plates. Do not change cell plating densities simply to accommodate excess cells.

6.4.2 IN PREPARATION FOR FUSION DAY

1. Last check on titer of mouse serum and last boost.
2. Last check on viability and count of myeloma cells. Viability must be at least 90% and approximately 10 million myeloma cells will be needed per spleen.
3. Feeder cells plated, 15 to 20 plates.
4. Enough media prepared, 1 l will suffice initially. Prepare early enough to confirm sterility.
5. Dissection instruments sterilized.
6. HAT and HT medium prepared and checked for sterility.
7. PEG prepared and previously tested by fusion.

6.4.3 FUSION DAY

All reagents, equipment, and cells should be checked prior to fusion, because once the animal is sacrificed, the fusion must proceed immediately. It is possible to freeze an excised spleen for later use, but this is not an ideal situation and never seems to work as well as expected. Quick movement is essential during the fusion; therefore, be sure to have all equipment, plasticware, centrifuge tubes, media, etc. conveniently available. Move all media to equilibrate at 37°C, including the PEG. Harvest the myeloma cells and dilute to 1×10^6 cells per ml in complete DMEM and place at 37°C.

6.4.4 FUSION PROTOCOL

1. Sacrifice the mouse by cervical dislocation or CO_2 asphyxiation.
2. Immediately withdraw blood from the heart for screening, using a 23-gauge needle/1 ml syringe.
3. Drench the mouse in 70% alcohol and blot excess.
4. Using a set of forceps and scissors, make a small incision and pull back the skin to expose the abdominal wall. Pull back the skin far enough to keep hair from getting in the way.
5. Switch to a new set of instruments and carefully make an incision in the peritoneal cavity to expose the spleen.
6. Remove the spleen to a Petri plate and transfer to a laminar flow hood.
7. Using a 10-ml syringe with a 23-gauge needle, vigorously inject 10 ml of PBS into the spleen causing the spleen cells to disperse. Repeat procedure.
8. Transfer spleen cells to 50-ml tube, bring volume to 40 ml with PBS, remove sample for cell count and centrifuge at $300 \times g$ for 5 min to collect cells.
9. Calculate number of spleen cells in pellet.
10. Add myeloma cells to spleen cell pellet at 10:1 (myeloma/spleen) ratio.
11. Centrifuge at $300 \times g$ for 5 min.
12. Pour off supernatant completely and tap to loosen pellet.
13. While swirling in 37°C water, slowly add 800 μl PEG over 1 min.
14. Let stand for 60 s and then add 5 ml DMEM over 3 min, starting very slowly and then increasing toward the end. Add an additional 10 ml DMEM over 3 min.
15. Centrifuge at $250 \times g$ for 5 min, bringing up to speed slowly.
16. Pour off supernatant completely and resuspend in DMEM + HAT to a concentration of 3×10^5 spleen cells/ml as determined by cell count above.
17. Plate out 100 μl/well in the macrophage-prepared 96-well plates.
18. Place in a humidified 37°C incubator at 5% CO_2 in air.

6.5 CULTURE AND PROPOGATION

After fusion the hybrids are in their most fragile state and must be cared for conscientiously. The first 10 days appear to be the most critical for survival. A mouse diploid cell contains 40 chromosomes; therefore, a hybrid can contain up to 80 chromosomes. However, within the first few days many of these chromosomes are lost from the cell simply due to the traumatic and unstable events of membrane fusion. Consequently, loss of certain chromosomes will result in cell death, cessation of cell growth, and loss of ability to synthesize immunoglobulin, resulting in "non-producing" hybrids. During these first several days, some hybrids will begin to divide, while others might take longer, and many will just die. The entire culture will display a large amount of cell death and a general unhealthy appearance caused by the fusion process. Due to this great variation in growth at this critical time it is extremely important to care for the hybrids within individual wells. Many contract monoclonal laboratories follow a strict schedule of maintenance for the entire fusion that will always result in a decreased yield of hybrids. Additionally, many manufacturers sell devices that will feed or screen an entire plate at once. Although these devices may have practical applications for high throughput and convenience, individual care at this point will absolutely increase the yield of hybridomas. A plate full of hybrids will never grow at the same rate and therefore will never need screening or feeding at exactly the same time. The hybrid cells are all individuals and, at this stage, must be cared for as such to maximize the results of all your hard work.

Each plate should be microscopically checked every day or two following the fusion for cell division, contamination, and other problems. No feeding will be necessary up to day 7, at which time wells with dividing cells should be fed with 100 µl of HT medium. After 7 days in HAT medium, all myeloma cells should be dead and aminopterin should be removed to allow the hybrids to abandon the salvage pathway. Culturing in HT medium should continue for at least 2 weeks to assure that all traces of aminopterin have been removed. This needs to be done very carefully as not to disturb the cells on the bottom of the well. Make sure to treat each well as an individual cell line and change pipet tips, etc., between each well when contact is made. At this point you should see small grape-like clumps of cells forming in the wells. As they continue to divide, the medium will change color from red to orange as the pH changes due to cell growth. This is a very quick way to identify wells which might need feeding. However, contamination with bacteria, fungi, and mycoplasma can also change the pH. Bacterial and fungal contamination is fairly obvious, but mycoplasma contamination at this point is extremely difficult to detect due to the already somewhat unhealthy appearance of the cells and the amount of cellular debris present from the fusion process. Identified contamination can be taken care of by adding a drop or two of bleach to that specific well and then removing and discarding as much liquid as possible from the well. Enough bleach will remain behind to inhibit any further growth.

Remember that many wells will show no growth at all and others may contain more than one hybrid. Since all the hybrids at this stage will begin division at different rates, care must be taken not to allow one hybrid to overtake another within the same well. In addition, the nonproducing hybrids will almost always outgrow the producing hybrids in the same well and eventually completely overtake them. Nonproducers are hybrid cells which may have received enough of the genetic information from both cells to survive the selection and remain viable but lack the information necessary for antibody production. Nonproducing hybrids are of no use since they do not produce immunoglobulin.

At approximately day 10, the screening process can begin with wells which have shown growth. Typically, one third of the well will be covered by cells; the color will be orange–yellow, and it will have been fed 2 to 3 days previously. Remove 50 to 100 μl for the screen and replace with HT medium. It is essential to screen the wells as soon as possible to avoid having nonproducers overtake potential producing hybrids. Also, when the wells are screened and eliminated from interest, they can be abandoned from further maintenance. However, each well should be negative through two screenings before being abandoned. Some hybrids may take longer to reach full production than others, and may not initially produce within the detection limits of the screen. In addition, it is quite possible to have a well initially appear to be slightly positive and then turn negative. This is most likely due to production of immunoglobulin from the unfused lymphocytes before dying off. Once medium has been removed and replaced, this well will now become negative. Any well that was positive from the first screen should be expanded to a second plate at the next feeding/screening. Gently remove the orange medium for screening, replace with fresh medium, and suspend the cells with gentle pipetting. Remove one half the volume to another well in a new plate. This action serves several purposes. The most critical objective is to help safeguard potential hybrids from various perils simply by growing them in two different physical locations. Also, this minimal dilution allows the cells to expand without decreasing cell density to the point where it might be deleterious.

6.6 CLONING AND CRYOPRESERVATION

A positive well should be cloned and cryopreserved as soon as possible. A well with two or three distinct-looking colonies may actually have resulted from disturbance of one colony. One distinct-looking colony may contain more than one hybrid due to proximity or the possibility of chromosome loss as previously discussed. Cells are cloned to ensure that hybrids are indeed monoclonal and to separate them from any nonproducing hybrids present. In general, cells should be cloned any time they undergo unusual stress or appear different, such as with increased cellular debris or slightly shrunken cells instead of large, round clusters, or when immunoglobulin production decreases. Freezing and thawing are very stressful. Therefore, cells should always be cloned following thawing. Cryopreservation is also accomplished at that time simply as a safeguard against any unforeseen occurrence to a specific well.

When a positively screened well is approximately 75% confluent, very gently resuspend the cells with a pipet, move them to a single well in a 24-well plate and feed them. Keep feeding the almost empty well as a safety measure if necessary. After a day or two of healthy growth, gently resuspend again and remove approximately half of the cells for cloning. Feed the other half and plan to cryopreserve the next day. When cryopreserving, at this point it is best to retain the supernatant for testing should the clone screening become negative.

6.6.1 CLONING

Cloning is basically the isolation and propagation of one hybridoma cell. This is absolutely necessary to ensure the hybridoma cells are clonal. Although a group of cells producing immunoglobulin and derived from one well may appear as one single cell line, it is quite possible that another producing or nonproducing cell line is present. Although chromosome loss primarily occurs within 7 days post-fusion, it can actually occur at any time in the culturing of hybridomas. Remember that hybridomas are not normal cells and therefore are much less stable and prone to stress. Cloning should take place as soon as hybrids of interest have been selected and cell numbers allow.

By far the most popular method of cloning is limited dilution in a liquid phase. However, some researchers still prefer limited dilution in agar, claiming that the possibility of cells shifting and appearing as one colony is greater in liquid. While this might be true, it can also be said that the possibility of having two different cells plated next to each other is the same with either method. The basic premise is to dilute the cells into wells until theoretically and statistically there is only one cell per well.

Cloning is preferably accomplished in 96-well microtiter plates using feeder cells such as macrophages as described earlier. Hybridomas plated at very high dilutions tend to die and therefore require feeder layers for acceptable survival. Cell count and viability need to be checked just prior to cloning. Due to the large dilution factor required, it is suggested to perform several smaller dilutions instead of only one dilution into a large volume. Statistically, an appropriate dilution to achieve one cell per well will result in 37% of the wells being empty. If, at this dilution, significantly fewer wells are empty, then it is reasonable to assume that monoclonality has not been achieved and the cloning should be repeated. To better assure monoclonality, a dilution achieving less than one cell per well may be used. If one third of the wells are empty at a dilution of one cell per well then any colonies formed at 0.5 cells per well, are very likely to be monoclonal.

6.6.2 CLONING PROCEDURE

1. Prepare one 96-well plate per clone with macrophages in HT medium.
2. Perform a cell count to do dilutions.
3. Do dilutions of 100, 30, 10, and 3 cells/ml in HT medium.
4. Plate out 100 µl of each dilution over the macrophages, using two rows per dilution.
5. Place in humidified incubator at 37°C with 5% CO_2 in air.
6. When colonies appear, feed and screen as done previously.
7. When the cells are approximately 80% confluent, resuspend in fresh medium and transfer to a 24-well plate to expand.
8. Although it is not always necessary, repeat cloning with the positive clones from the first round to confirm monoclonality.

Before transferring the cells, always handle the plates gently to avoid movement and potential confusion concerning the number of colonies present. After clones have been chosen, they need to be cryopreserved as soon as possible. Maintaining them in culture always runs the risk of contamination, and without an aliquot cryopreserved, that risk is bound to occur: even 2 to 3 vials frozen away initially will be acceptable.

6.6.3 CRYOPRESERVATION

To fully realize the potential of immortality the cell lines must be cryopreserved to allow for long-term storage. Although freezing and thawing cells results in damage and loss of viability, long-term culture runs the risk of contamination and mutation. It is easier to nurse a cell line back to health following thawing than reverse contamination and mutation. It is good practice to always have at least 5 to 10 vials frozen away at any time, and also to have aliquots prepared on different days, which takes into account the possibility of contamination on any particular day. A particularly valuable cell line should additionally be stored at another location in case of malfunction, power loss, fire, etc. The process of freezing the cells down to the temperature of liquid nitrogen (–196°C) must be done very carefully. Freezing at –80°C is not sufficient for long-term mammalian cell storage. As aqueous solutions freeze, sharp ice crystals that can cause severe damage to cells are formed. The addition of dimethylsulfoxide (DMSO) will greatly minimize the number and size of ice crystals formed during the freezing process. The ideal protocol would reduce the temperature 1 to 2°C per min but this requires expensive freezing equipment. A variety of inexpensive, successful techniques are available, of which one will be described as follows:

6.6.4 CRYOPRESERVATION PROTOCOL

1. Prepare freezing medium containing 15% DMSO, 20% FBS in DMEM.
2. Sterilize the complete DMEM before adding DMSO.
3. Cells must be in log-phase growth with viability greater than 80%.
4. Perform cell count and harvest into pellets containing approximately 5×10^6 cells per pellet.
5. To each pellet add 1 ml of cold freezing medium and resuspend quickly.
6. Transfer to a 1.5-ml cryopreservation vial and immediately place back on ice.
7. At this point it is critical that temperature changes only be downward. A rise in temperature at any point will result in cell death. Consequently, greatly minimize handling through the air.
8. Transfer vials to a –20°C freezer (not frost-free) for several hours, and then to a small pre-chilled styrofoam box and place in a –80°C freezer overnight. The styrofoam box will allow the temperature change to be somewhat gradual. The next day the vials can be moved directly into liquid nitrogen. Transfer on dry ice will minimize the possibility of a temperature increase.

6.6.5   THAWING

Unlike cryopreservation of cell lines, thawing must occur very quickly to minimize damage to the cells. Two predominant methods are utilized, and both will be described here. The idea is to bring the cell lines to 37°C quickly and remove them from the effects of the DMSO in the freezing medium since it is toxic to cells at this concentration.

6.6.6   THAW PROCEDURE 1

1. Remove vial from liquid nitrogen freezer and immediately immerse in a 37°C water bath.
2. When contents are just thawed, remove vial and alcohol swab exterior. Place in a laminar flow hood.
3. Transfer contents, generally 1 ml, to a T25 flask with 4 ml of 37°C complete DMEM.
4. Gently rock flask to mix contents and place in a CO_2 incubator with the flask resting at a slight angle from horizontal. This is to allow the cells to attach to the bottom of the flask and to maintain a reasonable cell density by tilting the flask instead of allowing the 5 ml of medium to cover the entire bottom of the flask.

6.6.7   THAW PROCEDURE 2

1. Remove vial from freezer and immediately immerse in a 37°C water bath.
2. When contents are just thawed, transfer to a 15-ml sterile tube with 9 ml of complete DMEM at room temperature.
3. Centrifuge at $400 \times g$ for 5 min.
4. Discard supernatant and resuspend pellet with 3 ml of 37°C complete DMEM.
5. Transfer to 3 wells of a 24-well microplate and place in a CO_2 incubator.

Within 3 to 6 days the cells should recover from the freeze/thaw process and should immediately be cloned to assure perpetuation of the original hybridoma. Some cell lines may require longer recovery periods prior to cloning; the cloning process is somewhat stressing. A balance between enough time for recovery and not enough time for potential nonproducers to take over the culture should be achieved. This small precaution will guarantee maintenance and production of the original hybridoma.

REFERENCES

1. Kohler, G. and Milstein, C., Continuous culture of fused cells secreting antibody of predefined specificity, *Nature*, 256, 495, 1975.
2. Radka, S. F., Kostyu, D. D., and Amos, B. D., A monoclonal antibody directed against the HLA-Bw6 epitope, *J. Immunol.*, 128, 6, 2804, 1982.

3. Kayano, T., Motoda, R., Usui, M., Ando, S., Matuhasi, T., and Kurimoto, M., Growth of rat–mouse hybridoma cells in immunosuppressed hamsters, *J. Immunol. Tech.*, 130, 25, 1990.

4. Moran, T. M., Usuba, O., Shapiro, E., Rubinstein, L. J., Ito, M., and Bona, C. A., A novel technique for the production of hybrid antibodies, *J. Immunol. Tech.*, 129, 199, 1990.

5. Fazekas de St. Groth, S. and Scheidegger, D., Production of monoclonal antibodies: strategy and tactics, *J. Immunol. Methods*, 35, 1, 1980.

6. Paul, J., *Cell and Tissue Culture*, Churchill Livingstone, New York, 1975, Appendix 1.

7. Bazin, R. and Lemieux, R., Increased proportion of B cell hybridomas secreting monoclonal antibodies of desired specificity in cultures containing macrophage derived hybridoma growth factor (IL-6), *J. Immunol. Methods*, 116, 245, 1989.

8. Littlefield, J. W., Selection of hybrids from matings of fibroblasts *in vitro* and their presumed recombinants, *Science*, 145, 709, 1964.

9. Esser, C. and Radbruch, A., Immunoglobulin class switching: molecular and cellular analysis, *Ann. Rev. Immunol.*, 8, 717, 1990.

10. Berek, C. and Ziegner, M., The maturation of the immune response, *Immunol. Today*, 14, 400, 1993.

11. Alt, F. W., Oltz, E. M., Young, F., Gorman, J., Taccioli, G., and Chen, J., VDJ recombination, *Immunol. Today*, 13, 306, 1992.

12. Gefter, M. L., Margulies, D. H., and Scharff, M. D., A simple method for polyethylene glycol promoted hybridisation of mouse myeloma cells, *Somatic Cell Genetics*, 3, 231, 1977.

7 Screening Techniques

Gamal E. Osman and Warren E. Ladiges

CONTENTS

7.1 INTRODUCTION

Seven to 10 days after fusion, a large number of fast growing B-cell hybridoma colonies will be ready to test. Usually, asuccessful fusion will produce 500 to 1000 hybrid colonies. However, the frequency of hybridomas producing monoclonal antibodies of the desired specificity can be as rare as 1 in 500 or as many as 5 of 10 growing B-cell hybrids.

Handling 500 to 1000 fast growing B-cell hybrid colonies can be laborious and requires more than one person to maintain. Therefore, the early identification of monoclonal antibodies with the desired specificities is the most critical step in monoclonal antibody (mAb) production. In addition to the rapid identification of hybridomas producing specific mAbs, many screening assays have to be done during the second phase of hybridoma production (i.e., cloning, subcloning, and expansion of the selected antibody-producing hybridomas). The choice of a reliable screening method is extremely important. Before constructing a reliable screening assay, criteria to consider should include sensitivity, speed, cost, throughput, and labor. Therefore, we advise the researcher to carefully examine and validate the potential screening method before fusion. This can be done by using hyperimmunized mouse sera as a source of specific antibodies to establish the screening method.

Generally, screening assays use labeled reagents for detecting antibodies. These assays are performed in solid phase and assay antibodies using reagents labeled with either radioisotopes (radioimmunoassay) or enzymes (enzyme-linked immunosorbent assay, ELISA). Radioimmunoassay and ELISA are the most widely used techniques of all immunological assays, since a large number of assays can be performed in a relatively short period of time. However, in recent years, ELISA, originally described by Engvall and Perlmann in 1971, has become more popular among immunologists. ELISA does not require the use of radioactive isotopes, and hence potential problems as a consequence of radioactive handling can be avoided. Positive wells containing the desired mAbs can be identified by the naked eye. To reflect on the increased use of this technique, this chapter will focus on three ELISA-based methods for assaying antibodies directed against either soluble antigens or cell-surface molecules.

7.2   ANTIBODY-CAPTURED ELISA TO DETECT SPECIFIC ANTIBODIES

This method is simple to set up and is used to detect specific antibodies in antisera or hybridoma supernatants. First, the soluble antigen is allowed to absorb to the wells of the microtiter plate. Diluted antisera or hybridoma supernatants are added to the wells and incubated. After washing away the unbound antibodies, those that are bound can be detected by a secondary reagent. Examples include akaline phosphatase conjugated to goat anti-mouse Ig antibodies or to proteins A and G (bacterial cell wall proteins which have high afffinities for the Fc portions of some Ig molecules). After incubation and washing, a solution containing the substrate is added (see Figure 7.1A). The amount of substrate hydrolysis is proportional to the number of antibodies in the test solution. Qualitatively, the positive wells can be identified by eye, due to a color change in the substrate. Alternatively, an ELISA reader can be used to quantify the number of the antibodies in the test solution.

7.2.1   Antigen Absorption (Coating) to the Plate

1. Dilute the antigen in phosphate-buffered saline (PBS) containing 0.02% NaN$_3$ (5 to 10 µg/ml) and dispense 50 µl into each well of a 96-well microtiter plate using a multipipette/dispenser. (Microtiter plates vary in their ability to bind antigen. In our experience, MaxiSorp plates from Nunc-Immuno were the best as far as the nonspecific absorption of antibodies or secondary reagents. We recommend that each researcher test for the plates of choice for their specific antigen.) Seal plates with adhesive plate sealer and incubate overnight at 4°C or 2 to 3 h at 37°C (coated plates can be prepared and stored in the refrigerator for several weeks).

2. Wash the plate three times with PBS using the Nunc-Immuno wash device (this device simultaneously delivers and aspirates fluid) and block any residual binding capacity by adding 50 µl of a blocking buffer (PBS

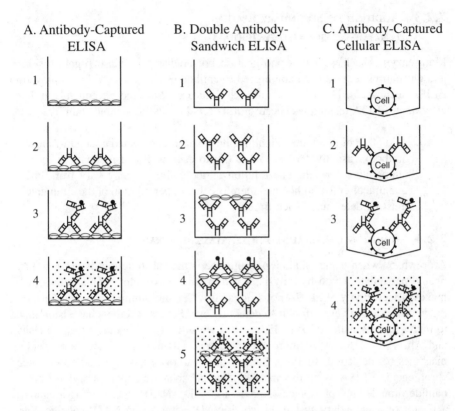

A. Antibody-Captured
   ELISA

B. Double Antibody-
   Sandwich ELISA

C. Antibody-Captured
   Cellular ELISA

FIGURE 7.1 A schematic representation of three ELISA-based methods for assaying antibodies directed against either soluble antigens or cell surface molecules. (A) Antibody-Captured ELISA. The assay involves the following steps: 1, coat well with antigen; 2, add hybridoma supernatant or diluted antiserum and incubate; 3, add antibody-enzyme conjugate and incubate; and 4, add substrate and detect color change. (B) Double Antibody-Sandwich ELISA. The assay involves five steps: 1, coat well with capture antibody; 2, add hybridoma supernatant or diluted antiserum and incubate; 3, add antigen and incubate; 4, add antibody-enzyme conjugate and incubate; and 5, add substrate and detect color change. (C) Antibody-Captured Cellular ELISA. The assay involves four steps: 1, add cells to the well; 2, add hybridoma supernatant or diluted antiserum and incubate; 3, add antibody-enzyme conjugate and incubate; and 4, add substrate, resuspend cells, and detect color change.

   containing 5% BSA, 0.02% NaN$_3$) to each well. Incubate the plate for 1
   h at room temperature.
3. Wash the plate three times with PBS.

7.2.2 ADDITION OF HYBRIDOMA SUPERNATANT (ANTIBODIES)

4. Transfer 50 μl of the hybridoma supernatant into each well and incubate
   for 1 h at room temperature. For a positive control, add 50 μl of serially
   diluted positive sera from hyperimmunized mice to each well. After incubation, wash the plate three times with PBS.

7.2.3   ADDITION OF SECONDARY REAGENT
(ENZYME-CONJUGATED ANTIBODIES)

Many enzymes such as alkaline phosphatase, horseradish peroxidase, β-galactosidase, and glucoamylase have been conjugated to antibodies and successfully employed in ELISA techniques. However, alkaline phosphatase is the most frequently utilized enzyme in ELISA techniques because of its rapid catalytic rate and stability.

5. Add 50 μl of the diluted alkaline phosphatase-conjugated goat anti-mouse antibody (usually 1:1000 to 1:2000) to each well and incubate at room temperature for 1 h. The dilution of the conjugate may vary from one manufacturer to another, and therefore the proper dilution of the conjugate must be determined each time.

7.2.4   ADDITION OF ALKALINE PHOSPHATASE SUBSTRATE

A drawback when using alkaline phosphatase is the substrate that is used, p-nitrophenyl phosphate. Upon hydrolysis, a yellow product develops. This yellow color makes the sensitivity of ELISA not as great as with radioimmunoassay. Furthermore, the yellow color is very difficult to detect by eye. Several attempts have been made to increase the sensitivity of ELISA, e.g., the use of a fluorogenic substrate (Ishaq and Ali, 1983). However, fluorogenic substrates require expensive plate reading machines for detection. In 1988, Stanley and his coworkers reported an enhanced chromogenic ELISA assay in which alkaline phosphatase dephosphorylates nicotinamide dinucleotide phosphate (NADP) to NAD^+. NAD^+ then acts as a catalytic activator of a secondary system in which NAD^+ activates an NAD^+-specific redox cycle, yielding an intense red color (Stanley et al., 1985).

6. Wash wells four times with Tris-buffered saline (0.05 M Tris.Cl, pH 7.5 containing 0.15 M NaCl) and immediately add 50 μl of the substrate (Gibco BRL ELISA Amplification System, Life Technologies, Grand Island, NY) to each well.
7. Incubate at room temperature for 15 min and then add 50 μl of the Gibco BRL ELISA amplifier substrate to each well and incubate for 5 to 10 min at room temperature.
8. Terminate the reaction by adding 50 μl of 0.3 M H_2SO_4 to each well.
9. Since the degree of hydrolysis of the substrate is proportional to the number of antibodies in the hybridoma supernatants, plates can be read by naked eye or quantified by measuring the absorbance at 490 nm using an ELISA microplate reader.

7.3   DOUBLE ANTIBODY-SANDWICH ELISA

This technique is more sensitive than the above technique and requires very small quantities of antigen. It is very useful *in situ*ations where the purified antigens are limited (nanograms). However, it requires the presence of specific antibodies, as shown in Figure 7.1B.

7.3.1 Conjugating Antibodies to Alkaline Phosphatase

1. Centrifuge 5 mg of alkaline phosphatase suspension (supplied as a suspension in 65% $(NH_4)_2SO_4$) in a microfuge for 5 to 10 min. Resuspend the enzyme pellet in a total volume of 1 ml PBS containing 10 mg of the antibody to be labeled.
2. Dialyze overnight against 0.1 M sodium phosphate buffer, pH 6.8 to remove any contaminating free amino groups.
3. In a fume hood, slowly add 50 µl of 1% glutaraldehyde solution while stirring for 5 min. Incubate at room temperature for 2 to 3 h, add 100 µl of 1 M ethanolamine, pH 7, and then incubate for additional 2 h at room temperature.
4. Dialyze overnight against PBS and remove any insoluble materials by centrifugation at 40,000 × g for 30 min.
5. Store the conjugate (supernatant) in the presence of 50% glycerol, 1 mM $MgCl_2$, 1 mM $ZnCl_2$, and 0.02% NaN_3 at 4°C.

7.3.2 Antibody Adsorption (Coating) to the Plate

1. Dilute either goat or rabbit anti-mouse Ig antibodies in PBS containing 0.02% NaN_3 (5 to 10 µg/ml), and dispense 50 µl into each well of a 96-well microtiter using the Eppendorf multipipette/dispenser. Seal plates with adhesive plate sealer and incubate overnight at 4°C or 2 to 3 h at 37°C.
2. Wash the plate three times with PBS and block the residual binding capacity by adding 50 µl of blocking buffer to each well. Incubate the plate for 1 h at room temperature.
3. Wash three times with PBS.

7.3.3 Addition of Hybridoma Supernatant (Antibodies)

4. Transfer 50 µl of the hybridoma supernatant or diluted ascites fluid (1:100) into each well and incubate at room temperature for 1 h. For a positive control, add 50 µl of serially diluted positive sera from hyper-immunized mice to each well. After incubation, wash the plate three times with PBS.

7.3.4 Addition of Antigen

5. Add 50 µl of the diluted antigen in blocking buffer (50 to 500 ng/ml) to each well and incubate at room temperature for 2 h.
6. Wash plates three times with PBS.

7.3.5   ADDITION OF ANTIBODY-ALKALINE PHOSPHATASE CONJUGATE

7. Add 50 µl of specific antibody conjugated to alkaline phosphatase (50 to 500 ng specific Ab/ml) diluted in blocking buffer to each well and incubate at room temperature for 1 h.
8. Wash plates three times with PBS.

7.3.6   ADDITION OF ALKALINE PHOSPHATASE SUBSTRATE

9. Wash wells four times with Tris-buffered saline (0.05 M Tris.Cl, pH 7.5 containing 0.15 M NaCl) and immediately add 50 µl of the substrate (Gibco BRL ELISA Amplification System, Life Technologies, Grand Island, NY) to each well.
10. Incubate at room temperature for 15 min and then add 50 µl of the Gibco BRL ELISA amplifier substrate to each well and incubate for 5 to 10 min at room temperature.
11. Terminate the reaction by adding 50 µl of 0.3 M H_2SO_4 to each well.
12. Since the degree of hydrolysis of the substrate is proportional to the number of antibodies in the hybridoma supernatants, plates can be read by naked eye or quantified by measuring the absorbance at 490 nm using an ELISA microplate reader.

7.4   ANTIBODY CAPTURE ON CELL SURFACE

This assay can be used to detect antibodies specific for cell surface molecules (see Figure 7.1C). However, many cell types exhibit high levels of endogenous peroxidase (macrophages and myeloid cells) or alkaline phosphatase (preB and B cells). To determine whether the cells bearing the surface molecules of interest express endogenous alkaline phosphatase, add the substrate directly to the cells and observe any color change. If cells express high levels of the enzyme, alternative enzymes such as those produced by bacteria, e.g., β-galactosidase can be used.

1. Dispense 100 µl of the cell suspension (5 to 10×10^6 cells/ml) in PBS into each well of V-shaped microtiter plate.
2. Centrifuge the plate at $500 \times g$ for 30 s and discard the supernatant by tapping the plate while it is held above a sink.
3. Resuspend the cells in 50 µl blocking buffer containing anti-FcγII/III antibody (anti-CD16/32 monoclonal antibody, Pharmingen, San Diego, CA) using the microtiter plate mixer and incubate at room temperature for 30 min.
4. Wash cells three times with PBS and resuspend in 100 µl hybridoma supernatant or 5 to 10 µg/ml control antibody. Incubate cells at 37°C for 30 min and then wash cells three times with PBS.

5. Wash cells four times with Tris-buffered saline (0.05 M Tris.Cl, pH 7.5 containing 0.15 *M* NaCl) and immediately add 50 μl of the substrate (Gibco BRL ELISA Amplification System, Life Technologies, Grand Island, NY) to each well.
6. Incubate at room temperature for 15 min and then add 50 μl of the Gibco BRL ELISA amplifier substrate to each well and incubate for 5 to 10 min at room temperature.
7. Terminate the reaction by adding 50 μl of 0.3 *M* H_2SO_4 to each well.
8. Since the degree of hydrolysis of the substrate is proportional to the number of antibodies bound to the cell surface molecules of interest, plates can be read directly by naked eye.

REFERENCES

1. Engvall, E. and Perlmann, P., Enzyme-linked immunosorbent assay (ELISA). Quantitative assay of immunoglobulin G, *Immunochemistry*, 8, 871–874, 1971.
2. Ishaq, M. and Ali, R., Enzyme-linked immunosorbent assay (ELISA) for detection of antibodies to extractable nuclear antigens in systemic lupus erythematosus, with nylon as solid phase, *Clin. Chem.*, 29, 823–827, 1983.
3. Stanley, C.J., Johannsson, A., and Self, C.H., Enzyme amplification can enhance both the speed and the sensitivity of immunoassays, *J. Immunol. Methods*, 83, 89–95, 1985.

8 Antibody Production by Ascites Growth

Kristi R. Harkins

CONTENTS

8.1 INTRODUCTION

In vivo production of ascites fluid rich in antibodies can be useful for producing 50- to 100-mg quantities of antibodies for use in the research laboratory. However, the use of mice and rats for this purpose is closely regulated in both the United States and Europe. The use of animals for ascites production has almost been eliminated in favor of *in vitro* methods. In Europe, two laws exist for the protection of laboratory animals (Council Directive 86/609/EEC and European Convention for the Protection of Vertebrate Animals Used for Experimental and Other Scientific Purposes, ETS 123). An excellent overview of these regulations can be found at http://www.nal.usda.gov/awic/pubs/antibody/ecvam.htm on the Internet. In the United States, researchers that receive funding from, or have collaborations with, institutions who receive funding from government service organizations such as the NIH must show that a project has failed to produce sufficient antibodies through the use of *in vitro* methods before approval will be given to proceed with *in vivo* production of ascites fluid.[1]

Ascites production in mice provides a relatively economical and fast method of antibody production. The main disadvantage, as discussed previously, is the need to use animals. Other disadvantages to this method include the presence of other mouse antibodies (nonspecific) that are not related to the antibodies produced by the hybridoma cell line (50 to 90% of the antibody can be nonspecific). Finally, other biological agents such as mouse viruses, bacteria, or mycoplasma may contaminate the fluid collected from the mouse. This chapter outlines methods used in the production of mouse and rat monoclonal ascites fluid and mouse polyclonal ascites fluid.

8.2 ASCITES PRODUCTION IN MICE (MONOCLONAL ANTIBODY)

8.2.1 PRIMING

Several papers in the literature document the comparison of Pristane with Freund's incomplete for priming the animals prior to implanting the hybridoma cells. Basically, it has been observed that Freund's incomplete will provide a high volume yield of ascites fluid with a similar antibody titer when compared to priming with Pristane.[2–4] Unfortunately, the use of Freund's adjuvant has come into question recently because of the tendency for animals to form lesions at the site of injection and to form granuloma tumors after intraperitoneal injections.[5] Both agents are listed in the procedures outlined with Freund's incompiete as the preferred reagent. The next consideration in methodology is the time between priming and implantation and the efficacy of multiple priming steps.[6] We routinely perform a single priming step no more than 3 weeks and no less than 2 days prior to implantation.

8.2.2 ANIMALS

It was once thought that castrated male mice provided a high antibody yield in ascites production when compared to females.[7] It has since been shown that normal male or female mice will work equally well for *in vivo* antibody production.[4] *Nude (nu/nu)* mice contain a mutation that prevents the development of a mature thymus (cortical epithelium) and therefore prevents the maturation of T lymphocytes. *Scid (scid/scid)* mice contain a mutation that prevents lymphocyte maturation. Both mouse types can be used for ascites fluid production if the parent mouse or rat strains are not available.[8,9] However, these mice cost approximately four times the cost of BALB/c mice and need to be housed in a very clean environment.

8.2.3 HYBRIDOMA

It is important verify the titer of the hybridoma cell line prior to implantation. Hybridoma cell lines can be inherently unstable and when maintained in culture for extended periods of time may become overgrown with non-secreting cells leading to a drop in the antibody titer. Verification of the titer prior to implantation will help to ensure the success of the production process. Additionally, note the generation of a proper negative control for assays that utilize ascites fluid is the implantation of the non-secreting myeloma cell line used as the progenitor of the hybridoma cell line and collection of this negative ascites fluid.

8.2.4 Tapping

Factors that may affect the yield and antibody titer during fluid collection or tapping have been recently evaluated.[10] The concentration of antibody and volume collected appears to be predominantly dependent upon the cell line used. There is an inverse correlation between the number of cells implanted and the time to first tap. However, evidence indicates that implantation of too many cells can lead to premature death of the animal before collection can begin. Clinical evaluation of the mice also is important during the tapping process. Typically, no more than three taps are recommended for each mouse, assuming the mouse shows minimal or no signs of physical duress.

8.2.4.1 Ascites Production — Priming and Implanting Procedure

Materials:

> Mice — cage of four mice, 6 to 8 weeks old:
>> Balb/c mice or syngeneic mice related to host cell lines
>> (Charles River Laboratories, Charles River, MA)
>> *nude* mice (Charles River Laboratories)
>> *scid* mice (Taconic Farms, Germantown, NY)
> Pristane (Sigma T-7640) or Freund's incomplete (Sigma)
> Tuberculin syringe with 25-gauge needle
> Phosphate-buffered saline (sterile)
> Hybridoma cells in log phase growth
> 3 cc syringe with 18-gauge needle and 20-gauge needle

Equipment:

> Hemacytometer (Z35, 962–9) with trypan blue (T8154), Sigma
> Coulter counter (Beckman Coulter, Miami, FL)
> Centrifuge

Time required: Priming a cage of four mice takes approximately 10 min and should be completed a minimum of 2 days prior to implantation. Preparation of the cells and subsequent implantation take approximately 45 min. Mice must be checked every few days after the implantation process to determine if production of ascites fluid has started. Production begins 1 to 2 weeks after implantation, typically. Tapping for each mouse must be completed within 7 days from the collection of the first tap. A maximum of three taps may be collected from each mouse during the 7-day time period.

Procedure:

1. The mice should be primed with Pristane (2, 6, 10, 14-tetramethyl-pentadecane) or Freund's incomplete (FIC) adjuvant at least 2 days and up to 3 weeks prior to implanting. Priming involves injecting 0.5 ml of the Pristane or FIC into the peritoneal cavity with a 25-gauge needle. Injections work best if the needle first pierces the skin (subcutaneous) and then is angled away from the point of penetration before piercing the abdominal wall. This way, when the needle is removed, the priming agent is less likely to leak out of the abdomen. The injection should be made in the lower abdomen to the left or right of the gut midline and between the nipples.

2. Split the hybridoma cells 1:1 (v/v) with fresh medium the day before implanting.

3. Count the cells and evaluate viability using a standard hemacytometer with trypan blue staining. Dilute the cells 1:1 in the trypan blue solution, wait 15 min and place a drop of the stained sample on a hemacytometer for counting. Count the number and average the count per square (10 squares). Multiply this count by the dilution factor and by 10^4 to calculate the number of cells/ml. Alternatively, dilute 50 µl into 10 ml of saline in a counting cup and determine the live and dead count using a Coulter counter. Cells should be 90 to 100% viable.

4. Centrifuge the cells at $200 \times g$ for 5 min at room temperature.

5. Remove the supernatant and resuspend the cells in sterile PBS.

6. Centrifuge cells at $200 \times g$ for 5 min at room temperature.

7. Remove the supernatant and resuspend the cells in sterile PBS to a final concentration of 2×10^6 cells/ml.

8. Pull the cells through an 18-gauge needle into a sterile syringe. Replace the 18-gauge needle with a 20-gauge needle and inject 0.5 ml of cell suspension intraperitoneally (IP) into each primed mouse following the injection method outlined in step 1. The injection should be made in the lower abdomen to the left or right of the gut midline and between the nipples.

9. Ascites collection usually starts 10 to 14 days after injection. When collection begins each mouse can be tapped three times within a 7-day period.

8.2.4.2   Ascites Production — Collecting Fluid

Materials:

Test tube (sterile, 10 to 15 ml)
Syringe
Sterile needle (18-gauge)
Sure-Sep II (Organon Teknika Corp., Durham, NC)

Equipment:

Centrifuge

Procedure:

1. Ascites collection usually starts 10 to 14 days after implanting the hybridoma cells. When collection begins each mouse can be tapped three times within a 7-day period. The mouse must be exsanguinated at the end of the 7-day period. For the best yield in fluid, begin the first tap when the mouse body weight has increased by 20% or when the abdomen is very distended.
2. Immobilize the mouse by grasping the loose skin behind the ears and tucking the tail between your fingers, thus exposing the abdomen.
3. (Option 1) An 18-gauge needle is inserted into the abdominal cavity (1 to 2 cm) to the left or right of the gut midline and the fluid is allowed to drip from the hub of the needle into a test tube. Gentle massaging of the abdomen can also increase the yield volume from each tap. A good tap can produce up to 10 ml of ascites fluid per mouse. Occasionally, fluid flow will stop prematurely because of tissue obstruction around the needle point. It may be necessary to gently move the needle up, down, and side to side within the abdomen to reestablish flow.
4. (Option 2) An 18-gauge needle is inserted into the abdominal cavity and then removed. The fluid will drip from the insertion point and is collected into a test tube. This method should only be used when the ascites flows around the needle point of insertion in the abdomen and begins to run down the needle, making it difficult to collect the fluid.
5. Pool all the ascites fractions collected from the four mice and allow the ascites fluid time for fiber/blood clot formation to occur (1 h at room temperature). Next, place a Sure-Sep II serum separation device on top of the test tube. Centrifuge the test tube at $500 \times g$ for 10 min. Collect the fluid about the silicon-based gel pellet. Aliquot the fluid into volumes that will be useful and rapid freeze using a dry-ice methanol bath. Store at $-70°C$. Avoid repeated freezing and thawing.
6. Before antibody purification, clarify the thawed ascites fluid by centrifugation at $14,000 \times g$ for 30 min and assay the titer. Removal of lipids can be accomplished by pouring the fluid through glass wool placed in a funnel. Collect the lipid-free fluid in a test tube. Filter the ascites through 0.45- and 0.22-μm syringe filters and proceed with the purification steps.

For documentation purposes, each mouse that is tapped within a cage of four is marked with a different colored marking pen along the back. The date and color of the mouse is marked on the cage card for each tap to allow the animal care takers to monitor the health and proper use of the mice in the cage.

Results: Volumes achieved on a per mouse basis average around 7 ml with an antibody concentration that ranges from 1 to 10 mg/ml. A cage of four mice typically yields a total of 25 to 30 ml of ascites fluid. In some cases not all the mice in a cage will produce ascites fluid.

Problems: Among the most common problems associated with ascites production are production of solid tumors, lack of ascites fluid production, and production of bloody fluid which is indicative of tissue damage and can lead to the animal's premature death before the project is complete. We have observed that cell lines that produce solid tumors will do so consistently and are not good candidates for *in vivo* production methods. If fluid can be collected from a mouse injected with this type of cell line, these cells can be serially passaged to a second and third mouse for further production at concentrations comparable to the original implantation.[11,12] Similarly, cells that do not produce any ascites fluid in mice will continue to fail, regardless of the number of cages of mice used for this purpose, and should be produced via *in vitro* methods. The use of an outcross F1 hybrid mouse for implantation has been shown to overcome this problem with some cell lines.[11,12] If the first tap is very bloody for a given cell line, it will probably be necessary to tap the mice on a daily basis. The health of these mice tends to decline rapidly[13] and should be monitored closely for signs of distress (respiratory distress, cold to the touch, lethargy, hunched back). The mice should be euthanized according to outlined procedures.

It is important to be careful when injecting and tapping the mice not to pierce the animals' internal organs, especially the bladders. Injections should be made in the lower quadrant of the abdomen, offset from the midline of the gut between the nipples, and the needle should not pierce too far into the abdominal cavity. Pristane will tend to leak out of the injection site if the needle gauge is too large. The needle should be placed in at a 45-degree angle from the wall of the gut to encourage the puncture wounds to rapidly reseal as the needle is withdrawn.

Monitor the growth rate and titer of the hybridoma culture. An increased growth rate indicates that non-secreting cells may be taking over the culture. Cells that don't secrete grow more rapidly than secreting cells. It is also important to keep a historical record of cell line production of ascites. Keep track of the volume collected, the antibody concentration, and the final titer. If the ascites volume increases or the antibody titer is reduced, the cells should be evaluated for secretion and possibly re-cloned before the next large-scale ascites production.

It is important to know of how the final product will be used. Keep in mind the product may not be free of virus or mycoplasma, as this information may be important and dictate the final use of the product.

8.3 ASCITES PRODUCTION IN MICE (POLYCLONAL ANTIBODY)

When a limited quantity of antigen is present and a larger volume of polyclonal antibody is desired, it is possible to generate polyclonal ascites fluid in mice following the procedure of Luo and Lin.[14] For optimal use of the animal, it is recommended that the spleen from the mouse be harvested after the last tap and exsanguination. The red blood cells are then lysed and the isolated lymphocytes can then be cryopreserved and stored in liquid nitrogen for generation of a possible hybridoma fusion at a later date.[15]

Materials:

Pristane (Sigma)
Balb/c mice (Charles River Laboratory, Charles River, MA)
Purified antigens (300 µg)
Freund's complete and incomplete adjuvants (Sigma)
SP2/0 mouse myeloma cell line (ATCC, Rockville, MD)
3-cc syringe with 25-gauge needle

Time required: Immunization regime will take approximately 6 weeks. Sera samples are collected and the titer measured (1 to 2 days). After the implantation of the myeloma cells, production of ascites fluid should take an additional 2 to 3 weeks.

Procedures:

1. Mice are primed with an intraperitoneal injection of Pristane (0.5 ml/mouse) 1 to 2 weeks before immunization.
2. Purified antigen (50 µg/100 µl) is mixed 1:1 with Freund's complete adjuvant to a final volume of 0.2 ml/mouse and 0.1 ml is injected to a single subcutaneous site and a single intramuscular site using a 25-gauge needle.
3. A second antigen injection is given 2 weeks after the first antigen exposure. Purified antigen (50 µg/100 µl) is mixed 1:1 with Freund's incomplete adjuvant to a final volume of 0.2 ml/mouse and injected into the peritoneal cavity (IP) using a 25-gauge needle. Follow injection technique outline in Section 8.2.4, step 1.
4. A third antigen injection is given 2 weeks after the second antigen exposure, as outlined in step 3.
5. Blood (200 µl) is collected via the lateral tail vein 10 days after the last injection. To collect blood, the mouse is warmed under a heat lamp for approximately 20 min and then immobilized in a 50-cc test tube with the bottom removed and holes in the lid (ring stand used to hold the test tube). A rubber stopper with a V-cut in the side is used to prevent the mouse from backing out of the tube and allows the tail to extend through the V-cut. A scalpel blade is used to nick one of the lateral tail veins and blood is collected into a microfuge test tube. Pressure is applied to the site to stop the blood flow and the mouse is returned to the cage. The blood is held at room temperature for 1 h and then centrifuged at $14,000 \times g$ for 1 min to separate the serum. The serum is tested for antibody titer and if the titer is poor, step 4 is repeated, and blood is collected again after 10 days for testing. Alternatively, one may abandon the antigen as non-antigenic in this mouse strain.

6. If the titer is acceptable (>1:1000), split the myeloma cells 1:1 with fresh medium the day prior to implanting and proceed with steps 3 through 9 from Section 8.2.4.1 (Implanting) and steps 1 through 6 from Section 8.2.4.2 (Collecting).

7. Additionally, blood should be collected from the mouse after the last tap and exsanguination following CO_2 asphyxiation. This can be accomplished by inserting the needle from a tuberculin syringe into the heart, just below the mouse sternum. If the needle is in the proper position, blood should begin accumulating in the syringe as the plunger is pulled. Artificial chest compression can be applied by placing the index and middle fingers on either side of the rib cage and gently squeeze to pump blood into the heart chamber. Approximately 1 ml of blood can be collected from an exsanguinated mouse using this method.

Results: Volume yields will be comparable to ascites production for monoclonal antibodies or approximately 25 to 30 ml/cage of four mice. The titer is comparable to that observed in the sera from the same mice with antibody concentrations ranging from 1 to 10 mg/ml.

Problems: Problems similar to those outlined at the end of Section 8.2..4.2 may be observed.

8.4   ASCITES PRODUCTION IN RATS (MONOCLONAL)

Production of ascites fluid in rats follows a method similar to that used for mice. A combination of Pristane and Freund's incomplete is used in the priming step and each rat is implanted with 50 fold increase of hybridoma cells.[16] The timing is similar to that followed for mouse production. Additionally, nude rats[17] have been used for production of heterohybridoma cell lines.[8] (See Reference 18 for a good overview on handling rats for these procedures.)

8.4.1   ASCITES PRODUCTION — PRIMING
AND IMPLANTING PROCEDURE

Materials required:

Rats (6 to 8 weeks of age) compatible with rat cell line, typically Louvain rats or *nu/nu* rats (Taconic Farms, Germantown, NY)
Pristane (Sigma 40)
Freund's incomplete (Sigma)
3-cc syringe with needles (18- and 20-gauge)

Time required: Ascites fluid can be collected within 14 to 21 days after injection.

Equipment:

Hemacytometer with trypan blue (Sigma)
Coulter counter (Beckman Coulter, Miami, FL)
Centrifuge

Procedures:

1. Use rats that will be genetically compatible with your hybridoma cells or use nude rats. The rat is primed with a 1:1 mixture of Pristane (2, 6, 10, 14-tetramethyl-pentadecane) and Freund's incomplete adjuvant just before the implantation of the hybridoma cells. Priming involves injecting 2 ml of the mixture into the peritoneal cavity with a 25-gauge needle. Injections are made in the lower left or right abdominal quadrant.
2. Split the cells 1:1 with fresh media the day prior to implanting.
3. Count the cells and evaluate viability using a standard hemacytometer with trypan blue staining. Dilute the cells 1:1 in the trypan blue solution, wait 15 min and place a drop of the stained sample on a hemacytometer for counting. Count the number and average the count per square (10 squares). Multiply this count by the dilution factor and by 10^4 to calculate the number of cells/ml. Alternatively, dilute 50 µl into 10 ml of saline in a counting cup and determine the live and dead count using a Coulter counter. Cells should be 90 to 100% viable.
4. Centrifuge the cells at $200 \times g$ for 5 min.
5. Remove the supernatant and resuspend the cells in sterile PBS.
6. Centrifuge cells at $200 \times g$ for 5 min.
7. Remove the supernatant and resuspend the cells in sterile PBS to a final concentration of 5×10^7 cells/ml.
8. Pull the cells through an 18-gauge needle into a syringe. Replace the 18-gauge needle with a 20-gauge needle and inject 1 ml of cell suspension intraperitoneally (i.p.) into each primed rat on the side opposite of the priming injection.
9. Ascites collection usually starts 14 to 21 days after injection.

8.4.2 ASCITES PRODUCTION — COLLECTING FLUID

Collection procedures are similar to those outlined for mice in Section 8.2.4.2 with a few modifications. A second person may be required to restrain the rat during the collection of ascites fluid. A single tap from a rat can yield 30 to 40 ml of fluid.

Problems: Problems similar to those outlined at the end of Section 8.2.4.2 may be observed.

REFERENCES

1. National Institutes of Health (1997), Production of monoclonal antibodies using mouse ascites method, OPRR Reports, Animal Welfare, no. 98–01.
2. Hoogenradd, N.J. and Wraight, C.J. (1986), The effect of Pristane on ascites tumor formation and monoclonal antibody production, *Methods Enzymol.*, 121, 375–381.
3. Gillette, R.W. (1987), Alternatives to Pristane priming for ascitic fluid and monoclonal antibody production, *J. Immunol. Methods*, 99, 21–22.
4. Jones, S.L, Cox, J.C., and Pearson, J.E. (1990), Increased monoclonal antibody ascites production in mice primed with Freund's incomplete adjuvant, *J. Immunol. Methods*, 129, 227–231.
5. Broderson, J.R. (1989), A retrospective review of lesions associated with the use of Freund's adjuvant, *Lab. Anim. Sci.*, 39, 400–405.
6. De Deken, R., Brandt, J., Ceulemans, F., Geerts, S., and Beudeker, R. (1994), Influence of priming and inoculation dose on the production of monoclonal antibodies in two age groups of BALB/c mice, *Hybridoma*, 13, 53–57.
7. Brodeur, B.R., Tsang, P., and Larose, Y. (1984), Parameters affecting ascites tumor formation in mice and monoclonal antibody production, *J. Immunol. Methods*, 71, 265–272.
8. Noeman, S.A., Misra, D.N., Yankes, R.J., Kunz, H.W., and Gill, T.J., III (1982), Growth of rat–mouse hybridomas in nude mice and nude rats, *J. Immunol. Methods*, 55, 319–326.
9. Truitt, K.E., Larrick, J.W., Raubitschek, A.A., Buck, D.W., and Jacobson, S.W. (1984), Production of human monoclonal antibody in mouse ascites, *Hybridoma*, 3, 195–199.
10. Jackson, L.R., Trudel, L.J., Fox, J.G., and Lipman, N.S. (1999), Monoclonal antibody production in murine ascites. II. Production characteristics, *Lab. Anim. Sci.*, 49, 81–86.
11. Stewart, F., Callander, A., and Garwes, D.J. (1989), Comparison of ascites production for monoclonal antibodies in Balb/c and Balb/c derived cross-bred mice, *J. Immunol. Methods*, 119, 269–275.
12. Mattes, C.E., Sridhara, S., Periman, P., and Morrow, K.J. (1991), Ascites production in recalcitrant hybridomas by backcrossing to the parental myeloma, *J. Immunol. Methods*, 144, 241–245.
13. Jackson, L.R., Trudel, L.J., Fox, J.G., and Lipman, N.S. (1999), Monoclonal antibody production in murine ascites. I. Clinical and pathological features, *Lab. Anim. Sci.*, 49, 70–80.
14. Luo, W. and Lin, S.H. (1997), Generation of moderate amounts of polyclonal antibodies in mice, *Biotechniques*, 23(4), 631–632.
15. Marusich, M.F. (1988), Efficient hybridoma production using previously frozen splenocytes, *J. Immunol. Methods*, 114, 155–159.
16. Kints, J.P., Manouvriez, P., and Bazin, H. (1989), Rat monoclonal antibodies. VII. Enhancement of ascites production and yield of monoclonal antibodies in rats following pretreatment with Pristane and Freund's adjuvant, *J. Immunol. Methods*, 119, 241–245.
17. Schuurman, H.J., Rozing, R., Van Loueren, H., Vassen, L.M.B., and Kampinga, J. (1989), The athymic nude rat, in *Immune-Deficient Animals in Experimental Medicine*, Wu & Zheng, Eds., S. Karger, Basel, p. 54.
18. Erb, K. and Hau, J. (1994), Monoclonal and polyclonal antibodies, in *Handbook of Laboratory Animal Science: Selection and Handling of Animals in Biomedical Research*, Per Svendsen and Jann Hau, Eds., CRC Press, Boca Raton, FL, pp. 293–310.

9 Growth of Cell Lines in Bioreactors

Beverly J. Norris, Michael J. Gramer,
and Mark D. Hirschel

CONTENTS

9.1 INTRODUCTION

The discovery more than 20 years ago by Köhler and Milstein[1] of the techniques for creation of monoclonal antibody-secreting hybridoma cell lines has led to the development of many technologies. Monoclonal antibodies (MAbs) are now versatile and valuable tools in biomedical research, and in the diagnosis and treatment of human and animal diseases. Bioreactor technologies have emerged to provide high-quality, cost-effective antibody production ranging from the small-scale needs of a research laboratory to the large-scale need of therapeutic antibody manufacturing.

A bioreactor, simply defined, is a vessel designed for the mass culture of cells. A bioreactor can be animal, vegetable, or mineral. Propagation of cells in animal ascites is still a viable method for small- to mid-scale (mg to g quantities) production of monoclonal antibodies[2]. Transgenic plants[3–5] and animals[6] are also bioreactors, in the broader sense, for the large-scale (kg) production of recombinant antibodies. More conventional types of mechanical bioreactors encompass a variety of technologies with varying production and scale-up capabilities.

9.2   COMMON BIOREACTOR THEMES

This chapter focuses on growth of hybridomas in mechanical bioreactors. While the technologies vary substantially, a number of common practices are used for all technologies. The temperature is almost always controlled at 37°C. Small variations in temperature (±0.5°C) seem to have little effect on cell growth, while larger variances can have positive and negative effects.[7] The medium pH is usually buffered to a small extent by phosphate in the medium, and to a larger extent by bicarbonate in an atmosphere containing usually 5 to 10% carbon dioxide. In a bioreactor where the pH is not controlled, the pH starts at about 7.2 to 7.4, and drops thereafter, primarily due to the production of lactic acid from glucose. The bicarbonate neutralizes the acid, and leaves the medium in the form of gaseous carbon dioxide. Where pH is not controlled, phenol red is generally added to the medium as a pH indicator. A medium color of orange to red indicates the optimum pH range, while purple is too basic and yellow too acidic. In more automated bioreactors, the pH is usually controlled between 7.0 and 7.2; a pH lower than about 6.9 and higher than about 7.5 is detrimental to cell growth.[8] As acid is produced, the percentage of carbon dioxide in the gas phase is lowered to drive the bicarbonate from the medium, raising the pH. In some cases, reducing the carbon dioxide concentration to zero is not sufficient to control pH, and additional buffer is automatically added to the bioreactor as needed.

The medium used to support cell growth can have a large effect on growth and antibody productivity. The most common medium for growth of hybridoma cells includes a base medium of nutrients such as DME, DME/F12, IMDM, or RPMI (basal medium) which is supplemented with about 10% fetal bovine serum. Serum-free media that support good cell growth are available from a number of suppliers; these media contain serum proteins such as insulin, transferrin, and albumin.[9] Totally defined protein-free media are also available. Serum-free and protein-free media can be just as expensive as serum-supplemented media, and not all cell lines adapt well to serum-free and protein-free media. As a result, serum-supplemented media are still widely used for the production of nontherapeutic antibodies.

While a number of variables are important for bioreactor optimization, the single most important parameter for scale-up of these bioreactors is oxygen delivery. Glucose and oxygen consumption rates are typically on the same order of magnitude (0.1 to 0.3 pmol/cell/h).[9-11] However, the concentration of glucose is usually on the order of 20 mM, while the solubility of oxygen in medium is only about 0.2 mM. As a result, the continual supply of ample oxygen is a major design consideration for large-scale bioreactors. Growth of cells at tissue densities (10^8 to 10^9/ml) requires an oxygenation source not more than about 100 µm from each cell.

9.3   BATCH CULTURE

Devices for low-density batch culture are the least complicated, and the least efficient. Cells are inoculated at about 5×10^4 to 5×10^5 cells/ml of culture fluid, and reach viable population densities ranging up to about 2×10^6 cells/ml. Antibody titers vary from about 1 to 50 µg/ml. At the low end of the bioreactor scale are

T flasks that provide cell culture volumes of about 5 to 100 ml. T flasks lie horizontally so that the medium forms a layer not more than about 2 to 3 mm thick. Oxygenation occurs by passive diffusion through the surface of the medium.

The next step up is spinner-flask culture for volumes on the order of 100 ml to a few liters. Spinner flasks are glass or disposable plastic cylinders sized so that the height is about one or two times the diameter of the vessel. The vessels are outfitted with paddle assemblies that are driven by magnetic stir bars. Oxygenation of the cell culture fluid is still accomplished by surface aeration, as in T flasks, but the lower surface-to-volume ratio is compensated for by stirring the pot and bringing more of the volume to the surface. Cell lines requiring higher concentrations of dissolved oxygen can be stirred faster, up to a point. Shear forces generated by the spinning paddles and, perhaps more importantly, by entrained air increase with higher speeds and can be destructive to the cells.[12, 13] The oxygen transfer limits cell growth at the lower end of paddle speed while the shear forces limit cell growth at the higher end of paddle speed. Since cell lines vary in their need for oxygen and sensitivity to shear forces, the optimum paddle speed may differ for different cell lines. Typical stirring speeds range from 50 to 150 rpm.

One can scale up a low-density culture further by growing cell lines in fermentation tanks with capacities ranging from tens to thousands of liters. At this scale, surface aeration will not deliver sufficient oxygen to sustain mass cell culture. Extra gas-transfer area is introduced by sparging (bubbling) the culture with air, or an oxygen-enriched gas. Sparging may cause damage to cells either at the sparger, at the paddle/gas interface, or the surface of the vessel as the bubble ruptures.[14] Gas-permeable tubing, such as silicone or porous polypropylene, can be placed in the tank to provide extra gas-transfer area without sparging, but this becomes impractical for tanks larger than about 10 to 100 L.

There are advantages and disadvantages to using low-density cell culture for the scale-up and production of monoclonal antibodies. The primary advantage is that stirred-tank fermenter technology is widely used, understood, and accepted by regulatory agencies. It is easier to maintain homogeneous conditions with low-density cultures, which may be important for consistent production and product quality. However, design challenges to maintain a homogeneous bioreactor still exist for very large stirred-tank fermenters.[15] The major disadvantage for this method of large-scale MAb production is that the cost of production can be very high compared to other available technologies. Since the cells are grown in suspension at low density, costly media components such as fetal bovine serum or defined serum substitutes are required in larger volumes. Another consequence of the low cell density is that product concentrations are low, leading to higher costs for processing a larger volume-to-yield purified final product. Furthermore, equipment and facility costs for operation of stirred-tank fermenters on a grand scale require a large capital outlay, making them economically suitable only for proven biopharmaceuticals with a large market.

9.4 FED BATCH CULTURE

The cell density and antibody titer in a batch culture are typically limited by nutrient depletion. As mentioned earlier, oxygen availability is the primary scale-up concern.

Once this is taken care of, depletion of other nutrients becomes the limiting factor. Simply adding extra nutrients at the start of culture is generally not optimal since the increased medium osmolarity tends to inhibit cell growth. To deal with this problem, a stirred-tank bioreactor can be operated in a fed-batch mode.[16] Cells are inoculated and grown as usual in the bioreactor through the exponential growth phase. Additional concentrated nutrients are added near the end of the growth phase, which increase the viable cell density attained (to about 10^7 cells/ml), and maintain the cells for a longer period in the stationary phase, resulting in potential antibody titers in the mg/ml range.[17-20] Optimization of fed-batch cultures can be a complicated, iterative process. Variables to consider are what, when, and how much nutrient concentrate to add. Generally, samples are taken to determine the rate and stoichiometry of nutrient depletion during a first run, and a nutrient formulation is created based on these findings. In a second run, the medium concentrate is added before the time of nutrient depletion, and the process continues. A general procedure for blind optimization has been proposed where no metabolite analysis is performed.[20] Operation in a fed-batch mode increases the productivity and reduces the cost of production in a stirred-tank system. However, the need for repeat batches and extensive metabolite analyses reduce the utility of fed-batch cultures for antibodies that are only produced in a few batches per year.

9.5   PERFUSION CULTURE

Fed-batch cultures are limited by the accumulation of unused nutrients (from unbalanced formulas) and metabolic waste products that build to toxic concentrations. To deal with this problem, bioreactors can be operated in a perfusion mode. There are numerous types of perfusion system designs, though all of them are variations on a single theme to add fresh medium and remove spent medium while retaining cells in the bioreactor. The types of bioreactors differ principally in the way that the cells are immobilized and product is harvested. With perfusion systems, cell densities can be maintained in the 10^7 to 10^8 range for weeks or months.

A stirred-tank fermenter is converted to a perfusion system by including a means to retain cells in the bioreactor. A number of technologies are available to remove cells from the spent medium stream including dialysis,[21,22] centrifugation,[23,24] tangential flow filtration,[25,26] spin filters,[27,28] sedimentation devices,[29,30] and acoustical cell separators.[31,32] Each of these devices has problems with scale-up or fouling, so that no single method has become a standard in the industry. Alternatively, hybridoma cells can be retained in the bioreactor by physical entrapment in larger particles that are easily separated from the product stream. One such example is the Celligen Plus system, where cells become entrapped in porous polyester disks.[33] The disks are large enough to be retained in the bioreactor inside a basket cage.

Another set of perfusion bioreactors uses circulating medium as opposed to stirring to provide nutrients to the cell mass. Medium is circulated from a reservoir, through a gas-exchange cartridge, to oxygenate the medium and adjust the pH, and then is perfused through the cell mass and is returned to the reservoir. Fresh medium is added and removed on a batch or continual basis. Ceramic core,[34] fluidized bed,[35] and fixed bed technologies[36-39] all rely on physical entrapment to retain the hybridoma cells in the bioreactor. Membrane systems (flat sheet and hollow fiber) bioreactors immobilize cells by passing the circulating medium on one side of a membrane while retaining cells on the other side of the membrane. The membrane typically has a molecular weight cutoff which does not allow passage of molecules larger than about 10 kDa. As a result, the large molecular weight growth factors required by the cells (serum components) are retained on the cell side of the membrane. The majority of nutrients are supplied through the membrane from inexpensive basal medium on the non-cell side of the membrane. The total amount of medium used to produce a given amount of antibody is similar for membrane and non-membrane systems. However, tremendous cost savings are achieved in membrane systems since the expensive cell-side medium is consumed at a rate of about 100 times less than that of the inexpensive non-cell-side medium. The antibody is also retained on the cell side of the membrane so that antibody concentrations of 1 to 10 mg/ml are common. This simplifies and reduces the cost of purification since the initial antibody purity is higher and concentration steps are not required prior to antibody purification.

The most commercially successful high-density perfusion systems for the production of antibodies utilize hollow fiber technology. Commercial hollow fiber bioreactor systems are available which support cell culture volumes ranging from about 2 ml to about 2 L. Cell densities and volumetric productivities in hollow fiber systems are typically about 100 times higher than for typical batch production systems. Loosely speaking, the productivity of a 2 L cell culture space in a hollow fiber system would be equivalent to harvesting a 200 L batch culture on a daily basis.

A few novel membrane bioreactors incorporate an additional oxygenation membrane so that medium recirculation is not required, significantly simplifying the operation of these systems. These include the Tecnomouse[40] and CELLine from Integra Biosciences and the Mini-Perm[41] from Heraeus Instruments. Sized for use in research laboratories, they will provide up to a few hundred milligrams of antibody in a month in the mg/ml concentration range.

The higher volumetric productivity and continuous production in perfusion systems provide cost savings through lower start-up and production costs relative to low-density systems. However, the use and validation of perfusion systems have lagged behind those of simple batch systems. Cell culture technologies were initially targeted at the high-value therapeutic market. However, manufacturers of therapeutic products have generally opted to stick with the more conservative approach of using well-known, albeit inefficient, low-density cell culture. Since the therapeutic products have high value, the cost of production has been less important than time to market. The breakthrough to perfusion systems is primarily driven by the *in vitro* diagnostic markets, where the cost of antibody production is critical to competitiveness. Many of the concerns regarding issues such as reproducibility, consistent long-term productivity, product quality, and validatability are being laid to rest. For example, Cytogen recently received a license from the FDA for ProstaCint, a hollow-fiber bioreactor-produced monoclonal antibody used for *in vivo* imaging and diagnosis of prostate cancer.[42] A number of manufacturers producing therapeutic monoclonal antibodies from hollow fiber systems are currently in clinical trials.

9.6 HOLLOW-FIBER BIOREACTOR

After discussing basic understanding of the design features and primary control parameters of bioreactors, it is perhaps most instructive to present a prototypical production run of an automated bioreactor culture for MAb production. The example provided here is the cultivation of a hybridoma in a commercial hollow-fiber system. A general description of procedures will be given first, followed by a specific example illustrating the growth of a murine hybridoma.

9.6.1 GENERAL DESCRIPTION

A simplified diagram of an automated hollow-fiber system (AcuSyst *MAXIMIZER*®, Cellex Biosciences) is shown in Figure 9.1. The hollow fibers are typically encased in a cylindrical tube and are potted at either end to define an intracapillary (IC) space (inside the fibers) and an extracapillary (EC) space (outside the fibers). For clarity, the IC and EC fluid circuits are shown separately in Figure 9.1. Cells are placed in the EC space which provides better cell retention. Cell culture medium is circulated from the IC chamber through a gas-exchange cartridge and is pumped into the bioreactor IC compartment. From inside the fibers, nutrients such as oxygen and glucose diffuse across the 10 kDa molecular weight cutoff fiber membrane into the EC space where the cells reside. Likewise, metabolic wastes produced by the cells, such as lactate and carbon dioxide, diffuse back across the membrane into the hollow fibers and are carried back to and diluted in the medium reservoir. To monitor the metabolic demand and optimize cell growth, accessory instruments able to produce off-line sample data quickly and conveniently are recommended (especially for large-scale systems) and include a blood-gas analyzer and a glucose analyzer. Basal medium is continually added to and removed from the IC circuit to supply

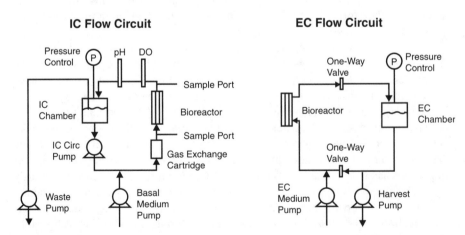

FIGURE 9.1 Simplified flow diagram of an automated hollow-fiber system (Acusyst Maximizer, Cellex Biosciences). The IC flow circuit (left) and EC flow circuit (right) are shown separately for clarity. Additional pumps and sample ports are available on the system, but are not shown here.

fresh low molecular weight nutrients and remove low molecular weight wastes. The IC medium addition rate is most commonly adjusted according to data from off-line glucose analysis. A general rule is to increase the medium addition rate if the glucose concentration falls to less than half of the original value. The IC circulation rate is set based on oxygen demand; the IC circulation rate is increased if the dissolved oxygen concentration at the bioreactor outlet drops below about 80 to 100 mmHg. The pH is automatically controlled by adjusting the percent of carbon dioxide gas passing through the gas-exchange cartridge and by adding additional base if neces-sary. Both the pH and dissolved oxygen (DO) probe are calibrated off-line by injecting bioreactor samples into a blood-gas analyzer. Fresh growth medium is continually added to the EC circuit to supply high-molecular weight growth factors, while conditioned EC medium is continually removed to harvest the antibody. As a general rule, the rate of EC medium addition or removal is kept around 100 times slower than the current IC medium addition rate. The slow rate of medium flow through the EC results in flow channeling and suboptimal productivity. To compen-sate for this problem, the bioreactor is operated in a cycling mode. Cycling is accomplished by pressurizing the IC chamber, which forces medium across the fibers into the EC chamber. The situation is reversed by pressurizing the EC chamber to force the medium back across the fibers into the IC chamber. The amount of medium cycled is monitored and controlled based on an ultrasonic level indicator in the EC chamber. One-way check valves are placed in the EC circuit to provide unidirectional flow. Cells that wash out and collect in the EC chamber are removed periodically. The conditioned medium harvested by this extra cell removal is also saved as product.

The first step in running a hollow-fiber system is to scale up the hybridoma cell culture to prepare the inoculum for the bioreactors. This is done using traditional cell culture methods in T flasks and spinner flasks, depending upon the scale of the system. To ensure reproducibility of production runs, the inoculum should be pre-pared each time from a new vial taken from a well-characterized cryopreserved cell bank. Preparation and testing of master cell banks and a manufacturer's working cell bank created from the master cell bank should take place as early as practical in the life cycle of a monoclonal antibody product. Cell banks should be tested for the presence of contaminating microorganisms, and a reference lot of MAb should be retained and characterized from an early production run for comparison to future manufactured lots to verify that the cell line and manufacturing process are producing a stable, safe, and effective product. The amount of inoculum to prepare will, of course, vary with the type and scale of the system employed, and will also vary according to the growth characteristics of a particular cell line, such as doubling time and typical density during logarithmic growth phase. The optimal amount of inoculum to use can be determined experimentally using a small-scale device and extrapolating results to the larger scale, which is recommended if multiple manu-factured lots of a single product are required. Otherwise, sufficient cell numbers should be procured to propel the culture straight into a logarithmic growth phase once introduced into the bioreactor. Inoculating with insufficient cell numbers may create a long lag phase before real growth begins, slowing the MAb production, or even cause complete failure of the culture to thrive in the bioreactors. As a general rule, hollow fiber bioreactors should be inoculated at about 5×10^6 cells/ml of cell culture space.

Several days prior to the inoculation, the sterile cultureware set should be installed in the instrument in the place where it is to be operated. The cultureware must be aseptically filled and flushed with sterile cell culture media so that any cytotoxic residues remaining from manufacture or sterilization will be rinsed away. In addition, it is wise to run the instrument in operational mode for at least a day or two before inoculating the cells to be sure that the sterility of the system remains uncompromised and that it has no mechanical problems.

As with any cell culture system, all operations must be performed aseptically. Although these instruments do not need to be completely contained within a sterile field, procedures such as inoculation, changing sterile feed and waste containers, sampling, and harvesting secreted product are all potential ports of entry for contaminating microorganisms. Careful aseptic technique and a clean environment are essential prerequisites for success with any type of cell culture, but with a long-term culture, the consequences of a loss due to microbial infection are far more costly than the loss of a T flask or two in an incubator.

It cannot be stressed too strongly, or too often, that a rigorous program of infection control must be followed. The room in which the instruments are to be set up should be kept uncluttered and free of dust. Surfaces such as floors and countertops should be wiped down with a disinfectant weekly. The room should not have doors or windows opening directly to the outdoors. Care should be taken to prevent facilitating spots where mold could grow and release spores, especially in warm and humid climates or seasons. In particular, nothing should be stored in cardboard containers, since cardboard harbors millions of spores and molds quickly if it gets damp. Any water baths or humidifier trays in incubators should contain antimicrobial agents at appropriate concentrations. Personnel entering the laboratory should be appropriately attired in lint-free lab coats and should wear gloves rubbed down with isopropyl alcohol while handling cell cultures. Hair nets and face masks can provide extra protection for critical procedures. Food and beverages should be strictly prohibited in a cell culture laboratory. Some additional measures which can be taken are to install tacky mats at the entryway to the instrument room and to install HEPA filters in the ceiling.

When a sufficient number of cells have been accumulated in culture to inoculate the system, the cells can be harvested and concentrated for injection into the bioreactor. The cell culture should be at a density which correlates near mid-log phase on a growth curve and near peak viability at harvest. Cells can be concentrated by aseptic centrifugation, and then the pellet can be resuspended gently in a convenient volume of growth medium.

Cells are inoculated into the extracapillary space by injection with a syringe or by pumping the cell suspension from a sterile bottle. Following inoculation of cells into the bioreactor, the growth phase begins. During this phase, the primary objective is to get the cells to divide and occupy the extracapillary space. It is important during this phase to monitor pre- and post-bioreactor pH and concentrations of metabolites such as glucose and dissolved oxygen. Nutrients should not become limiting during this phase, so media feed rates and circulation rates should be increased at appropriate intervals to keep pace with cell growth. The cell culture medium car , optimized for each cell line in T-flask culture prior to initiating the bioreactor culture so that metabolic requirements are met, and also so that minimum costs are incurred. Inclusion of phenol red as part of the media formulation provides an easy way to monitor production when access to more sophisticated assay data is not readily available, although it is often preferable to omit phenol red later on at the larger scales required for product manufacture, since it is one more component to be removed during purification.

The stationary production phase is reached after the cells have formed large masses of colonies within the bioreactor extracapillary space, and the media feed rates required to maintain glucose setpoints begin to plateau. Stable production may last anywhere from several weeks to several months, depending upon the growth characteristics of the cell line in question and how well culture conditions are selected and optimized for that cell line. During this time, media consumption rates for the intracapillary (or IC) medium usually remain fairly stable. Factor feed rates for the extracapillary (or EC) medium will need to be increased in step with increased harvest rates, although total concentrations of serum or serum proteins required in the EC space may be substantially reduced compared to growth phase once the cells are at high density. Harvest rates are tied to product concentration; MAbs secreted by the cells should be harvested at a rate such that total yield of purified product from a single run is maximized and processing costs are minimized. Some experimentation may be required with the first few cultures to establish a good process. In general, a continuous harvest method has been found for many cell lines to produce a greater total quantity of MAb than harvesting discrete batches periodically. The rate of harvest of fluid from the extracapillary space should be tailored to make collection and processing of harvest volumes convenient. Harvests should be collected aseptically into collection vessels and kept refrigerated or cooled with ice packs. This low-temperature storage enhances stability of the MAbs and protects them from degradation by proteases, particularly if the pH of the harvested fluid is neutral or acidic. When a collection container is full, it should be aseptically removed from the system and replaced with a new sterile collection vessel. From this point, any container to which product is transferred during processing should be carefully and consistently labeled, especially if more than one MAb is produced in the same laboratory.

The first step in processing the harvested material is to separate the cells and cell debris from the supernatant containing the secreted MAb. It is usually desirable to use a two-step process to clarify the supernatant. The first step is a crude refinement to remove the largest particles by centrifugation or filtration using a membrane with a relatively large pore size. The second step would be a filtration step with a finer pore size to remove smaller colloidal particles in the 0.2- to 0.5-μm size range. This step removes most of the column-fouling particles from the fluid prior to purification processes utilizing column chromatography. It has the additional advantage of providing a filter sterilization of the harvest material, which by now is a very high-value-added biological fluid. Once processed, the harvests can be stored refrigerated or frozen, depending upon the stability of the MAb activity at different storage temperatures over established time intervals.

In general it is desirable to store all of the harvests until the end of the production run, testing each one for sterility and MAb activity along the way. Then after production all acceptable harvest material can be pooled prior to purification. It helps in the development of a more uniform and predictable purification process to have all of the starting material of the same composition, particularly if purification requires multiple runs of a single process to purify all of the material produced.

9.6.2   CELL CULTURE EXAMPLE

To better illustrate antibody production in a bioreactor, a specific example is given here using an AcuSyst *MAXIMIZER* 1000 (Cellex Biosciences) hollow fiber system (see Figure 9.1). The hollow-fiber bioreactor used for this run had a molecular weight cutoff of 10 kDa, a fiber surface area of 2.6 m^2 (based on fiber ID), and an EC volume of 270 ml. A murine hybridoma secreting an IgG MAb was thawed 1 week prior to inoculation. The cells were scaled up in a 2-L spinner in DME/F12 medium containing 10% fetal bovine serum. The cultureware was set up and flushed with 10 L of basal medium 1 day prior to inoculation. The IC medium consisted of DME/F12 supplemented with 4 mg/ml ethanolamine, 4 mM glutamine, 3.4 g/L sodium bicarbonate, 4.15 g/L glucose, 0.066 g/L penicillin G, and 0.144 g/L streptomycin sulfate (final concentrations). The EC medium consisted of IC medium supplemented with 10% fetal bovine serum. Several hours prior to inoculation, the EC compartment was filled with 10% serum-supplemented medium. A total of 1×10^9 cells at 8×10^5 cells/ml were pelleted by centrifugation at 275 g and resuspended in 15 ml of serum-supplemented medium. The cells were injected into the bioreactor EC compartment, followed by an additional 5 ml of fresh serum supplemented medium to flush the lines.

The rate of basal IC fresh medium addition/waste removal was initially set at 25 ml/h. This rate was increased to meet the increase in glucose demand as the cells expanded in the bioreactor (Figure 9.2). On day 6, the medium pump was set to the maximum rate (800 ml/h) which resulted in lower glucose concentrations as the cells continued to expand. On days 11 to 13, the pH dropped from the setpoint of 7.2 to 6.8 due to inadequate buffering; adjustment of the initial medium pH from 7.2 to 7.6 resolved that problem. The glucose utilization rate topped out at about day 14 and reduced somewhat as the culture entered the stationary production phase.

The oxygen uptake rate steadily increased in step with the glucose uptake rate (see Figure 9.3). To meet the increased oxygen demand, the IC circulation rate was increased from 250 ml/min initially to the maximum of 1000 ml/min on day 7. The bioreactor outlet dissolved oxygen concentration reduced somewhat thereafter due to continued cell expansion, and leveled off during the stationary production phase.

The EC medium feed/harvest rates were initially set at zero. After 3 days, cycling was initiated and the feed/harvest rates were set at 1 ml/h. The feed/harvest rates were kept at about 100 times slower than the IC medium addition rate (Figure 9.4). The antibody concentration steadily increased to about 2 mg/ml and was fairly stable from day 15 through day 60. Cells were removed from the EC chamber about 2 times per week, and this medium (50 to 100 ml) was pooled with the harvest. The total amount of antibody produced over the 60-day period was 25 g.

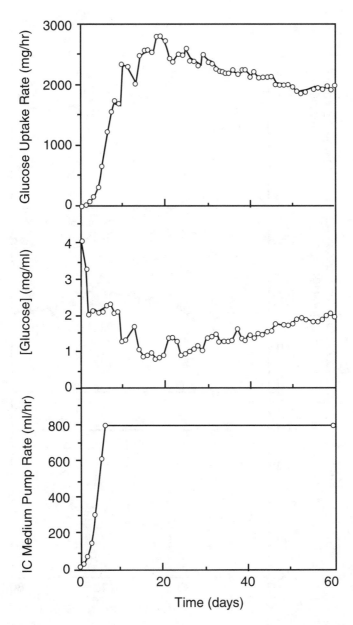

FIGURE 9.2 Control of IC medium feed rate. As the glucose demand increases during the growth phase, the IC medium pump is increased to keep the glucose concentration from dropping below 2 g/L. When the maximum rate of medium addition is attained (800 ml/hr), the glucose concentration falls below the set point and levels off during the stationary production phase.

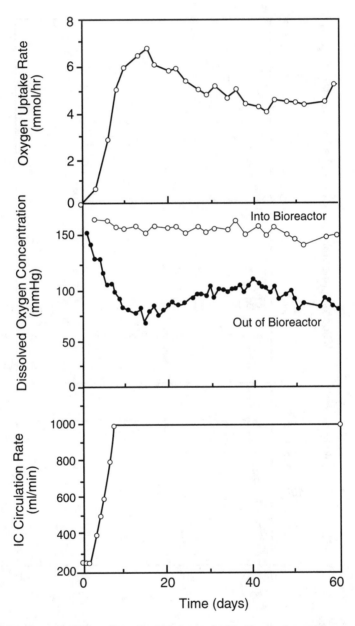

FIGURE 9.3 Control of IC medium circulation rate. As the oxygen demand increases during the growth phase, the rate of IC medium circulation is increased to keep the concentration of dissolved oxygen above 100 mmHg. When the maximum rate of medium addition is attained (1000 ml/min), the dissolved oxygen concentration falls below the set point and levels off during the stationary production phase.

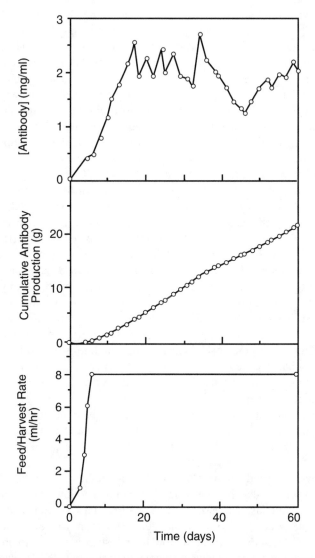

FIGURE 9.4 Control of EC feed/harvest rate. The feed/harvest rates were initially at zero so that cells could get established in the bioreactor. On day 3 and thereafter, the EC feed/harvest rates were kept about 100 times lower than the IC medium addition rate.

9.7 SUMMARY: CHOOSING A TECHNOLOGY

Choosing a technology depends on factors such as scale, frequency of production, product end use, available capital, and time available to produce the antibody. On a research scale (<200 mg), the choices include spinner flasks, small high-density perfusion systems (hollow fiber and flat sheet) and mouse ascites. The total costs of antibody production in these different systems are similar enough that convenience rather than cost is the primary consideration for choosing a technology. The growth and productivity of a hybridoma are usually characterized first in a T flask or small spinner flask. For quick one-time production with no surprises, an appropriately sized spinner flask is most often chosen. The productivity of a hybridoma in a T flask does not necessarily correlate to the productivity that will be seen in perfusion systems and mouse ascites, and the production in small perfusion systems and mouse ascites (about 2 to 4 weeks) generally takes a little longer compared to a spinner flask (about 1 to 2 weeks). The major driving force for using perfusion systems and mouse ascites is that the antibody concentration typically reaches 1 to 10 mg/ml (compared to 1 to 50 µg/ml in spinners) so that antibody concentration and purification may not be necessary for use in a research application.

The production choices at the intermediate scale (200 mg to 2 g) are essentially identical to those of the research scale, except that cost becomes more of a factor for choosing a technology. A stirred-tank system operated in batch mode is the conservative and predictable option. However, the initial capital costs and cost of production in that system will be much higher compared to other methods. One option is to operate the tank in fed-batch mode. Another option is mouse ascites; this is the upper range of usefulness for mouse ascites, and many antibody manufacturers are turning to perfusion systems at this scale. Growth of a hybridoma for the first time in a perfusion system may yield unpredictable results, better or worse than expected, based on T-flask data. However, perfusion systems can be operated for months at a time so that lower-than-expected performance can be compensated for by running the system for a longer period of time while still achieving cost savings over a batch stirred tank. Hollow-fiber perfusion systems are typically less expensive and easier to operate than to stirred-tank perfusion systems. However, cells tend to grow faster in a stirred-tank perfusion system leading to shorter production times. One approach to optimize production is to incorporate both technologies; use the hollow-fiber system for cost savings and convenience when the manufacturing lead time is 1 to 2 months, and use the perfusion tank for the production of antibodies with shorter lead times.

For large-scale production of monoclonal antibodies (>2 g), the choices are a stirred-tank batch, fed-batch or perfusion bioreactor, a hollow-fiber system, or transgenic plants or animals. The issues between stirred-tank systems and hollow-fiber systems are the same as cited in the previous paragraph. However, the capacity of the largest commercially available hollow fiber system is limited to about a kg per year, while very large stirred tanks have potential for about 100 kg/year production. Transgenic plants and animals are very recent developments in the field of protein production. At present, the large initial cost of generating a transgenic animal is only justified by the commercial potentials of products with estimated market sizes higher than 10 kg/year.[6] Transgenic antibodies are economically produced in plants, but details regarding the large-scale purification of functional antibodies from plants have not been addressed.[4] For therapeutic antibodies, differences in protein glycosylation can affect antibody function. As a result, questions prevail regarding functions of antibodies produced from transgenic animals (pigs, cows, and sheep can add an antigenic sugar linkage) and especially transgenic plants, which may attach immunogenic sugars to the antibody.[43]

REFERENCES

1. Köhler, G. and Milstein, C., Continuous culture of fused cells secreting antibody of predefined specificity, *Nature*, 256, 495, 1975.
2. Jackson, L. R., Trudel, L. J., Fox, J. G., and Lipman, N. S., Evaluation of hollow fiber bioreactors as an alternative to murine ascites production for small scale monoclonal antibody production, *J. Immunol. Methods*, 189, 217, 1996.
3. Whitelam, G. C., Cockburn, W., and Owen, M. R. L., Antibody production in transgenic plants, *Biochem. Soc. Trans.*, 22, 940, 1994.
4. Holzmann, D., Agracetus grows monoclonals in soybean and corn plants, *Genetic Eng. News*, 14, 1, 1994.
5. Ma, J. K. C. and Hein, M. B., Plant antibodies for immunotherapy, *Plant Physiol.*, 109, 341, 1995.
6. Young, M. W., Okita, W. B., Brown, E. M., and Curling, J. M., Production of biopharmaceutical proteins in the milk of transgenic dairy animals, *BioPharm.*, 10, 34, 1997.
7. Chuppa, S., Tsai, Y., Yoon, S., Shackleford, S., Rozales, C., Bhat, R., Tsay, G., Matanguihan, C., Konstantinov, K., and Naveh, D., Fermenter temperature as a tool for control of high-density perfusion cultures of mammalian cells, *Biotechnol. Bioeng.*, 55, 328, 1997.
8. Ozturk, S. S. and Palsson, B. O., Growth, metabolic, and antibody production kinetics of hybridoma cell culture: 2. Effects of serum concentration, dissolved oxygen concentration, and medium pH in a batch bioreactor, *Biotechnol. Prog.*, 7, 481, 1991.
9. Glassy, M. C., Tharakan, J. P., and Chau, P. C., Serum-free media in hybridoma culture and monoclonal antibody production, *Biotechnol. Bioeng.*, 32, 1015, 1988.
10. Ozturk, S. S., Riley, M. R., and Palsson, B. O., Effects of ammonia and lactate on hybridoma growth, metabolism, and antibody production, *Biotechnol. Bioeng.*, 39, 418, 1992.
11. Banik, G. G. and Heath, C. A., Hybridoma growth and antibody production as a function of cell density and specific growth rate in perfusion culture, *Biotechnol. Bioeng.*, 48, 289, 1995.
12. Kunas, K. and Papoutsakis, E., Damage mechanisms of suspended animal cells in agitated bioreactors with and without bubble entrainment, *Biotechnol. Bioeng.*, 36, 476, 1990.
13. Abu-Reesh, I. and Kargi, F., Biological responses of hybridoma cells to hydrodynamic shear in an agitated bioreactor, *Enzyme Microb. Technol.*, 13, 913, 1991.
14. Chalmers, J. J., Cells and bubbles in sparged bioreactors, *Cytotechnology*, 15, 311, 1994.
15. Humphrey, A., Shake flask to fermentor: What have we learned? *Biotechnol. Prog.*, 14, 3, 1998.
16. Bibila, T. A. and Robinson, D. K., In pursuit of the optimal fed-batch process for monoclonal antibody production, *Biotechnol. Prog.*, 11, 1, 1995.
17. Xie, L. and Wang, D. I. C., High cell density and high monoclonal antibody production through medium design and rational control in a bioreactor, *Biotechnol. Bioeng.*, 51, 725, 1996.
18. Zhou, W., Chen, C., Buckland, B., and Aunins, J., Fed-batch culture of recombinant NSO myeloma cells with high monoclonal antibody production, *Biotechnol. Bioeng.*, 55, 783, 1997.

19. Bushell, M. E., Bell, S. L., Scott, M. F., Spier, R. E., Wardell, J. N., and Sanders, P. G., Enhancement of monoclonal antibody yield by hybridoma fed-batch culture, resulting in extended maintenance of viable cell population, *Biotechnol. Bioeng.*, 44, 1099, 1994.

20. Bibila, T. A., Ranucci, C. S., Glazomitsky, K., Buckland, B. C., and Aunins, J. G., Monoclonal antibody process development using medium concentrates, *Biotechnol. Prog.*, 10, 87, 1994.

21. Harigae, M., Matsumura, M., and Kataoka, H., Kinetic study on HB-s-MAb production in continuous cultivation, *J. Biotechnol.*, 34, 227, 1994.

22. Amos, B., Al-Rubeai, M., and Emery, A.N., Hybridoma growth and monoclonal antibody production in a dialysis perfusion system, *Enzyme Microb. Technol.*, 16, 688, 1994.

23. Johnson, M., Lanthier, S., Massie, B., Lefebvre, G., and Kamen, A., Use of the Centritech lab centrifuge for perfusion culture of hybridoma cells in protein-free medium, *Biotechnol. Prog.*, 12, 855, 1996.

24. Tokashiki, M., Arai, T., Hamamoto, K., and Ishimaru, K., High density culture of hybridoma cells using a perfusion culture vessel with an external centrifuge, *Cytotechnology*, 3, 239, 1990.

25. Mercille, S., Johnson, M., Lemieux, R., and Massie, B., Filtration-based perfusion of hybridoma cultures in protein-free medium: reduction of membrane fouling by medium supplementation with DNase I, *Biotechnol. Bioeng.*, 43, 833, 1994.

26. Smith, C., Guillaume, J., Greenfield, P., and Randerson, D., Experience in scale-up of homogeneous perfusion culture for hybridomas, *Bioproc. Eng.*, 6, 213, 1991.

27. Emery, A. N., Jan, D. C.-H., and Rubeai, M., Oxygenation of intensive cell-culture system, *Appl. Microbiol. Biotechnol.*, 43, 1028, 1995.

28. Deo, Y., Mahadevan, M., and Fuchs, R., Practical considerations in operation and scale-up of spin-filter based bioreactors for monoclonal antibody production, *Biotechnol. Prog.*, 12, 57, 1996.

29. Hansen, H., Damgaard, B., and Emborg, C., Enhanced antibody production associated with altered amino acid metabolism in a hybridoma high-density perfusion culture established by gravity separation, *Cytotechnology*, 11, 155, 1993.

30. LaPorte, T., Shevitz, J., Kim, Y., and Wang, S., Hybridoma perfusion system using a sedimentation device, *Biotechnol. Techn.*, 9, 837, 1995.

31. Trampler, F., Sonderhoff, S., Pui, P., Kilburn, D., and Piret, J., Acoustic cell filter for high density perfusion culture of hybridoma cells, *Bio/Technology*, 12, 281, 1994.

32. Doblhoff-Dier, O., Gaida, T., Katinger, H., Burger, W., Groschl, M., and Benes, E., A novel ultrasonic resonance field device for the retention of animal cells, *Biotechnol. Prog.*, 10, 428, 1994.

33. Wang, G., Zhang, W., Jacklin, C., Freedman, D., Eppstein, L., and Kadouri, A., Modified Celligen-packed bed bioreactors for hybridoma cell cultures, *Cytotechnology*, 9, 41, 1992.

34. Lydersen, B. K., Perfusion cell culture system based on ceramic matrices, in *Large Scale Cell Culture Technology*, Lydersen, B. K., Ed., Hanser Publishers, New York, 1987, 169.

35. Dean, R. C., Jr., Karkare, S. B., Phillips, P. G., Ray, N. G., and Runstadler, P. W., Jr., Continuous cell culture with fluidized sponge beads, in *Large Scale Cell Culture Technology*, Lydersen, B. K., Ed., Hanser Publishers, New York, 1987, 145.

36. Moro, A., Rodrigues, M., Gouvea, M., Silvestri, M., Kalil, J., and Raw, I., Multiparametric analyses of hybridoma growth on glass cylinders in a packed-bed bioreactor system with internal aeration. Serum-supplemented and serum-free media comparison for MAb production, *J. Immunol. Methods,* 176, 67, 1994.
37. Bohmann, A., Portner, R., Schmieding, J., Kasche, V., and Markl, H., The membrane dialysis bioreactor with integrated radial-flow fixed bed — a new approach for continuous cultivation of animal cells, *Cytotechnology,* 9, 51, 1992.
38. Griffiths, J., Looby, D., and Racher, R., Maximisation of perfusion systems and process comparison with batch-type cultures, *Cytotechnology,* 9, 3, 1992.
39. Bliem, R., Oakley, R., Matsuoka, K., Varecka, R., and Taiariol, V., Antibody production in packed bed reactors using serum-free and protein-free medium, *Cytotechnology,* 4, 279, 1990.
40. Schlapfer, B. S., Scheibler, M., Anke-Peggy, H., Van Nguyen, H., and Pluschke, G., Development of optimized transfectoma cell lines for production of chimeric antibodies in hollow fiber cell culture systems, *Biotechnol. Bioeng.,* 45, 310, 1995.
41. Falkenberg, F. W., Weichert, H., Krane, M., Bartels, I., Palme, M., Nagels, H., and Fiebig, H., *In vitro* production of monoclonal antibodies in high concentration in a new and easy to handle modular minifermenter, *J. Immunol. Methods,* 179, 13, 1995.
42. Danheiser, S. L., Hollow fiber bioreactor gets boost from injectable antibody approval, *Genet. Eng. News,* 16, 1, 1996.
43. Goochee, C. F., Gramer, M. J., Andersen, D. C., Bahr, J. B., and Rasmmussen, J. R., The oligosaccharides of glycoproteins: bioprocess factors affecting oligosaccharide structure and their effect on glycoprotein properties, *Bio/Technology,* 9, 1347, 1991.

10 Phage Display

Peter Amersdorfer and James D. Marks

CONTENTS

0-8493-9445-7/00/$0.00+$.50
© 2000 by CRC Press LLC

10.1 INTRODUCTION

The ability of monoclonal antibodies (MAb) to bind specifically to antigen and to block antigen function or synthesis has led to their increasing importance as laboratory reagents, diagnostics, and therapeutics. The modular structures of antibodies have also made it possible to construct smaller antibody fragments, such as the Fab and single chain Fv (scFv) which retain the antigen-binding properties of the IgG from which they were derived (see Figure 10.1). Besides having different pharmacokinetic properties which can be useful,[1,57] Fab and scFv can be expressed in functional form in *E. coli*, allowing rapid protein engineering to reduce immunogenicity, increase affinity, or alter specificity.[22] scFv has proven particularly useful, since they can be encoded in a single gene and yield a single polypeptide chain. Compared to heterodimeric IgG or dimeric Fab, scFv facilitates construction of fusion proteins, such as immunotoxins[35] and viral or nonviral gene therapy vectors.[21,52] scFv can also be expressed intracellularly in eukaryotic cells to achieve phenotypic knockout of the antigen they bind.[7]

Mabs are classically obtained from mice immunized with a purified antigen (hybridoma technology).[33] The V genes of Mabs can be used to construct recombinant Fab or scFv antibody fragments. While this approach has yielded many useful antibodies for research and diagnosis, it has limitations. The process is time consuming and inefficient; only a relatively small number of antibodies are typically produced against a few dominant immunogenic epitopes. This may result in failure to isolate the precise specificity desired for a particular aim. Furthermore, production

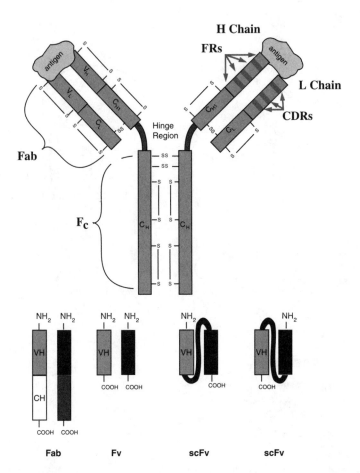

FIGURE 10.1 Structures of immunoglobulins and derived fragments. (Top) The basic immunoglobulin molecule is Y-shaped and is composed of two heavy and two light chains. The antigen-binding sites are located at the tips of the Y in regions of variable protein sequence, called the Fv fragment. Each Fv consists of a heavy chain variable domain (V_H) and a light chain variable domain (V_L). Within each variable domain are regions of more-conserved sequences (framework regions, FR) that serve as a scaffold for three regions of hypervariable sequences (complementarity determining regions, CDRs). (Bottom) Schematic structures of monovalent antibody fragments. Fab and Fv fragments contain the antigen binding site (V_H and V_L) and Fab have additional constant regions (C_H1 and C_L). Fv fragments can be stabilized by connecting the V_H and V_L via a flexible peptide linker forming a single chain Fv (scFv).

of antibodies against proteins conserved between species is difficult or impossible. Use of MAbs to construct recombinant antibody fragments can be limited by difficulties amplifying the heavy (V_H) and light (V_L) chain variable regions,[46] problems cloning the V genes, or low levels of expression in bacteria.[32] Limitations of hybridoma technology can be partially overcome by taking advantage of recent advances to produce scFv or Fab directly in bacteria (reviewed in References 27, 37, and 56). Antigen-specific antibody fragments are directly selected from antibody-fragment

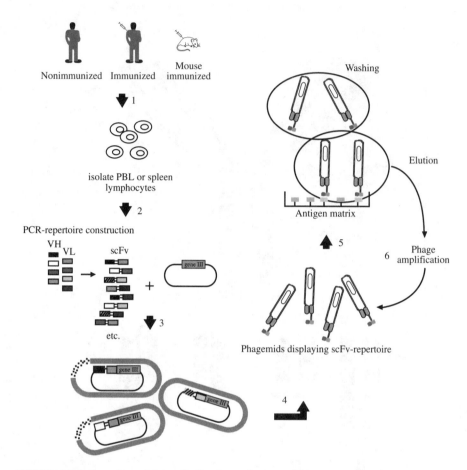

FIGURE 10.2 Overview of the antibody phage display technique. Lymphocytes are isolated from mice or humans (step 1) and the V_H and V_L genes amplified using PCR (step 2). scFv gene repertoires are created by PCR assembly of V_H and V_L genes. The scFv repertoire is cloned into a phage display vector and the ligated DNA used to transform *E. coli* (step 3). Phage displaying scFv are prepared from transformed *E. coli* (step 4). Phage are incubated with immobilized antigen (Step 5), nonspecifically bound phage removed by washing, and antigen-specific phage eluted by acid or alkali. Eluted phage are used to infect *E. coli*, to produce more phage for the next round of selection (step 6). Repetition of the selection process results in the isolation of antigen-specific phage antibodies present at low frequencies.

gene repertoires expressed on the surface of bacteriophage, which infect bacteria (phage display)[26,39] (see Figure 10.2). The technique can be used to bypass conventional hybridoma technology by using the V genes from immunized mice or humans. Using this approach, murine and human antibodies have been made against hepatitis B surface antigen,[58] hepatitis C,[12] respiratory syncytial virus,[3] HIV-1 gp120,[4] hemophilus influenza,[45] and botulinum neurotoxins.[2] Many different antibody fragments are produced with affinities (10 nM to 1 nM) that compare favorably to the affinities of monoclonal antibodies produced using hybridoma technology. Phage display can also be used to make antibodies without prior immunization by displaying very large and diverse V-gene repertoires on phage[23,37,49,55] and results in the ability to isolate antibodies with any desired specificity from a single phage display library. Antibody fragments produced in this manner almost invariably express at high level in bacteria.[36,55] Higher affinity antibody fragments can be selected from phage antibody libraries created by mutating the V genes of initial isolates.[24,37]

This chapter will focus on creation and manipulation of single-chain Fv phage antibody libraries. The techniques described will also work for Fab libraries, although different primers and vectors are required.[31] Our laboratory prefers to work with scFv due to generically higher expression levels and the single gene nature of scFv antibodies.

10.2 GENERATION OF HUMAN AND MURINE SCFV GENE REPERTOIRES

10.2.1 DESCRIPTION

This section describes the amplification of human or murine V genes and their assembly by PCR to create diverse scFv gene repertoires. mRNA can be prepared from different sources of B cells (bone marrow, peripheral blood lymphocytes, spleen, or tonsil cells) of a normal healthy human, or an immunized person or mouse, depending on whether a "naive" or immune phage display library will be made (see Figure 10.2). cDNA is prepared by reverse transcription of total RNA with oligonucleotides that prime in the immunoglobulin heavy and light chain constant regions. Preparation is straightforward, since the sequences of exons for human and murine constant domain are known.[30] As an alternative, cDNA can also be made by standard methods such as oligo dT or random hexamer priming.

For creation of human V-gene repertoires, V_H and V_L genes are amplified from first strand cDNA using family specific V-gene and J-gene primer sets as described in Table 10.1B.[38] To maximize gene repertoire diversity and the efficiency of amplification, PCR primers were designed based on the consensus sequence of each V_H and V_L gene family.[38] For design of PCR primers at the 5' end of the V_H gene (V_H back primers), 66 human V_H sequences were extracted from the Kabat database (30) and the EMBL database. For design of the PCR primers at the 5' end of the V_λ (V_λ back primer), 36 germ line and rearranged human V_λ were extracted from the Kabat database[30] and the EMBL database. For design of the PCR primers at the 5' end of the V_κ (V_κ back primer), 42 germ line and rearranged human V_κ were extracted from the Kabat database[30] and the EMBL database. The V-gene sequences were classified according to family and the frequency of the most common nucleotide at each position used to derive the sequences of a set of family-based primers.[36,38] Amplification primers at the 3' end of the V gene (forward primer) were designed based on each of the sequences of the 6 J_H,[30] 5 J_κ,[30] or 4 J_λ,[30] genes that comprise the 3' terminal of the V gene. Recently, all human V, D, and J genes have been updated and catalogued in the V-BASE database.[54] The combination of the forward and back primers results in the amplification of the complete V_H, V_κ, or V_λ genes. Restriction sites were incorporated into the forward (*Sfi* I and *Nco* I) and back primers (*Not* I) to facilitate cloning into phage or phagemid vectors as shown in Table 10.1C. (see reference 36 and Chapter 10, Section 3).

Similarly for murine V-gene repertoires, V_H- and V_L genes are amplified from first strand cDNA using universal V gene and J gene primer sets as described by Orlandi et al., 1989[41] and family specific primers.[2,14]

Single chain Fv is constructed by sequential cloning of V_H and V_L genes[8,29] or by PCR, where the assembly of the V_H, V_L, and linker fragments is driven by homologies at the ends of the various fragments. The 3′ end of the V_H is comple-

---

TABLE 10.1
Oligonucleotide Primers Used for PCR of Human Immunoglobulin Genes

A. First-Strand cDNA Synthesis

Human heavy chain constant region primers

HuIgG1-4 CH1 forward	5′ GTC CAC CTT GGT GTT GCT GGG CTT 3′
HuIgM forward	5′ TGG AAG AGG CAC GTT CTT TTC TTT 3′

Human K constant region primer

HUC$_K$ forward	5′ AGA CTC TCC CCT GTT GAA GCT CTT 3′

Human λ constant region primer

HUC$_λ$ forward	5′ TGA AGA TTC TGT AGG GGC CAC TGT CTT 3′

B. Primary PCRs

Human V_H back primers

VH1	5′ CAG GTG CAG CTG GTG CAG TCT GG 3′
VH2	5′ CAG GTC AAC TTA AGG GAG TCT GG 3′
VH3	5′ GAG GTG CAG CTG GTG GAG TCT GG 3′
VH4	5′ CAG GTG CAG CTG CAG GAG TCG GG 3′
VH5	5′ GAG GTG CAG CTG TTG CAG TCT GC 3′
VH6	5′ CAG GTA CAG CTG CAG CAG TCA GG 3′

Human J_H forward primers

JH1–2	5′ TGA GGA GAC GGT GAC CAG GGT GCC 3′
JH3	5′ TGA AGA GAC GGT GAC CAT TGT CCC 3′
JH4-5	5′ TGA GGA GAC GGT GAC CAG GGT TCC 3′
JH6	5′ TGA GGA GAC GGT GAC CGT GGT TCC 3′

Human V_K back primers

Vk1	5′ GAC ATC CAG ATG ACC CAG TCT CC 3′
Vk2	5′ GAT GTT GTG ATG ACT CAG TCT CC 3′
Vk3	5′ GAA ATT GTG TTG ACG CAG TCT CC 3′
Vk4	5′ GAC ATC GTG ATG ACC CAG TCT CC 3′
Vk5	5′ GAA ACG ACA CTC ACG CAG TCT CC 3′
Vk6	5′ GAA ATT GTG CTG ACT CAG TCT CC 3′

Human J_K forward primers

Jk1	5′ ACG TTT GAT TTC CAC CTT GGT CCC 3′
Jk2	5′ ACG TTT GAT CTC CAG CTT GGT CCC 3′
Jk3	5′ ACG TTT GAT ATC CAC TTT GGT CCC 3′
Jk4	5′ ACG TTT GAT CTC CAC CTT GGT CCC 3′
Jk5	5′ ACG TTT AAT CTC CAG TCG TGT CCC 3′

TABLE 10.1 (CONTINUED)
Oligonucleotide Primers Used for PCR of Human Immunoglobulin Genes

Human V_λ back primers

Vλ1	5' CAG TCT GTG TTG ACG CAG CCG CC 3'
Vλ2	5' CAG TCT GCC CTG ACT CAG CCT GC 3'
Vλ3a	5' TCC TAT GTG CTG ACT CAG CCA CC 3'
Vλ3b	5' TCT TCT GAG CTG ACT CAG GAC CC 3'
Vλ4	5' CAC GTT ATA CTG ACT CAA CCG CC 3'
Vλ5	5' CAG GCT GTG CTC ACT CAG CCG TC 3'
Vλ6	5' AAT TTT ATG CTG ACT CAG CCC CA 3'

Human J_λ forward primers

Jλ1	5' ACC TAG GAC GGT GAC CTT GGT CCC 3'
Jλ2-3	5' ACC TAG GAC GGT CAG CTT GGT CCC 3'
Jλ4-5	5' ACC TAA AAC GGT GAG CTG GGT CCC 3'

C. Reamplification with Primers Containing Restriction Sites

Human V_H back primers

VH1Sfi1	5' GTC CTC GCA ACT GCG GCC CAG CCG GCC ATG GCC CAG GTG CAG CTG GTG CAG TCT GG 3'
VH2Sfi1	5' GTC CTC GCA ACT GCG GCC CAG CCG GCC ATG GCC CAG GTC AAC TTA AGG GAG TCT GG 3'
VH3Sfi1	5' GTC CTC GCA ACT GCG GCC CAG CCG GCC ATG GCC GAG GTG CAG CTG GTG GAG TCT GG 3'
VH4Sfi1	5' GTC CTC GCA ACT GCG GCC CAG CCG GCC ATG GCC CAG GTG CAG CTG CAG GAG TCG GG 3'
VH5Sfi1	5' GTC CTC GCA ACT GCG GCC CAG CCG GCC ATG GCC CAG GTG CAG CTG TTG CAG TCT GC 3'
VH6Sfi1	5' GTC CTC GCA ACT GCG GCC CAG CCG GCC ATG GCC CAG GTA CAG CTG CAG CAG TCA GG 3'

Human J_K forward primers

Jk1Not1	5' GAG TCA TTC TCG ACT TGC GGC CGC ACG TTT GAT TTC CAC CTT GGT CCC 3'
Jk2Not1	5' GAG TCA TTC TCG ACT TGC GGC CGC ACG TTT GAT CTC CAG CTT GGT CCC 3'
Jk3Not1	5' GAG TCA TTC TCG ACT TGC GGC CGC ACG TTT GAT ATC CAC TTT GGT CCC 3'
Jk4Not1	5' GAG TCA TTC TCG ACT TGC GGC CGC ACG TTT GAT CTC CAC CTT GGT CCC 3'
Jk5Not1	5' GAG TCA TTC TCG ACT TGC GGC CGC ACG TTT AAT CTC CAG TCG TGT CCC 3'

Human J_λ forward primers

Jλ1Not1	5' GAG TCA TTC TCG ACT TGC GGC CGC ACC TAG GAC GGT GAC CTT GGT CCC 3'
Jλ2-3Not1	5' GAG TCA TTC TCG ACT TGC GGC CGC ACC TAG GAC GGT CAG CTT GGT CCC 3'
Jλ4-5Not1	5' GAG TCA TTC TCG ACT TGC GGC CGC ACY TAA AAC GGT GAG CTG GGT CCC 3'

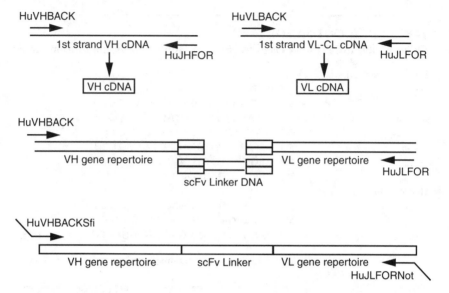

FIGURE 10.3 PCR amplification of antibody variable regions and assembly into scFv genes by one-step cloning. mRNA is primed with immunoglobulin heavy- and light-chain constant region specific primers and 1st-strand cDNA synthesized. V_H and V_L gene repertoires are amplified from first-strand cDNA using family-specific V-gene primers and J-gene primers. The separately amplified V_H and V_L genes are combined in a second PCR amplification containing linker DNA that overlaps the C terminus of the V_H and the N terminus of the V_L genes. This reaction mixture is subjected to temperature cycling followed by amplification. The resulting scFv gene repertoires are reamplified with flanking primers providing restriction sites for cloning.

mentary to the 5′ end of the linker and the 3′ end of the linker is complementary to the 5′ end of the light chain (see Figure 10.3).[14,36] We will describe in this method section the PCR assembly of equimolar mixtures of separately amplified linker $(Gly_4Ser)_3$ with human and murine V genes.

10.2.2 REAGENTS

Denaturing solution:

> Stock solution: add 17.6 ml of 0.75 M sodium citrate, pH 7.0 and 26.4 ml of 10% (w/v) N-lauryl sarcosine to 293 ml of water. Add 250 g guanidine thiocyanate and stir at 60°C to dissolve (store at RT for a maximum of 3 months).
> For working solution: add 0.35 ml β-mercaptoethanol to 50 ml of stock solution (store no longer than 1 month at RT).

Lysis buffer:

> 5 M guanidine monothiocyanate, 10 mM ethylenediaminetetraacetic acid (EDTA), 50 mM Tris HCl, pH 7.5, 1 mM dithiothreitol (DTT)

RNA solubilization buffer:

0.1% SDS, 1 mM EDTA, 10 mM Tris-HCl, pH 7.5

10 × 1st strand cDNA buffer:

500 mM Tris pH 8.1, 1.4 M KCl, 80 mM MgCl$_2$

10 × Vent DNA polymerase buffer:

10 mM KCl, 10 mM (NH$_4$)$_2$SO$_4$, 20 mM Tris-HCl, pH 8.8, 0.1% Triton X-100, 20 mM MgSO$_4$

10 × Taq DNA polymerase buffer:

500 mM KCl, 100 mM Tris-HCl, pH 9.0, 1% Triton χ-100, 15 mM MgCl$_2$
Chloroform/isoamyl alcohol (49:1)(v/v)
Water-saturated phenol
4 M and 3 M lithium chloride
Ficoll Paque (Pharmacia 10-A-001-07)
Diethyl pyrocarbonate (DEPC), 0.2% (v/v)
Methacryloxypropyltrimethoxysilane (Silane)
AMV reverse transcriptase and Vent DNA polymerase (New England Biolabs, NEB)
RNAsin (Promega)
Taq DNA polymerase (Promega)
Geneclean (Bio 101, Inc.)

10.2.3 EQUIPMENT

Glass Teflon homogenizer
Silane/DEPC-treated Eppendorf tubes and PCR tubes
PCR thermo-cycler
30 ml Corex tube, product number 8445 (Corning)

10.2.4 TIME REQUIRED

Day 1: Total RNA preparation and first-strand cDNA synthesis
Day 2: Primary PCR of V$_H$, V$_\kappa$, and V$_\lambda$ gene repertoires
Day 3: PCR assembly

10.2.5 METHODS

As with any RNA preparative procedure, special care must be taken to ensure that solutions and glassware are free of ribonucleases. Therefore, any water or salt solution should be treated with diethylpyrocarbonate (DEPC), which inactivates ribonucleases by covalent modification. We usually prefer disposable plasticware at this stage. Where glassware is used, we incubate with 0.2% DEPC solution for 1 h. In addition, Eppendorf tubes for the PCR reaction should be treated with silane, to avoid sticking of RNA to the plastic walls. We recommend wearing gloves during experiments, in order to minimize contamination with Rnase. Avoidance of contamination is critical when performing PCR, particularly when the products are to be cloned for phage display. Be sure to include negative controls in each amplification step.

10.2.5.1 Total RNA Preparation from Spleen, Tissue, and Tissue Culture Cells (Guanidine Method)

1. For tissue: add 1 ml denaturing solution per 100 mg tissue and homogenize with a few strokes in a glass Teflon homogenizer. For cultured cells: after centrifuging suspension cells, discard the supernatant and add 1 ml denaturing solution per 10^7 cells and pass the lysate through a pipet seven to ten times.
2. Transfer the homogenate to a 5 ml polypropylene tube. Add 0.1 ml of 2 M sodium acetate, pH 4.0, and mix thoroughly by inversion. Add 1 ml water-saturated phenol, mix thoroughly, and add 0.2 ml of 49:1 (v/v) chloroform/isoamyl alcohol. Mix thoroughly and incubate the suspension for 15 min at 4°C.
3. Centrifuge for 20 min at 10,000 × g at 4°C. Transfer the upper aqueous phase (containing RNA) to a new tube; DNA and proteins are left behind in the interphase and phenol layer.
4. Precipitate RNA by adding 1 ml of 100% isopropanol. Incubate the sample for 30 min at –20°C.
5. Centrifuge for 10 min at 10,000 × g at 4°C and discard supernatant. Dissolve the RNA pellet in 0.3 ml denaturing solution and transfer to a 1.5 ml microcentrifuge tube.
6. Precipitate the RNA with 0.3 ml of 100% isopropanol for 30 min at –20°C.
7. Centrifuge for 10 min at 10,000 × g at 4°C and discard supernatant. Dissolve RNA pellet in 2 ml 75% ethanol, vortex, and incubate 10 to 15 min at room temperature to dissolve any residual amounts of guanidine, which may be contaminating the pellet.
8. Centrifuge for 5 min at 10,000 × g at 4°C and discard supernatant. Air dry the RNA pellet.
9. Dissolve the RNA pellet in 100 to 200 μl DEPC-treated water and store RNA at –70°C either as an aqueous solution or as an ethanol precipitate.

Note: This single-step method for isolating RNA has been developed by Chomczynski et al., 1987.[13] From a mouse spleen the yield is $5 \times 10^7 - 2 \times 10^8$ white blood cells (WBC) of which 35 to 40% are B cells and lymphocytes.

10.2.5.2 Total RNA Preparation from Human Peripheral Blood Lymphocytes (PBL)

1. Dilute 20 ml of heparinized blood with an equal volume of PBS. Divide the diluted blood into two 20-ml fractions and overlay each with 15

ml Ficoll Paque (Pharmacia) to separate the lymphocytes from the red blood cells.

2. Centrifuge for 30 min at $200 \times g$ at room temperature.
3. The PBLs are found at the interface as a whitish band. Carefully remove the upper plasma layer with a Pasteur pipette and collect the lymphocyte layer combined to a 50-ml Falcon tube. Wash the PBLs with an equal volume of ice-cold PBS and spin again at $200 \times g$ for 5 min at 4°C.
4. Add 7 ml lysis buffer (will lyse approximately 5×10^8 PBLs) and vortex vigorously to lyse the cells.
5. Add 7 volumes (49 ml) of 4 M lithium chloride and incubate at 4°C for 15 to 20 h.
6. Transfer the suspension to 30 ml Corex tubes (acid-washed, silanized) and spin at $7000 \times g$ for 2 h at 4°C.
7. Pour off the supernatant and dissolve pellet in 2 ml of RNA solubilization buffer. Freeze solution at –20°C.
8. Thaw by vortexing for 20 s every 10 min for a total of 45 min.
9. Extract once with an equal volume of phenol and once with an equal volume of chloroform.
10. Precipitate the RNA by adding 1/10 volume 3 M sodium acetate pH 4.8 and 2 volumes of –20°C ethanol. Mix thoroughly and leave overnight at –20°C.
11. Spin RNA at $24,000 \times g$ for 30 min. Resuspend pellet in 200 µl DEPC-treated water and store RNA at –70°C either as an aqueous solution or as an ethanol precipitate.

This method for RNA preparation from peripheral blood lymphocytes has been developed by Cathala et al., 1983.[11] In human blood there are approximately 4 to 11×10^6 white blood cells (WBC) per ml of which approximately 30% are B cells and lymphocytes.

10.2.5.3 First-Strand cDNA Synthesis

1. For first-strand cDNA synthesis, prepare the following reaction mix in a pretreated 1.5-ml Eppendorf tube. For the generation of naive human library use HuIgM forward primer, and for immune human libraries use HuIgG1-4 CH1 forward primer, respectively.

$10 \times$ 1st strand cDNA buffer	5 µl
$20 \times$ dNTPs (5 mM each)	5 µl
0.1 M DTT	5 µl
HuIgM (or HuIgG1 to 4 CH1) forward primer (10 pm/µl)	1 µl
HuC$_\kappa$ forward primer (10 pm/µl)	1 µl
HuC$_\lambda$ forward primer (10 pm/µl)	1 µl

The primers for the first-strand cDNA synthesis of human heavy chain constant region and human κ or λ constant region primers are listed in Table 10.1A. For a murine library, use the respective forward primers for the amplification of V_H and V_κ immunoglobulin genes as described by Orlandi et al., 1989[41] or Amersdorfer et al., 1997.[2]

2. Take an aliquot (1 to 4 μg) of RNA in ethanol, place into pretreated 1.5 ml Eppendorf tube and spin 5 min in microcentrifuge. Wash the RNA pellet once with 70% ethanol, air dry in the hood and resuspend in 28 μl of DEPC-treated water.

3. Heat at 65°C for 5 min to denature, quench on ice 2 min, and spin down immediately in microcentrifuge for 5 min. Take the supernatant and add to first-strand reaction mixture.

4. Add 2 μl (5000 u/ml) AMV reverse transcriptase (Promega) and 2 μl (40,000 u/ml) RNAsin (Promega) and incubate at 42°C for 1 h.

5. Boil the reaction mixture for 5 min, quench on ice 2 min, and spin down in microcentrifuge for 5 min. Take the supernatant and heat at 65°C for 5 min to denature, quench on ice 2 min, and spin down immediately in micro centrifuge for 5 min. Take the supernatant, containing the first-strand cDNA and proceed with the primary PCR amplification.

10.2.5.4 Primary PCR

1. Use for each V-gene repertoire an equimolar mixture of the designated forward/back primer sets at a final concentration of 10 pm/μl total (V_H back-J_H forward, V_κ back-J_κ forward, and V_λ back-J_λ forward), and prepare the following reaction mixture, e.g., human V_H gene repertoire:

Water	31.5 μl
10 × Vent buffer	5 μl
20 × dNTPs (5 mM each)	2.0 μl
Acetylated BSA (10 mg/ml)	0.5 μl
V_H 1 to 6 back mix (10 pm/μl)	2.0 μl
J_H 1 to 6 forward mix (10 pm/μl)	2.0 μl
cDNA reaction mix	5.0 μl

For human libraries, V_H, V_κ and V_λ genes are amplified in separate PCR reactions using the appropriate back and forward primers (see Table 10.1B). Back primers are an equimolar mixture of either 6 V_H back, 6 V_κ back, or 6 V_λ back primers at a final concentration of 10 pm/μl total. Forward primers are an equimolar mixture of either 6 J_H, 5 J_κ, or 5 J_λ primers at a final concentration of 10 pm/μl total. For murine libraries, V_H and V_κ genes are amplified in separate PCR reactions using the appropriate back and forward primers as described previously.

The Vent DNA polymerase buffer already contains 2 mM $MgSO_4$ when the buffer is diluted to its final 1× form. However, for optimal primer extensions we usually titrate the $MgSO_4$ concentration (ranging from 2 to 6 mM) for optimal results.

2. Overlay with paraffin oil, unless you have a thermo-cycler with a heated lid.
3. Heat to 94°C for 5 min in a PCR thermo-cycler to denature the DNA ("hot-start"). This improves amplification results by preventing extension of primers that have misannealed.
4. Add 1.0 µl (2 units) Vent DNA polymerase under the oil. Cycle 30 times to amplify the V genes at 94°C for 1 min, 60°C for 1 min, and 72°C for 1 min.
5. Purify the PCR fragments by electrophoresis on a 1.5% agarose gel and extract the 350 bp band corresponding to the V_H genes and 300 bp band corresponding to the V_L genes using Geneclean.

10.2.5.5 PCR Splicing of V_H and V_L Genes

The purified V_H and V_L genes (V_κ or V_λ) are combined in a second PCR reaction containing DNA which encodes the scFv linker (93 bp). To make the linker DNA, 52 separate 50 µl PCR reactions are performed using each of the 4 reverse J_H primers in combination with each of the 6 V_κ or 7 V_λ reverse primers as described by Marks et al., 1991.[38] The template is pSW2scFvD1.3,[39] yielding the $(Gly_4Ser)_3$ linker described by Huston et al., 1988.[29] The PCR reaction and purification from the agarose gel are as described in Section 10.2.5.6 on Reamplification of scFv Gene Repertoires with Primers Containing Appended Restriction Sites, except for the use of the appropriate primers. For successful assembly of the V_H and V_L gene repertoire by the $(Gly_4Ser)_3$ linker, it is crucial to use equimolar ratios of the DNA fragments. This corresponds to a mass ratio of V_H/linker/V_L of 3:1:3, since the approximate ratio of sizes of V_H (350 bp) and V_L (300 bp) to linker (90 bp) is 3:1. We recommend running different dilutions of the DNA fragments on an agarose gel and comparing their intensities with a marker of known size and concentration.

1. Prepare 25 µl PCR reaction mixes containing the following:

Water	7.5 µl
10 × Vent buffer	2.5 µl
20 × dNTP's (5 mM each)	1.0 µl
scFv linker (80 ng)	2.0 µl
V_H repertoire (240 ng)	5.0 µl
V_L repertoire (240 ng)	5.0 µl

2. Overlay with paraffin oil, unless you have a thermo-cycler with a heated lid.
3. Heat to 94°C for 5 min in PCR thermo-cycler.
4. Add 1.0 µl (2 units) vent DNA polymerase.
5. Cycle seven times without amplification at 94°C for 1 min and 72°C for 1.5 min to randomly join the fragments.
6. After 7 cycles, hold at 94°C while adding 2 µl of each flanking primer. For the human library, use an equimolar mixture of the 6 V_H back primers and an equimolar mixture of the 5 J_κ forward or 5 J_λ forward primers (10 pm/µl).

7. Cycle 30 times to amplify the assembled fragments at 94°C for 1 min and 72°C for 2 min.
8. Gel-purify the assembled scFv gene repertoires (approximately 800 bp) on a 2% agarose gel and further purify the DNA by Geneclean. Resuspend the product in 25 µl of water.

10.2.5.6 Reamplification of scFv Gene Repertoires with Primers Containing Appended Restriction Sites

1. Prepare 50 µl PCR reaction mixes containing the following:

Water	37 µl
20 × dNTPs (5 mM each)	2.0 µl
10 × Taq buffer	5.0 µl
Back primers (10 pm/µl)	2.0 µl
Forward primers (10 pm/µl)	2.0 µl
scFv gene repertoire (10 ng)	1.0 µl

Note: For the human library, use an equimolar mixture of the 6 V$_H$ back *Sfi* I primers and an equimolar mixture of the 5 J$_\kappa$ forward *Not* I or 5 J$_\lambda$ forward *Not* I primers at a final concentration of 10 pm/µl. For the murine library, use an equimolar mix of 11 V$_H$ back *Sfi* I primers and an equimolar mixture of 5 J$_\kappa$ forward *Not* I primers at a final concentration of 10 pm/µl.

2. Overlay with mineral oil, unless you have a thermo-cycler with a heated lid.
3. Heat to 94°C for 5 min in a PCR thermo-cycler.
4. Add 1.0 µl (5 units) Taq DNA polymerase under the oil. We recommend using Taq DNA polymerase rather than the Vent product at this stage, because the associated 5′ to 3′ exonuclease activity of Vent DNA polymerase will degrade the primer DNA.
5. Cycle 30 times to amplify the assembled V genes at 94°C for 1 min, 55°C for 1 min, and 72°C for 1 min.
6. Gel-purify the assembled scFv gene repertoires (approximately 800 bp) on a 2% agarose gel and further purify the DNA by Geneclean. Resuspend the product in 25 µl of water.

10.3 LIBRARY CONSTRUCTION

10.3.1 DESCRIPTION

This section describes the cloning of scFv gene repertoires to create large phage antibody libraries. To display antibody fragments on the surface of phage, a scFv gene cassette is inserted as a fusion to the gene encoding a phage surface protein, resulting in the expression of the antibody on the phage surface (Figure 10.4). In the first example of phage display, filamentous bacteriophage fd was used to express

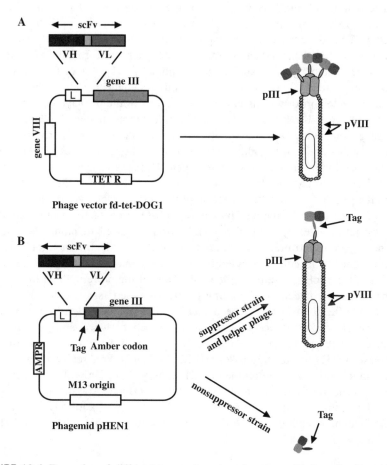

FIGURE 10.4 Examples of different types of vectors for phage display of scFv antibody fragments. Insertion of an scFv gene in frame with bacteriophage gene III results in expression of a scFv-pIII fusion protein, which is incorporated into the phage surface. The gene encoding the scFv is contained within the phage. Thus, the phage serves as a vehicle which physically links genotype with phenotype. (A) In phage vectors, 3 to 5 copies of the scFv fragment are displayed (one on each of the pIII molecules). (B) In phagemid vector, fewer than 3 copies are displayed, because pIII from the helper phage competes with the fusion protein for incorporation into the phage surface. Phagemid vectors can contain an amber codon between the antibody fragment gene and gene III. This makes it possible to easily switch between displayed and soluble antibody fragment simply by changing the host bacterial strain. L: leader exon; V_H: heavy variable region; V_L: light variable region; gene III: encoding the minor coat protein pIII; gene VIII: encoding the major coat protein pVIII; AMP_R: ampicillin resistance gene; TET_R: tetracycline resistance gene.

peptides fused to the N-terminus of the phage minor coat protein (pIII) by inserting synthetic DNA encoding the peptide into the 5′ end of gene III.[42,51] Today, phage and phagemid based libraries utilize the genetic linkage of protein to either gene III[5,18,19,26,34,39] or gene VIII.[28,31]

The number of antibody fragments expressed on the surface of the phage is largely determined by the choice of either the minor coat protein pIII or major coat protein pVIII and the use of phage or phagemid vectors (reviewed in Reference 37). Advantages of the phagemid based libraries are higher transformation efficiency and better genetic stability compared to phage libraries. Also for pIII fusions, phage vectors carry three to five copies of the antibody fragments per phage, whereas with phagemid vectors most virions have 1 copy or less of the displayed protein, which greatly influences the kinetic values of the selected antibodies.[15] When selecting with phage, the multivalent presentation of antibody increases the percentage of low affinity binders due to the avidity effect, which can be, in some cases, undesirable. For the selection of high-affinity binders, gene III fused phagemid vectors, such as pHEN-1 are the preferred choices.

In the pHEN-1 vector, transcription of the scFv cassette is driven by the lacZ promoter, which can be induced by isopropyl β-D-thiogalactopyranoside (IPTG). The restriction sites *Sfi* I or *Nco* I and *Not* I are used to clone the antibody fragment gene repertoire. The export of native antibody fragments to the periplasmic space of *E. coli* is directed by the pelB signal leader sequence at the N-terminus of the scFv protein. At the C-terminus of the protein, the c-myc peptide tag permits easy detection of binding in ELISA-based assays recognized by the monoclonal 9E10 antibody.[20] The presence of an amber codon between the tag and gene III makes it possible to easily switch between antibody fragment displayed on the phage surface and soluble antibody fragment by use of either suppressor (TG1) or nonsuppressor (HB2151) strains. Practically, the translation of the amber codon as a glutamine in TG1, is only about 70% efficient, producing antibody-gene III fusion proteins and soluble antibody fragments at the same time. The vector can therefore be used for the display of antibody fragments on the surface of phagemid pHEN-1, as well as for soluble expression. This is described in Section 11.5.

10.3.2 REAGENTS

Water-saturated phenol/chloroform
Nco I, *Not* I, *Sfi* I restriction enzymes (NEB)
T4 DNA ligase (NEB)
Electrocompetent TG1 bacteria
Diethyl ether

SOB media: (per liter): To 950 ml deionized H_2O add 20 g Bacto-tryptone (Difco), 5 g yeast extract (Difco), and 0.5 g NaCl. Add 10 ml of a 250 mM KCl solution. Adjust the pH to 7.0 with 5 N NaOH and adjust the volume of the solution to 1 liter with deionized H_2O. Sterilize by autoclaving for 20 min. Just before use, add 1 ml of a sterile solution of 1 M $MgCl_2$ and 1 ml 1 M $MgSO_4$ each, otherwise it will precipitate out. SOC media is identical to SOB media except that it contains 20 mM glucose. After the SOB media has been autoclaved, allow it to cool down to 60°C or less, and then add 10 ml of a sterile 20% solution of glucose.

2xTY media: (per liter): To 900 ml of deionized H_2O add the following:

Bacto-tryptone	16 g
Bacto-yeast extract	10 g
NaCl	5 g

Adjust the pH to 7.0 with 5 N NaOH and adjust the volume of the solution to 1 liter with deionized H_2O. Sterilize by autoclaving for 20 min and allow the solution to cool to 60°C. Add 10 ml of 20% glucose per 100 ml of medium and the appropriate antibiotics.

TYE plates (per liter): For agarose plates, add 15 g of Difco agar per liter of 2xTY media. Sterilize by autoclaving for 20 min and allow the solution to cool to 60°C. Add 10 ml of 20% glucose per 100 ml of medium and the appropriate antibiotic.

Medium and agarose plates are prepared according to the formula described in Sambrook et al., 1989.[47]

10.3.3 EQUIPMENT

Small agar plates (100 × 15 mm) (Fisherbrand)
Large agar plates (150 × 15 mm) (Fisherbrand)
37°C incubator (New Brunswick Scientific)
Electroporator (Biorad Gene Pulser™)
16°C water bath
PCR thermo-cycler

10.3.4 TIME REQUIRED

Day 1: Restriction digests of scFv repertoires and phagemid vector, digest overnight

Day 2: Electroelution of phagemid vector and ligation with scFv repertoire overnight

Day 3: Transformation into *E. coli*

10.3.5 METHODS

10.3.5.1 Restriction Digest and Ligation of scFv Gene Repertoires

1. For optimal digestion, the restriction digest of the PCR-generated scFv repertoires is performed using the buffer supplied by the manufacturer. We also recommend overdigestion of the PCR products due to the poor efficiency with which PCR fragments are digested. For cloning of human scFv and Fab fragments into pHEN-1, the rare cutting enzymes *Nco* I and

Not I are used, except mouse variable genes are cloned as *Sfi* I–*Not* I cassettes (*Nco* I cuts frequently in murine V genes).

Prepare 200 µl reaction mix to digest scFv repertoires with *Nco* I:

scFv DNA (1 to 4 µg)	100 µl
water	74 µl
10 × NEB 4 buffer	20 µl
Nco I (10 u/µl)	6.0 µl

2. Incubate at 37°C overnight.
3. Phenol/chloroform extract with 100 µl of each, ethanol precipitate, wash with 70% ethanol, air dry and resuspend in 100 µl water.
4. Prepare 200 µl reaction mix to digest scFv repertoires with *Not* I:

scFv DNA	100 µl
Water	72 µl
Acetylated BSA (10 mg/ml)	2.0 µl
10 × NEB 3 buffer	20 µl
Not I (10 u/µl)	6.0 µl

5. Incubate at 37°C overnight.
6. Phenol/chloroform extract with 100 µl of each, ethanol precipitate, wash with 70% ethanol, air dry, and resuspend in 100µl water. Determine DNA concentration by analysis on a 1.5% agarose gel with markers of known size and concentration.
7. Approximately 4 µg of cesium chloride purified pHEN-1 is digested with the appropriate restriction enzymes exactly as described above (for human library, *Nco* I and *Not* I; for mouse library, *Sfi* I and *Not* I). The digested vector DNA is purified on a 0.8% agarose gel, extracted from the gel and ethanol precipitated. For optimal digestion, the restriction digest is carried out overnight and vector DNA is gel purified prior to ligation. Efficient digestion is important because a small amount of undigested vector leads to a very large background of nonrecombinant clones.
8. In ligation experiments, the molar ratio of insert to vector should be 2:1. Since the ratio of sizes of assembled scFv (800 bp) to vector (4500 bp) is approximately 6:1, this translates into a ratio of insert to vector of 1:12 by weight.

Prepare 100 µl ligation mixture:

10 × ligation buffer	10 µl
Water	67 µl
Digested pHEN-1 (100 ng/µl)	10 µl
scFv gene repertoire (10 ng/µl)	8.0 µl
T4 DNA ligase (400 u/µl)	5.0 µl

9. Ligate overnight at 16°C.

10. Bring volume to 200 µl with H$_2$O, extract once with phenol/chloroform, twice with ether to remove traces of phenol, ethanol precipitate and wash with 70% ethanol. Cleaning up the ligation mixture by phenol/chloroform extraction and ethanol precipitation increases transformation efficiencies 10- to 100-fold.

11. Resuspend DNA in 10 µl of water and use 2.5 µl/transformation into 50 µl electrocompetent *E. coli* TG 1.[17] Set up a "no DNA" control for the electroporation to ensure the TG1 cells are not contaminated. Typical transformation efficiencies for *E. coli* TG1 cells are at least 10^9/µg plasmid DNA.

12. Set the electroporator at 200 ohms (resistance), 25 µFD (capacitance) and 2.5 kilovolts. After electroporation, the time constant should be approximately 4.5 s.

13. Grow bacteria in 1 ml SOC at 37°C for 1 h shake (250 rpm), and plate serial dilutions onto small TYE/amp/glu agar plates for determining the size of the library.

14. Centrifuge remaining bacteria solution at 1700 × *g* for 10 min at 4°C. Resuspend pellet in 250 µl and plate onto two small TYE/amp/glu plates. Incubate overnight at 37°C.

15. Scrape bacteria from large plates by washing each plate with 3 ml 2xTY/amp/glu. Make glycerol stocks by adding 1.4 ml of bacteria and 0.6 ml 50% glycerol in PBS (sterilized by filtration through 0.45 µm filter). Save library stock at –70°C.

10.4 PANNING

10.4.1 DESCRIPTION

This section describes different selection or "panning" procedures for enriching antigen-binding clones from phage antibody libraries. Panning was used in the 18th century to wash gold particles from river sediments. Generally, one round of selection consists of the following steps: binding of phage to the antigen, removing nonbinding phage by washing, and eluting bound phage by addition of alkali or acid. The eluted phage is used to reinfect bacteria to produce more phage for the next round of selection (see Figure 10.2).

Selection can be any method that enables separation of binding phage from background phage. The first phage antibody libraries were selected on columns of antigen immobilized on Sepharose,[39] or antigen adsorbed onto ELISA plate wells[9] and immunotubes.[36] Some proteins will partially or completely denature when adsorbed to the plastic surface, resulting in the selection of scFv, which binds to the antigen on the surface but not to its native form. This difficulty can be overcome by tagging the antigen with biotin,[24] followed by selection in solution. After incubation of phage with the biotinylated antigen, complexes of phages bound to the antigen are captured with streptavidin-coated magnetic beads and a magnet. One potential disadvantage of this method (in particular, when using nonimmune libraries) is the high background of phage binding to streptavidin. Alternation of streptavidin and avidin-coated magnetic beads in different rounds of selection will reduce the background.[49] In subsequent rounds of selection, the antigen concentration may be decreased to significantly less than the desired K_d to favor the enrichment of antibodies with a higher affinity.[48]

In theory, only one round of selection would be required to pull out a specific antibody, but in reality the enrichment factors for a single round of affinity selection can vary from 20- to 1,000,000-fold.[39] If, for example, the enrichment factor is as low as 100-fold, the eluted phage are reinfected in bacteria and subject to a second round of selection, which then increases the enrichment factor to 10,000. Thus, even with low enrichments, multiple rounds of selection can lead to the isolation of rare binders.

More recently, the focus has been directed to cell surface selection, which adds a useful application to the powerful selection procedures of phage display libraries.[10]

We are currently investigating the use of biotinylated cell lines, presenting novel surface markers for clinical and diagnostic purposes, in combination with magnetic columns for easy adsorption of the desired cell population.

10.4.2 REAGENTS

Minimal media plate: (per liter):

K_2HPO_4	10.5 g
KH_2PO_4	4.5 g
$(NH_4)_2SO_4$	1 g
Sodium citrate.2 H_2O	0.5 g
Agar	15 g

Adjust the volume of solution to 1.0 liter with deionized H_2O and sterilize by autoclaving for 20 min. Allow the solution to cool to 60°C, then add 1 ml of 1 M $MgSO_4 \cdot 7\ H_2O$, 0.5 ml of 1% B1 thiamin, and 10 ml of 20% glucose as a carbon source, and pour the plates.

2xTY/100 µg/ml kanamycin/(2xTY/kan)
M13K07 helper phage (Stratagene)
20% PEG 8000/2.5 M NaCl
PBS 2% powdered skim milk (MPBS)
Streptavidin-magnetic beads (Dynabeads, M-280, Dynal A.S., Oslo, Norway)
Avidin-magnetic beads (Controlled Pure Glan, Lincoln Park, New Jersey)

10.4.3 SPECIAL EQUIPMENT

Shaker-incubator (37 and 25°C)
Centrifuge (adapter for microtitre plates)
Immunotubes (Nunc)
Rotator for selection tubes

Magnetic rack (Dynal MPC-E, Cat.No. 120.04, Dynal A.S., Oslo, Norway)
Biotinylation kit (Pierce, NHS-LC-Biotin, Cat. No. 21335, Pharmacia, Recombinant Phage Selection Module)

10.4.4 TIME REQUIRED

One round of selection consists of the following steps:

Day 1: Rescuing phagemid libraries
Day 2: Phage preparation
Day 3: Selection of phage-antibody libraries

10.4.5 METHODS

10.4.5.1 Rescuing Phagemid Libraries for Selection

1. Calculate the number of bacteria per ml from your library glycerol stock (A_{600} of 1.00 corresponds to approximately 1×10^8 cells). Usually the optical density of your bacterial stock is around 100, or 10^{10} cells/ml. The input of cells for rescuing is dependent on the density of the original bacteria glycerol stock and should be in 10-fold excess of the number of different clones in the library, but should not exceed A_{600} of 0.05. This step ensures the diversity of the library for subsequent rounds of selections. For example, an immune library of 10^7 unique members requires 10^8 cells for starting the initial culture. The inoculum is therefore 10 μl from your glycerol stock into 20 ml of 2xTY/amp/glu.

2. Grow with shaking (250 rpm) at 37°C to an $A_{600} \sim 0.7$ (corresponds to 7×10^7 bacteria/ml) to get the cells into exponential phase so that they express the F pilus. Since not all repertoires will grow equally fast, check the optical density to prevent overgrowth. If the optical density is over 0.7 in approximately 2 h, dilute the inoculum with prewarmed 2xTY/amp/glu to 0.7.

3. Transfer 10 ml (7×10^8 bacteria total) to a 50 ml Falcon tube containing the appropriate number of helper phages. To ensure rescue of all clones in the library the ratio of helper phage to bacteria should be 10:1. Add 7×10^9 plaque-forming units (pfu) of helper phage (VCSM13, Stratagene) to the bacterial solution. Incubate at 37°C without shaking for 30 min. Again, this temperature is critical for infection.

4. Incubate at 37°C with shaking (250 rpm) for 30 min.

5. Plate 1 μl onto TYE/kan plate to check for infectivity. Incubate at 37°C overnight. The plate should be nearly confluent next day, indicating successful rescuing.

6. Centrifuge cells at $3000 \times g$, 4°C to remove glucose and resuspend in 50 ml TYE/amp/kan. Shake at 37°C for 30 min (220 rpm).

7. Grow with shaking (250 rpm) overnight at 25°C.

10.4.5.2 Phage Preparation

1. Remove bacteria by centrifugation at $4000 \times g$ 10 min at 4°C . Decant the clear supernatant containing phage particles (if cloudy, repeat centrifugation) into a 500 ml centrifuge bottle and add 10 ml 20% PEG/2.5 M NaCl per bottle. Mix and incubate on ice for 10 min.

2. Pellet phage by spinning for 15 min, $4000 \times g$ at 4°C. Discard the supernatant.

3. Resuspend the white phage pellet in 10 ml PBS. To remove remaining bacteria debris, we recommend spinning down in the centrifuge for 10 min, $4000 \times g$ at 4°C.

4. Transfer the supernatant in a 15 ml Falcon tube and repeat PEG precipitation with 2 ml 20% PEG/2.5 M NaCl. Incubate on ice for 15 min.

5. Centrifuge 10 min, $4000 \times g$ at 4°C and resuspend the white pellet in 2.5 ml PBS.

6. Filter supernatant through 0.45 μm syringe filter. The phage stock should be used at once for the next round of selection, but can be stored at 4°C approximately 1 week without much loss in binding activity.

7. Before starting selections, titer the phage preparation by diluting 10 μl of the eluted phage stock into 1 ml 2xTY (10^2 dilution), vortex briefly, and transfer 10 μl into 1 ml 2xTY (10^4 dilution). Vortex again and transfer 10 μl into 1 ml of exponentially growing $E.\ coli$ TG1 ($A_{600} \sim 0.7$) (10^6 dilution), prepared according to methods discussed in Section 10.4.5.3 on selection of phage antibody libraries in immunotubes. It is important to have at least a ten-fold excess of bacteria over phage, to guarantee that every phage particle can infect bacteria (10^6 phage vs. 10^7 bacteria). Incubate at 37°C without shaking for 30 min. Transfer 10 μl into 1 ml 2xTY (10^8 dilution). Vortex again and plate 1 μl onto a small 2xTY/amp/glu plate and incubate at 37°C overnight. Multiply the number of counted colonies by the factor of 10^{11}, which represents the phage preparation titer/ml. This protocol usually gives rise to 1 to 10×10^{12} phage (TU)/ml per 50-ml culture.

10.4.5.3 Selection of Phage Antibody Libraries in Immunotubes

1. Prior to selection, streak out $E.coli$ TG1 on a minimal media plate and incubate overnight at 37°C. This will select only male TG1 bacteria displaying the F pili. Toothpick one clone off the plate and incubate in 2 ml TYE media at 25°C, shaking overnight. Next day, make 1/100 dilution in 2xTY media and grow bacteria at 37°C to exponential phase. Proceed to step 9.

2. Coat Nunc immunotube with 1 ml antigen in PBS, pH 7.4 or 100 mM sodium bicarbonate, pH 9.6 overnight. Antigen concentration should be at least around 50 to 100 μg/ml for the first round of selection (sometimes coating for 2 h at 37°C can be used as an alternative).

3. Wash the tube with PBS (simply pour solution in and out immediately) and add 4 ml 2% MPBS to block (fill the tube to the top). Incubate at room temperature for 1 h.

4. Wash the tube three times with PBS.
5. Add 10^{12} to 10^{13} TU phage in 2% MPBS (less than 4 ml volume total), cap the tube, and rock for 30 min to 1 h at room temperature. Then let tube stand without rocking for 30 to 45 min at room temperature.
6. Wash 20 times with PBS-Tween-20 (0.1%), then 20 times with PBS (Tween will inhibit growth of *E. coli*, so the order of wash is important). Each wash step is performed by gently filling to the top with wash solution, then vigorously flicking out the liquid into the sink.
7. Add 1 ml 100 mM triethylamine (make fresh: 140 µl of stock/10 ml H_2O, pH must be 12). Recap the immunotube. Be sure to use a new cap to prevent cross-contamination with phage left on the cap. Rock for no more than 10 min.
8. Transfer the eluted phage solution to an Eppendorf tube containing 0.5 ml of 1 M Tris, pH 7.4 and mix by inversion. It is necessary to neutralize the phage eluate immediately after elution. Save on ice until time to infect exponentially growing TG1 bacteria.
9. Add 0.75 ml of the phage stock to 10 ml of exponentially growing TG1 (A_{600} ~ 0.7). Store the remaining phage mix at 4°C.
10. Incubate at 37°C for 30 min without shaking. Do not let the temperature drop below 37°C or the bacterial F pilus will retract and infection efficiency of *E. coli* will decrease.
11. Titer TG1 infection by plating 1 and 10 µl onto small TYE/amp/glu plates (10^4 and 10^3 dilutions, respectively) and incubate at 37°C overnight.
12. Centrifuge the remaining bacteria solution at $1700 \times g$ for 10 min at 4°C.
13. Resuspend pellet in 250 µl 2xTY media and plate onto two large TYE/amp/glu plates. Incubate overnight at 37°C.
14. Add 3 ml of 2xTY/amp/glu media to each plate, then scrape the bacteria from the plate with a bent glass rod. Make glycerol stocks by mixing 1.4 ml of bacteria and 0.6 ml 50% glycerol in PBS (filtered). Save stock at −70°C.

For large "naive" libraries (complexity > 10^8), the selection titer from the first round of selection should be 10^4 to 10^6 TU. If the titer is larger than 10^7, it is likely that the washing steps have been inadequate. Repeat the first round of selection with increased washing steps. If the titer is below 10^4, you have washed too many times, or the antigen has been poorly adsorbed to the polystyrene surface. In that case, try to use a higher antigen concentration or different buffer for coating and/or reduce the number of washes.

10.4.5.4 Selection of Phage Antibody Libraries on Biotinylated Antigen

The ability to use soluble antigen for selections implies a greater degree of control over the selection process. Phage are allowed to bind to biotinylated antigen and are recovered with streptavidin magnetic beads. Biotinylation may be carried out using

NHS esters of biotin (Pierce, NHS-LC-Biotin) or according to the instructions of Pharmacia (Recombinant Phage Selection Module) to modify primary amino groups.

1. Prior to selection, block 50 μl streptavidin magnetic beads with 1 ml 5% MPBS for 1 h at 37°C in 1.5 ml Eppendorf tube. Spin down the beads briefly at $800 \times g$ for 30 s and remove blocking buffer.

2. Block 1.5 ml Eppendorf tube with 5% MPBS for 1 h at 37°C and discard the blocking buffer. Incubate biotinylated antigen (10 to 500 nM), prepared according to the manufacturer's instructions, with 1 ml of polyclonal phage (approximately 10^{12} TU) in 1% MPBS (final concentration) by rocking at room temperature for 30 to 60 min.

3. Add 100 μl streptavidin magnetic beads to the phage-antigen mix and incubate on rotator at room temperature for 30 min. Briefly spin the tube to dislodge particles in the cap at $800 \times g$ for 30 s and then place tube in a magnetic rack for 20 s. Beads will migrate toward the magnet.

4. Aspirate tubes carefully, leaving the beads on the side of the Eppendorf tube. Wash beads (1 ml per wash) with PBS-Tween (0.1%) ten times, followed by PBS ten times. Transfer the beads after every second wash to a fresh Eppendorf tube to facilitate efficient washing. After the last washing step, transfer the beads into a new 1.5 ml Eppendorf tube, preblocked with 5% MPBS.

5. Elute phage with 500 μl 100 mM triethylamine for 10 min at room temperature. Place tube in magnetic rack for 20 s. Beads will migrate toward the magnet. Remove the supernatant containing eluted phage and neutralize with 1 ml of 1 M Tris, pH 7.4. Save on ice until time to infect exponentially growing TG1 bacteria.

6. For the infection of TG1 bacteria, follow steps 9 through 14 as described in Section 10.4.5.3 covering selection of phage antibody libraries in immunotubes.

We recommend alternating between avidin and streptavidin magnetic beads in successive selection cycles and preclearing the phage mix with the appropriate beads, which will prevent the selection for streptavidin/avidin phage binders. For the first round of selection, we typically use 100 nM of antigen, which is decreased fivefold in the following rounds. The actual amounts of phage and antigen will vary according to the affinities present in the library and the stage of panning. The final antigen concentration should be around or below the desired K_d of selected antibody fragments.

10.5 IDENTIFICATION OF ANTIGEN BINDING CLONES

10.5.1 DESCRIPTION

This section describes suitable methods for screening large numbers of selected scFv antibodies by ELISA. The specificity of binding clones is then confirmed by ELISA using the relevant antigen and a panel of irrelevant antigens. Individual clones can be analyzed by phage ELISA or soluble scFv ELISA. Generally we find that phage-based assays give more consistent results and higher sensitivity. The next step is to determine the number of unique clones by PCR fingerprinting. This method can be used to provide information on the diversity of a panel of clones between sequential rounds of selection or the diversity between clones prior to sequencing. The scFv gene is amplified directly from bacterial glycerol stocks using primers that flank the gene (LMB3 and fdseq 1[36]). The amplified scFv genes are then digested with the restriction enzyme BstN1, which cuts frequently in the human and murine V_H genes, resulting in a distinctive banding pattern.

10.5.2 REAGENTS

50% glycerol/5 mM MgSO$_4$
2xTY/amp/glu (see Section 10.3.2)
Nusieve agarose (3:1) (FMC Bio Products)
M13K07 helper phage (Stratagene)
PBS
PBS –0.1% Tween-20
1 mM IPTG
2% powdered skim milk in PBS (MPBS)
Biotinylated anti-M13-phage antibody (5Prime–>3Prime Inc., Boulder, CO)
9E10 antibody (Santa Cruz Biotechnology, CA)
Horseradish peroxidase conjugated anti-mouse IgG Fc monoclonal antibody (Sigma)
Horseradish peroxidase conjugated streptavidin (Pierce)
50 mM citric acid
50 mM sodium citrate
75 mM NaF
BstN 1 restriction enzyme (NEB)
Taq DNA polymerase (Promega)
10 × Taq buffer
500 mM KCl, 100 mM Tris-HCl pH 9.0, 1% Triton χ-100, 15 mM MgCl$_2$

10.5.3 SPECIAL EQUIPMENT

96-well round-bottomed plates, product no. 25850 (Corning)
96-well flat-bottomed microtiter plates, product no. 3912 (Falcon)
96-well transfer device
Plate sealer, product no. 3095 (Costar)
Shaker-incubator (37 and 25°C) (New Brunswick Scientific)
ELISA plate reader
DNA thermo-cycler
Multichannel pipette
Centrifuge holder for microtiter plates

10.5.4 TIME REQUIRED

Day 1: Grow master plates overnight
Day 2: Grow and rescue phagemid particles/soluble antibodies
Day 3: ELISA
Day 4: PCR fingerprinting

10.5.5 METHODS

10.5.5.1 Growth and Rescue of Phagemid Particles in 96-Well Microtiter Plates

1. Toothpick individual colonies (usually 94 clones per round of panning) into 150 µl 2xTY/amp/glu in 96-well round-bottom plates and grow with shaking (200 rpm) overnight at 37°C. This is the masterplate.
2. Next day, inoculate from the masterplate to a new 96-well round-bottom plate containing 150 µl 2xTY/amp/0.1% glu per well, using a 96-well transfer device (use three to four repeated transfers or pipette 2 µl per well from the masterplate). This is the expression plate. The method, based on that of DeBellis and Schwartz, 1990,[16] relies on the low level of glucose repressor present in the starting media to be metabolized by the time the inducer (IPTG) is added.
3. Grow bacteria in the newly inoculated expression plate to an A_{600}-0.7 for 2 to 3 h at 37°C (250 rpm). All the clones will not grow at the same rate, and you will have to estimate when most of the clones have the correct optical density.
4. To the wells of the masterplate add 50 µl of 50% glycerol/5 mM MgSO$_4$ per well. Cover the surface with a plate sealer and store at –70°C.
5. To each well of the expression plate add 50 µl helper phage (1.03×10^{10} TU/ml) diluted 1:1000 in 2xTY/amp. Incubate 30 min at 37°C (standing) and 30 min at 37°C shaking (250 rpm).
6. Add 50 µl 2xTY/amp/kan per well and shake (200 rpm) overnight at 30°C. Next morning, shake (250 rpm) 2 h at 37°C.
7. Spin down bacteria at $800 \times g$ for 10 min. Then transfer the supernatant containing phage particles to another plate. Use 50 µl per well for the phage ELISA.

10.5.5.2 Induction of Soluble Antibody Fragments in 96-Well Plates

1. Toothpick individual colonies (usually 94 clones per round of panning) into 150 µl 2xTY/amp/glu in 96-well round-bottom plates and grow with shaking (250 rpm) overnight at 37°C (the masterplate). Include one positive control and one negative control.
2. Next day, inoculate from the masterplate to a fresh 96-well round-bottom plate containing 150 µl 2xTY/amp/0.1% glu per well, using a 96-well

transfer device (use three to four repeated transfers or pipette 2 µl per well from the masterplate). This is the expression plate. The method is based on that of DeBellis and Schwartz, 1990[16] and relies on the low level of glucose repressor present in the starting media to be metabolized by the time the inducer (IPTG) is added.

3. Grow bacteria in the newly inoculated expression plate to an A_{600}-0.7 for 2 to 3 h at 37°C (250 rpm). All the clones will not grow at the same rate, and you will have to estimate when most of the clones have the correct optical density.

4. To the wells of masterplate add 50 µl of 50% glycerol/5 mM MgSO$_4$ per well. Cover the surface with a plate sealer and store at –70°C.

5. To each well of the expression plate add 50 µl 4 mM IPTG in 2xTY/amp (final concentration 1 mM) and continue shaking (250 rpm) at 25°C overnight.

6. Spin down bacteria debris at $800 \times g$ for 10 min. Then transfer the supernatant containing soluble antibody fragments to a new plate. Use 50 µl per well for antibody ELISA.

10.5.5.3 ELISA for Detection of Soluble or Phage Antibody Fragments

1. Coat a microtiter plate (Falcon 3912) with 50 µl/well of antigen at 1 to 10 µg/ml in PBS, pH 7.4. If insufficient antigen is adsorbed to the polystyrene plate, try coating in 100 mM sodium bicarbonate, pH 9.6. Leave overnight at 4°C.

2. Wash wells three times with PBS, then block with 200 µl/well of 2% skim milk powder in PBS (MPBS) for 1 h at room temperature. Wash by submersing the plate into buffer and removing the air bubbles in the wells by agitation. Tap the ELISA plates on a dry paper towel, to ensure that no buffer remains in the wells.

3. Wash wells three times with PBS and add 50 µl/well of soluble antibody fragment or phage antibody. Incubate for 1.5 h at room temperature.

4. Discard the solution and wash wells three times with PBS 0.1% Tween-20 and three times with PBS.

5a. For soluble antibody detection, add 50 µl/well of 9E10 antibody (Santa Cruz Biotechnology, CA) at 1 µg/ml in 2% MPBS and incubate at room temperature for 1 h.

5b. For phage antibody detection, add 50 µl/well of bio-anti-M13-phage antibody (5Prime–>3Prime Inc., Cat. No. 7-187156) at 2.5 µg/ml in 2% MPBS and incubate at room temperature for 1 h.

6. Discard antibody and wash wells three times with PBS 0.1% Tween-20 and three times with PBS.

7a. For soluble antibody detection, add 50 µl/well of horseradish peroxidase conjugated anti-mouse IgG Fc monoclonal antibody (Sigma A-2554) at 1 µg/ml in 2% MPBS. Incubate at room temperature for 1 h.

7b. For phage antibody detection, add 50 µl/well of horseradish peroxidase conjugated streptavidin (Pierce 21126) at 0.5 µg/ml in 2% MPBS. Incubate at room temperature for 1 h.

8. Discard antibody and wash wells three times with PBS (0.1%) Tween-20 and three times with PBS.

9. Prepare developing solution by adding one 10 mg ABTS (2, 2′- azino bis (3-ethylbenzthiazoline-6-sulfonic acid) tablet (Sigma) to 10 ml of 50 mM citric acid and 10 ml of 50 mM sodium citrate. Add 20 µl of 30% hydrogen peroxide to the ABTS solution immediately before dispensing 100 µl per well. Leave at room temperature for 20 to 30 min.

10. Quench reaction by adding 50 µl/well of 75 mM sodium fluoride. Read at 405 nm.

If you do not obtain any signals including signals from the positive control, we recommend checking the expression levels of soluble or phage antibodies by dot-blot, since levels can vary from one clone to another and range from 2 to 1000 µg/ml. Transfer 50 µl of the supernatant from step 5 onto a nitrocellulose filter and proceed exactly as described in steps 3 through 9 above. Develop the nitrocellulose in DAB-solution one (10 mg DAB (diaminobenzidine tetrahydrochloride) in 20 ml PBS and 20 µl of 30% hydrogen peroxide). Also check the activity of the hydrogen peroxide solution, which can lose potency after 1 month of storage in the refrigerator, and replace if necessary.

10.5.5.4 PCR Fingerprinting of Clones with Restriction Enzyme *BstN* I

1. Prepare master mix, with 20 µl PCR mix per clone, containing the following:

Water	14.8 µl
10 x Taq buffer	2.0 µl
dNTPs (5 mM each)	1.0 µl
LMB 3 primer (10 pm/µl)	1.0 µl
fdseq 1 primer (10 pm/µl)	1.0 µl
Taq DNA polymerase (5 u/µl)	0.2 µl

The denoted sequences for PCR screening oligonucleotides LMB 3 and fdseq 1 are as follows: LMB 3 (5′-CAG GAA ACA GCT ATG AC-3′ annealing upstream from the pelB leader sequence) and fdseq 1 (5′-GAA TTT TCT GTA TGA GG-3′ annealing at the 5′ end of gene 3).

2. Aliquot 20 µl of PCR reaction mix into wells of a 96-well PCR-compatible microtiter plate.

3. Touch with a sterile toothpick a single bacterial colony from an agar plate and twist about three times, taking care not to transfer an excess amount of bacteria, or use 1 µl of a bacterial glycerol stock.

4. Overlay the PCR reaction mixes with mineral oil. Insert the microtiter plate into a thermolcycler preheated to 94°C, and hold at that temperature for 10 min to lyse the bacteria.
5. Cycle 25 times at 94°C for 1 min; 42°C for 1 min; and 72°C for 1 min.
6. Check PCR reactions for full length inserts (scFv fragements run approximately at 900 base pairs) on a 1.5% agarose gel. Depending on the quality of the library, you may obtain a variable number of single-domain antibodies with either V_H or V_L genes.
7. Prepare a restriction enzyme mixture from the following:

Water	17.8 µl
10 x NEB buffer 2	2.0 µl
BstN 1 (10 u/µl)	0.2 µl

8. Add 20 µl of the above mix to each PCR-containing well under the mineral oil. Incubate the restriction digest at 60°C for 2 h.
9. Add 4 µl of 10 × agarose gel electrophoresis sample dye under the oil and analyze the restriction digest on a 4% Nusieve agarose gel cast containing 0.5 µg/ml ethidium bromide.

10.6 EXPRESSION AND PURIFICATION OF NATIVE ANTIBODY FRAGMENTS

10.6.1 DESCRIPTION

This section describes large-scale expression and purification of soluble scFv antibodies in *E. coli*. The first step is the functional expression of correctly folded scFv fragments by secretion in the periplasmic space[6,50]; the second is the *in vitro* refolding of protein obtained from inclusion bodies from the cytoplasm or the periplasm.[8,29] The method of choice depends mainly on the desired application of the antibodies. If a series of kinetic constants has to be analyzed on the Biacore, or a number of clones have to be tested for specificity by ELISA, secretion is the faster way. However, if one particular fragment is needed in very large quantities on a continuous base, the work of preparative folding may be considered as an alternative.[53] The cytoplasmic and periplasmic environments differ in a number of respects, which result in different folding status properties of the antibodies. The cytoplasm maintains a reducing milieu wherein cysteinyl residues cannot correctly form the intradomain disulfide bonds that are essential to obtain correctly folded antibodies. In order to target the periplasmic space, which has an oxidizing environment, and encourage the formation of disulfide bonds, researchers have attached a variety of bacterial signal sequences.[43,44] The signal sequence directs the expressed domains into the periplasmic space, where they fold correctly into functional heterodimeric Fv fragments. Better's group used two copies of a different signal sequence, pelB (pectate lyase), to express a functional Fab antibody fragment.[6]

The production of scFv antibodies in *E. coli* has to be carefully monitored, and important parameters such as growth temperature after induction, IPTG concentration, and induction time have to be determined empirically for each clone. Depending on the primary structure of the antibody fragments, we have exploited cell death and lysis of *E. coli* due to toxicity.

Detection of scFv expression and binding to antigen by ELISA are facilitated by fusion of a C- or N-terminal epitope tag, such as the c-myc epitope[36,40] or E-tag.[40] The epitope tags can also be used for affinity purification,[14,36] but require use of expensive antibody columns and stringent elution conditions that may damage the scFv. The current technique is to fuse a C-terminal hexa-histidine tag and purify the scFv from the bacterial periplasm using immobilized metal affinity chromatography (IMAC).[25]

10.6.2 REAGENTS

Overnight culture media: 2xTY/100 µg/ml carbenicillin/2% glucose (2xTY/carb/glu)

Growth media: 2xTY/100 µg/ml ampicillin/0.1% glucose (2xTY/amp/0.1% glu)

Periplasmic buffer (PPB): 200 mg/ml sucrose, 1 mM EDTA, 30 mM Tris-HCl, pH 8.0 and freshly added 0.5 mM Pefabloc

Osmotic shock buffer: 5 mM MgS0$_4$

Ni^{2+}- NTA agarose (Qiagen)

10.6.3 SPECIAL EQUIPMENT

2-L baffled shaker flask (Bellco Biotechnology)

37 and 25°C shaker-incubator (New Brunswick Scientific)

PolyPrep chromatography columns for IMAC (Biorad)

Superdex 75 column (Pharmacia)

High-pressure liquid chromatography system for gel filtration (BioCAD SPRINT)

Dialysis tubing, cut off 12,000 to 14,000 kDa (Spectrum)

Centricon-10 (Amicon)

Sorvall centrifuge (DuPont Instruments)

10.6.4 TIME REQUIRED

Day 1: Inoculum of bacteria overnight

Day 2': Growing bacteria, induction, periplasmic and osmotic shock preparation, dialysis overnight

Day 3: IMAC purification and gel filtration, and SDS-PAGE

10.6.5 METHODS

1. Grow a 5-ml overnight culture in 2xTY/carb/glu at 37°C (250 rpm).
2. Add 5 ml of the overnight culture to 500 ml 2xTY/amp/0.1% glu in a baffled flask and grow at 37°C. Shake at 250 rpm for approximately 2 h to A$_{600}$ of 0.7.

3. Induce with 250 μl 1 *M* IPTG (final concentration of 500 μ*M*) and grow at 25°C at 200 rpm for 4 h. Collect cells by centrifuging in a 500 ml plastic bottle at 4000 × *g* for 15 min.

4. For the periplasmic preparation, resuspend the bacterial pellet in 12.5 ml PPB buffer (use 1/40 of total growth volume) and keep on ice for 20 min. Spin down cells in centrifuge at 4000 × *g* for 15 min and collect the supernatant containing soluble scFv fraction into small, high-speed centrifuge tubes. Use the bacterial pellet for the osmotic shock preparation.

5. For the osmotic shock preparation, resuspend the pellet in 5 m*M* MgSO₄ buffer (use 1/40 of total growth volume) and incubate on ice for 20 min. Transfer samples to small, high-speed centrifuge tubes and spin preparations down at 25,000 × *g* for 15 min.

6. Pool the supernatants of the two preparations and dialyze against 4 L PBS overnight at 4°C to remove traces of EDTA (contained in the PPB buffer), which complexes Ni²⁺ ions.

7. The dialyzed sample is loaded onto a Ni²⁺-NTA agarose column (1 ml), pre-equilibrated with 2 × 5 ml of PBS, pH 7.5 and 1 × 5 ml of loading buffer (PBS pH 7.5 buffer containing 20 m*M* imidazole). The sample is allowed to pass through the column with a flow rate of approximately 0.5 ml/min.

8. After the sample has completely entered the gel bed, the column is washed with 10 ml of washing buffer (PBS pH 7.5 buffer containing 35 m*M* imidazole). For some scFv fragments, the imidazole concentration needs to be adjusted to avoid stripping the scFv from the column.

9. Elute scFv antibody fragments with 2 ml elution buffer (PBS pH 7.5 buffer containing 250 m*M* imidazole and 0.02% azide).

10. Concentrate samples to 0.5 ml using Centricon-10 at 5000 × *g* for 1 h and analyze sample by gel filtration and SDS-PAGE.

11. Ni²⁺-NTA agarose columns can be reused for the purification of the identical clone after stripping the column with 5 ml regeneration buffer (PBS pH 7.5 buffer containing 500 m*M* imidazole) and equilibration in 5 ml PBS, pH 7.5 containing 0.02% azide.

REFERENCES

1. Adams, G. P., J. E. McCartney, M. S. Tai, H. Oppermann, J. S. Huston, W. F. Stafford, M. A. Bookman, I. Fand, L. L. Houston, and L. M. Weiner, 1993, Highly specific *in vivo* tumor targeting by monovalent and divalent forms of 741F8 anti-c-erbB-2 single-chain Fv, *Cancer Res.*, 53, 4026–4034.

2. Amersdorfer, P., C. Wong, S. Chen, T. Smith, S. Desphande, R. Sheridan, R. Finnern, and J. D. Marks, 1997, Molecular characterization of murine humoral immune response to botulinum neurotoxin type A binding domain as assessed by using phage antibody libraries, *Infect. Immun.*, 65, 3743–3752.

3. Barbas, C., J. Crowe, D. Cababa, T. Jones, S. Zebedee, B. Murphy, R. Chanock, and D. Burton, 1992, Human monoclonal Fab fragments derived from a combinatorial library bind to respiratory syncytial virus F glycoprotein and neutralize infectivity, *Proc. Natl. Acad. Sci. U.S.A.*, 89, 10164–10168.

4. Barbas, C. F., T. A. Collet, W. Amberg, P. Roben, J. M. Binley, D. Hoekstra, D. Cababa, T. M. Jones, A. Williamson, G. R. Pilkington, N. L. Haigwood, E. Cabezas, A. C. Satterthwait, I. Sanz, and D. R. Burton, 1993, Molecular profile of an antibody response to HIV-1 as probed by combinatorial libraries, *J. Mol. Biol.*, 230, 812–823.

5. Barbas, C. F., A. S. Kang, R. A. Lerner, and S. J. Benkovic, 1991, Assembly of combinatorial antibody libraries on phage surfaces: the gene III site, *Proc. Natl. Acad. Sci. U.S.A.*, 88, 7978–7982.

6. Better, M., C. P. Chang, R. R. Robinson, and A. H. Horwitz, 1988, *Escherichia coli* secretion of an active chimeric antibody fragment, *Science*, 240, 1041–1043.

7. Biocca, S., P. Pierandrei-Amaldi, and A. Cattaneo, 1994, Intracellular immunization with cytosolic recombinant antibodies, *Biotechnology*, 12, 396–399.

8. Bird, R. E., K. D. Hardman, J. W. Jacobson, S. Johnson, B. M. Kaufman, S. M. Lee, T. Lee, S. H. Pope, G. S. Riordan, and M. Whitlow, 1988, Single-chain antigen-binding proteins, *Science*, 242, 423–426.

9. Burton, D. R., C. F. Barbas, M. A. A. Persson, S. Koenig, R. M. Chanock, and R. A. Lerner, 1991, A large array of human monoclonal antibodies to type 1 human immunodefficiency virus from combinatorial libraries of asymptomatic seropositive individuals, *Proc. Natl. Acad. Sci. U.S.A.,* 88, 10134–10137.

10. Cai, X. and A. Garen, 1995, Anti-melanoma antibodies from melanoma patients immunized with genetically modified autologous tumor cells: selection of specific antibodies from single-chain Fv fusion phage libraries, *Proc. Natl. Acad. Sci. U.S.A.,* 92, 6537–6541.

11. Cathala, G., J. Savouret, B. Mendez, B. L. Wesr, M. Karin, J. A. Martial, and J. D. Baxter, 1983. A method for isolation of intact, transcriptionally active ribonucleic acid, *DNA*, 2, 329.

12. Chan, S., J. Bye, P. Jackson, and J. Allain, 1996, Human recombinant antibodies specific for hepatitis C virus core and envelope E2 peptides from an immune phage display library, *J. Gen. Virol.,* 10, 2531–2539.

13. Chomczynski, P. and N. Sacchi, 1987, Single-step method of RNA isolation by acid guanidinium-thiocyanate-phenol-chloroform extraction, *Anal. Biochem.*, 162, 156–159.

14. Clackson, T., H. R. Hoogenboom, A. D. Griffiths, and G. Winter, 1991, Making antibody fragments using phage display libraries, *Nature*, 352, 624–628.

15. Clackson, T. and J. A. Wells, 1994, *In vitro* selection from protein and peptide libraries, *Tibtech*, 12, 173–184.

16. De Bellis, D. and I. Schwartz, 1990, Regulated expression of foreign genes fused to lac: control by glucose levels in growth medium, *Nucleic Acids Res.*, 18, 1311.

17. Dower, W. J., J. F. Miller, and C. W. Ragsdale, 1988, High efficiency transformation of *E. coli* by high voltage electroporation, *Nucleic Acids Res.,* 16, 6127–45.

18. Dubel, S., F. Breitling, P. Fuchs, M. Braunagel, I. Klewinghaus, and M. Little, 1993, A family of vectors for surface display and production of antibodies, *Gene*, 128, 97–101.

19. Engelhardt, O., R. Grabher, G. Himmler, and F. Ruker, 1994, Two-step cloning of antibody variable domains in a phage display vector, *Bio/Techniques*, 17, 44–46.

20. Evan, G., G. Lewis, G. Ramsay, and J. Bishop, 1985, Isolation of monoclonal antibodies specific for c-myc proto-oncogene product, *Mol Cell Biol.*, 5, 3610–3616.

21. Fominaya, J. and W. Wels, 1996, Target cell-specific DNA transfer mediated by a chimeric multidomain protein, *J. Biol. Chem.*, 271, 10560–10568.

22. Griffiths, A. D. and A. R. Duncan, 1998, Strategies for selection of antibodies by phage display, *Curr. Opinion Biotechnol.*, 9, 102–108.

23. Griffiths, A. D., S. C. Williams, O. Hartley, I. M. Tomlinson, P. Waterhouse, W. L. Crosby, R. E. Kontermann, P. T. Jones, N. M. Low, T. J. Allison, T. D. Prospero, H. R. Hoogenboom, A. Nissim, J. P. L. Cox, J. L. Harrison, M. Zaccolo, E. Gherardi, and G. Winter, 1994, Isolation of high affinity human antibodies directly from large synthetic repertoires, *EMBO J.*, 13, 3245–3260.

24. Hawkins, R. E., S. J. Russell, and G. Winter, 1992, Selection of phage antibodies by binding afinity: mimicking affinity maturation, *J. Mol. Biol.*, 226, 889–896.

25. Hochuli, E., W. Bannwarth, H. Dobeli, R. Gentz, and D. Stuber, 1988, Genetic approach to facilitate purification of recombinant proteins with a novel metal chelate adsorbent, *Bio/Technology*, 6, 1321–1325.

26. Hoogenboom, H. R., A. D. Griffiths, K. S. Johnson, D. J. Chiswell, P. Hudson, and G. Winter, 1991, Multi-subunit proteins on the surface of filamentous phage: methodologies for displaying antibody (Fab) heavy and light chains, *Nucleic Acids Res.*, 19, 4133–4137.

27. Hoogenboom, H. R., J. D. Marks, A. D. Griffiths, and G. Winter, 1992, Building antibodies from their genes, *Immunol. Rev.*, 130, 41–68.

28. Huse, W., T. Stinchcombe, S. Glaser, L. M. Starr, M, K. Hellstrom, I. Hellstrom, and D. Yelton, 1992, Application of a filamentous phage pVIII fusion protein system suitable for efficient production, screening, and mutagenesis of F(ab) antibody fragments, *J. Immunol.*, 149, 3914–3920.

29. Huston, J. S., D. Levinson, H. M. Mudgett, M. S. Tai, J. Novotny, M. N. Margolies, R. J. Ridge, R. E. Bruccoleri, E. Haber, R. Crea, and H. Oppermann, 1988, Protein engineering of antibody binding sites: recovery of specific activity in an anti-digoxin single-chain Fv analogue produced in *Escherichia coli, Proc. Natl. Acad. Sci. U.S.A.*, 85, 5879–5883.

30. Kabat, E., T.T. Wu, M. Reid-Miller, H.M. Perry, and K.S. Gottesmann, 1987, *Sequences of Proteins of Immunological Interest*, U.S. Department of Health and Human Services, U.S. Government Printing Office, Washington, D.C.

31. Kang, A., C. Barbas, K. Janda, and S. Benkovic, 1991, Linkage of recognition and replication functions by assembling combinational Fab libraries along phage surfaces, *Proc. Natl. Acad. Sci. U.S.A.*, 88, 4363–4366.

32. Knappik, A., C. Krebber, and A. Pluckthun, 1993, The effects of folding catalysis on the *in vivo* folding process of different antibody fragments expressed in *Escherichia coli, Bio/Technology*, 11, 77–83.

33. Kohler, G. and C. Milstein, 1975, Continous cultures of fused cells secreting antibody of predefined specificity, *Nature*, 256, 495–497.

34. Lah, M., A. Goldstraw, J. White, O. Dolezal, R. Malby, and P. Hudson, 1994, Phage surface presentation and secretion of antibody fragments using an adaptable phagemid vector, *Human Antibodies and Hybridomas*, 5, 48–56.

35. Lorimer, I. A., A. Keppler-Hafkemeyer, R. A. Beers, C. N. Pegram, D. D. Bigner, and I. Pastan, 1996, Recombinant immunotoxins specific for a mutant epidermal growth factor receptor: targeting with a single chain antibody variable domain isolated by phage display, *Proc. Natl. Acad. Sci. U.S.A.*, 93, 14815–20.

36. Marks, J. D., H. R. Hoogenboom, T. P. Bonnert, J. McCafferty, A. D. Griffiths, and G. Winter, 1991, By-passing immunization: human antibodies from V-gene libraries displayed on phage, *J. Mol. Biol.*, 222, 581–597.

37. Marks, J. D., H. R. Hoogenboom, A. D. Griffiths, and G. Winter, 1992, Molecular evolution of proteins on filamentous phage: mimicking the strategy of the immune system, *J. Biol. Chem.*, 267, 16007–16010.

38. Marks, J. D., M. Tristrem, A. Karpas, and G. Winter, 1991, Oligonucleotide primers for polymerase chain reaction amplification of human immunoglobulin variable genes and design of family-specific oligonucleotide probes, *Eur. J. Immunol.*, 21, 985–991.

39. McCafferty, J., A. D. Griffiths, G. Winter, and D. J. Chiswell, 1990, Phage antibodies: filamentous phage displaying antibody variable domains, *Nature*, 348, 552–554.

40. Munro, S. and H. R. Pelham, 1986, An Hsp-like protein in the ER: identity with the 78kd glucose regulated protein and immunoglobulin heavy chain binding protein, *Cell*, 46, 291–300.

41. Orlandi, R., D. H. Gussow, P. T. Jones, and G. Winter, 1989, Cloning immunoglobulin variable domains for expression by the polymerase chain reaction, *Proc. Natl. Acad. Sci. U.S.A.*, 86, 3833–3837.

42. Parmley, S. F. and G. P. Smith, 1988, Antibody-selectable filamentous fd phage vectors: affinity purification of target genes, *Gene*, 73, 305.

43. Pluckthun, A., 1991, Advances from the use of Escherichia coli expression systems, *Biotechnology*, 9, 545.

44. Pluckthun, A., 1992, Mono- and bivalent antibody fragments produced in *Escherichia coli*: engineering, folding, and antigen binding, *Immunol. Rev.*, 130, 151.

45. Reason, D., T. Wagner, and A. Lucas, 1997, Human Fab fragments specific for the *Haemophilis influenzae* B polysaccharide isolated from a bacteriophage combinatorial library use variable region gene combinations and express an idiotype that mirrors *in vivo* expression, *Infect. Immun.*, 65, 261–266.

46. Ruberti, F., A. Cattaneo, and A. Bradbury, 1994, The use of the RACE method to clone hybridoma cDNA when V region primers fail, *J. Immunol. Meth.*, 173, 33–39.

47. Sambrook, J., E. F. Fritsch, and T. Maniatis, 1989, *Molecular Cloning — A Laboratory Manual*, Cold Spring Harbor Laboratory, Cold Spring Harbor, NY.

48. Schier, R., J. M. Bye, G. Apell, A. McCall, G. P. Adams, M. Malmqvist, L. M. Weiner, and J. D. Marks, 1996, Isolation of high affinity monomeric human anti-c-erbB-2 single chain Fv using affinity driven selection, *J. Mol. Biol.*, 255, 28–43.

49. Sheets, M. D., P. Amersdorfer, R. Finnern, P. Sargent, E. Lindqvist, R. Schier, G. Hemingsen, C. Wong, J. C. Gerhart, and J. D. Marks, 1998, Efficient construction of a large nonimmune phage antibody library: the production of high affinity human single-chain antibodies to protein antigens, *Proc. Natl. Acad. Sci. U.S.A.*, 95, 6157–6162.

50. Skerra, A. and A. Pluckthun, 1988, Assembly of a functional immunoglobulin Fv fragment in Escherichia coli, *Science*, 240, 1038–1041.

51. Smith, G., 1985, Filamentous fusion phage: novel expression vectors that display cloned antigens on the virion surface, *Science*, 228, 1315.

52. Somia, N. V., M. Zoppe, and I. M. Verma, 1995, Generation of targeted retroviral vectors by using single-chain variable fragment: an approach to *in vivo* gene delivery, *Proc. Natl. Acad. Sci. U.S.A.*, 92, 7570–7574.

53. Tai, M., M. Mudgett-Hunter, D. Levinson, G. M. Wu, E. Haber, H. Oppermann, and J. Huston, 1990, A bifunctional fusion protein containing Fc-binding fragment B of staphylococcal protein A amino terminal to antidigoxin single-chain Fv, *Biochemistry*, 29, 8024–8030.

54. Tomlinson, I. M., S. C. Williams, S. J. Corbett, J. P. L. Cox, and G. Winter, 1995, *VBASE Sequence Directory*, MRC Centre for Protein Engineering, Cambridge, UK.

55. Vaughan, T. J., A. J. Williams, K. Pritchard, J. K. Osbourn, A. R. Pope, J. C. Earnshaw, J. McCafferty, R. A. Hodits, J. Wilton, and K. S. Johnson, 1996, Human antibodies with sub-nanomolar affinities isolated from a large non-immunized phage display library, *Nature Biotech.*, 14, 309–314.

56. Winter, G., A. Griffiths, R. Hawkins, and H. Hoogenboom, 1994, Making antibodies by phage display technology, *Annu. Rev. Immunol.*, 12, 433–455.

57. Yokota, T., D. Milenic, M. Whitlow, and J. Schlom, 1992, Rapid tumor penetration of a single-chain Fv and comparison with other immunoglobulin forms, *Cancer Res.*, 52, 3402–3408.

58. Zebedee, S. L., C. F. Barbas, Y.-L. Hom, R. H. Cathoien, R. Graff, J. DeGraw, J. Pyatt, R. LaPolla, D. R. Burton, and R. A. Lerner, 1992, Human combinatorial antibody libraries to hepatitis B surface antigens, *Proc. Natl. Acad. Sci. U.S.A.,* 89, 3175–3179.

11 Antibody Purification Methods

Kristi R. Harkins

CONTENTS

11.1 INTRODUCTION

There are many well-documented approaches to purifying antibody from a variety of sources (for reviews, see References 1 and 2). The method of choice will depend upon the antibody source, time available, cost considerations, and final use of the antibody. This chapter is organized to provide the reader with options that involve single steps for purifying IgG and IgM that will save time but will be less cost effective. Alternative two-step methods are also provided that will cost less in terms of supplies but will require more time to complete. In each section, a brief paragraph provides information on the advantages and disadvantages of each method and gives examples of when each method might be best utilized.

Begin by determining the use and final level of purity required for the antibody you have generated. Some form of purification will be required in instances were the antibody will be used for immunoassay, immunotags, and as immunoaffinity reagents. Purification is also required when background or nonspecific binding is observed in your assay negative controls. Consider the degree of purity needed and how the method of choice will effect the final yield, purity, and especially antibody activity. Are you purifying monoclonal or polyclonal antibody from ascites (1 to 10 mg/ml), sera (20 to 30 mg/ml), cell culture supernatant [static (50 µg/ml or bioreactor (0.1 to 10 mg/ml)] and what is the host species and isotype of the antibody? In general, the more expensive immunoaffinity chromatography methods are the primary methods of choice for purifying monoclonal antibody from ascites or bioreactor culture fluids. This method can also be used for purifying antibody from serum and ascites. The economical two-step methods are more commonly employed for purifying polyclonal antibody fluids. Factors such as the effect the purification method has on the antigen (Ag) binding affinity and/or Fc region and the time and cost may also influence the method selected. The following table provides a general summary of the pros and cons for each of the methods outlined in this chapter.

11.2 PRELIMINARY STEPS

11.2.1 CLARIFICATION

In most cases, antibody-rich fluids (serum, ascites fluid, and culture fluid) will be collected, pooled, and frozen for later purification. Contaminating cells and cellular debris should be removed before the fluids are pooled and frozen by centrifugation ($1500 \times g$ for 15 min). In the case of ascites fluid, it may also be necessary to remove lipids by filtering the ascites through glass wool prior to purification. Upon thawing, it is very important to further clarify your antibody solution by centrifugation at $20,000 \times g$ for 30 min before proceeding with any purification procedure. Centrifugation will remove any final cellular debris and protein/antibody aggregates that may have formed during the freezing and thawing process. A step filtration through a 0.45-µm filter and then a 0.22-µm sterile syringe filter prior to purification should follow.

TABLE 11.1
Overview of Methods of Antibody Purification

Method	Cost	Time	Yield	Purity	Comments
Source	Low <$100				
Ig class	High >$100				
Protein G	High	1 day	>95%	>95%	Potential reduced activity
Monoclonal and polyclonal IgG					
Protein L	High	1 day	>95%	>95%	Potential reduced activity, doesn't bind bovine Ig
Monoclonal and polyclonal IgG, IgM, IgY					
Immunoaffinity (anti-IgM)	High	1 day	>80%	>95%	Potential reduced activity
Monoclonal and polyclonal IgM					
Immunoaffinity (antigen antibody)	High	1 day	>80%	>95%	Potential reduced activity, improved specificity
Monoclonal and polyclonal IgG, IgM, IgY					
Thiophilic gel	Low	1 day	>80%	>90%	No effect on activity
Monoclonal and polyclonal IgG/IgY					
Ammonium sulfate	Low	1 day	50–80%	50–80%	No effect on activity, requires second step
Monoclonal and polyclonal IgG, IgM, IgY					
Caprylic acid	Low	1 day	50–80%	50–80%	May affect activity, requires second step
Polyclonal IgG/IgY					
Gel filtration	Low	1 day	90%	50–80%	No effect on activity, dilute product, requires a first step
Monoclonal and polyclonal IgM					
Anion exchange chromatography	Low	1 day	90%	>90%	May affect activity, requires a first step
Monoclonal and polyclonal IgG, IgY					

11.2.2 CHARACTERIZATION

Quantitation of the total protein in the sample is an important first step and can be accomplished using a protein assay kit (e.g., BCA kit from Pierce) or by measuring the absorbance at 280 nm using a UV spectrophotometer ($A_{280} \times 0.8 =$ mg/ml). Second, the level of antibody activity or antibody titer in the unpurified sample must be established as a point of reference for later evaluating the purified product. Finally, capture ELISA kits are available that measure the quantity of mouse and rabbit immunoglobulin in a sample (Pierce). The total starting protein concentration and the level of antibody reactivity at a given dilution or titer will provide a reference point for determining the yield and the potential for loss of antibody activity when purification is complete.

11.3 PURIFICATION OF IgG

11.3.1 ONE-STEP METHOD USING CHROMATOGRAPHY

11.3.1.1 Protein G and Protein L

Introduction: Protein G (30 to 35 kDa), isolated from β-hemolytic streptococci (group G) has a natural affinity for the constant region of the antibody heavy chain. This protein also has a binding site for albumin, which has been deleted in recombinant forms of Protein G (e.g., GammaBind® Plus, Pharmacia). Protein A affinity matrix can also be found on the market, but does not have a comparable binding affinity or diversity in subclass binding that can be found with Protein G. For this reason Protein G is preferred for its overall utility.[3,4]

Protein L, originally isolated from *Peptostreptococcus magnus*, binds to the kappa light chain and thus binds to all antibody classes, including IgM, and is the most versatile of the three proteins. Protein L is especially useful for purifying Fab and single-chain variable fragments (ScFV).[7] Also, because it does not bind bovine antibodies, it is useful in purifying monoclonal antibodies from hybridoma cell culture medium containing bovine serum. Protein L provides a better affinity for purifying mouse IgG3 when compared to Protein G. However, Protein L does not work as well as Protein G with rabbit, sheep, goat, or bovine polyclonal purification. Protein L is useful for purifying chicken IgG and IgY and porcine.[5-7]

This method of purification involves a higher initial expense, with chromatography gels costing over $200 for a 2-ml volume, but the columns can be reused multiple times, reducing the long-term costs of purification and is recommended for both polyclonal and monoclonal antibody purification.

Note: The procedure outlined is generally applicable for all immunoaffinity (one-step methods) provided in this chapter. Slight variations in the buffer compositions will be noted in each section when appropriate. Commercial resins also may be purchased with binding and elution buffers prepared by the manufacturer for immediate use and designed for optimal binding capacity and elution profiles.

TABLE 11.2
List of Some Commercial Immunoaffinity Products and Other Relevant Supplies[a]

Manufacturer	Product	Purpose
Bio-Rad (www.biorad.com)	Affi-gel® 10 and 15	Antigen coupling matrix
	MiniPROTEAN® II Gel System and supplies	Antibody purity evaluation
Pharmacia (www.apbiotech.com)	Protein G resin	Purify IgG
	GammaBind® Plus	Purify IgG
	CNBr Activated Sepharose®	Antigen coupling matrix
	HiTrapQ™	Purify IgG
Pierce (optional binding and elution buffers available)	Protein G resin	Purify IgG
	Protein A/G resin	Purify IgG
	T-gel® resin	Purify Ig
	Protein L resin	Purify Ig
Pierce (piercenet.com)	IgG (mouse and rabbit assay kit)	Quantify antibody concentration
Pierce	BCA protein assay kit	Quantify Total Protein
Clontech (www.clontech.com)	Protein L resin	Purify IgG, IgM, IgY
Southern Biotech/Fisher Scientific (www.fishersci.com)	Rat anti-mouse (kappa) HP conjugate	Mouse IgG quantitative ELISA
Sigma (www.sigma-aldrich.com)	Protein G resin	Purify IgG
	Anti-mouse IgM agarose	Purify IgM
	Anti-mouse IgG$_1$ agarose	Purify IgG$_1$
	Anti-mouse IgG$_3$ agarose	Purify IgG$_3$
	Goat anti-mouse Fc	Mouse IgG quantitative ELISA
	Mouse IgG (pure fraction)	Mouse IgG quantitative ELISA

[a] Other commercial sources may exist in addition to those listed here. The author does not recommend any one vendor.

Materials and solutions:

Commercial Protein G and Protein L Resins (select from list in Table 11.2)
Immunopure® Immobilized Protein L (Pierce, 2 ml, Cat. # 20510ZZ)
Protein L Agarose Beads (Clontech, 2 ml, Cat. # 3901–1)
GammaBind® Plus Sepharose®, 5 ml (Pharmacia, Cat. # 17-0886-01)

Buffers

Binding buffer, pH 7.0
　　0.01 M sodium phosphate, dibasic
　　0.15 M NaCl
Protein G elution buffer, pH 3.0 (adjust pH with ammonium hydroxide)
　　0.5 M acetic acid (14.37 ml glacial acetic acid + 485.63 ml H$_2$O)

Protein L elution buffer, pH 2.0 (0.1 M glycine) or 0.2 M citrate buffer (pH 2.8)
Neutralizing buffer, pH 9.0
    1.0 M Tris base
Cleansing buffer, pH 2.5
    1.0 M acetic acid (28.74 ml glacial acetic acid + 481.26 ml H_2O)
Storage buffer
    100 ml binding buffer
    0.05% w/v sodium azide

Equipment:

Kontes Flex-column (1.5 cm x 10 cm, 18 ml bed volume),
Fisher Scientific, Chicago, IL
3-Way stopcock (Fisher Scientific)
Column support system, input and outlet tubing, buffer reservoir
UV spectrophotometer with UV cuvettes
Fraction collector (optional)

Procedure:

1. Prepare the column according to manufacturer's instruction. Open column stopcock, letting the buffer drain out to the top of the resin. Don't let the column run dry.
2. Gently apply 5 ml of binding buffer with a Pasteur pipet, to the top of the bed without disrupting the resin's surface. Open column and let five column bed volumes (25 ml) of binding buffer wash through.
3. Prepare and label blank and fraction tubes as follows. A binding buffer blank will have 1.0 ml of binding buffer. Label one tube "runoff." The elution buffer blank will have 1.0 ml of elution buffer plus the volume of the neutralizing buffer necessary to change the pH to 7.0 (about 0.5 ml; test beforehand). Mark off the total volume of elution buffer plus neutralizing buffer on labeled elution tubes and number 1 to 10 (ten elution tubes needed to collect IgG fractions). Pipet the necessary volume of neutralizing buffer into each of the elution tubes.
4. Mix clarified and filtered antibody solution with binding buffer. Use 3 ml binding buffer for every 0.50-ml sample (final dilution 1:6 in binding buffer).
5. Using a Pasteur pipet, apply sample onto the column resin without disturbing the column bed. Allow the diluted sample to run into the column, and then shut off the column flow and let the column set for 15 min.
6. Wash the column with five column bed volumes of binding buffer. Collect an early fraction (about 3 to 4 ml into the elution run) of unbound serum proteins and label the 1.0 ml fraction "runoff." You can use the runoff fraction in a control lane on the SDS-PAGE analysis gel to determine the efficiency of Ig binding and to determine whether the column was overloaded. You don't want to see bands in the 25,000 and 55,000 molecular weight ranges for IgG purification.

7. Using a Pasteur pipet, apply two column bed volumes of the appropriate elution buffer for either Protein G or Protein L matrices onto the column resin. Open the column and start collecting 1.0-ml samples into your numbered fraction collection tubes with the neutralizing buffer already in the tube. Mix each tube so the pH of the fraction neutralizes as it is collected.

8. Wash the column with five column bed volumes of elution buffer followed by five column volumes of cleansing buffer to remove residual proteins from the column. Shut off the column.

9. Using a Pasteur pipet, apply on column volume of binding buffer onto the column resin. Open the column and wash the column with four column volumes of binding buffer. Apply two column volumes of storing buffer. Shut column off and store at 4°C.

10. Read the absorbance values for each fraction on the spectrophotometer.

Spectrophotometer use: Warm up the spectrophotometer. Use the binding buffer as the blank when measuring the absorbance of the "runoff" tube contents. Use the elution tube as the blank when measuring the elution tubes. Use quartz cuvettes or disposable cuvettes (e.g., Fisher Scientific UV semi-microcuvettes). The arrow of the cuvette faces the light source of the spectrophotometer. Read the absorbance at 280 nm and record. Pool the protein containing peak fractions.

Estimation of Ig concentration by UV absorbance: The concentration of a sample equals the absorbance value of the sample multiplied by the path length of the cuvette divided by the extinction coefficient. The extinction coefficient of IgG is 1.38. If you have a fraction that gives an absorption of 0.76 at 280 nm in a 1-cm cuvette path length, the concentration of that sample would be 0.55 mg/ml. The total amount of that fraction's IgG content is 0.55 mg/ml × fraction volume of 1.5 ml = 0.825 mg of IgG. Or you can simply multiply the absorbance of IgG by 0.72 for the IgG concentration in mg/ml. If you are purifying IgM, then multiply the absorbance of IgM at 280 nm by 0.84. Please note that this is only an estimate; any other contaminating proteins in your fraction will also add to your absorbance reading.

Results: Preparation of the column, washing, loading, eluting, and evaluation of the collected fractions take approximately 3 h. Assuming the column is not overloaded and the elution conditions are optimal, minimal loss of antibody should be observed (95% yield). No contaminating bands should be observed when evaluating the product on SDS PAGE.

Problems: It is especially important to verify the activity of the antibody (i.e., the antigen-binding capacity) of the purified product before and after purification. There have been instances where antibody activity is significantly reduced by the low elution pH. It has also been observed that the affinity ligand may leach off the column matrix to a small degree.[8] This low-level contamination may not be acceptable for the use of biotheraputic antibodies *in vivo*. Rat-derived monoclonal antibodies can be purified using the Protein G or Protein L chromatography, though there is some evidence to suggest that the elution conditions may be too harsh for the antibody to withstand. In this situation a step gradient of elution buffers beginning with pH 7 (sodium phosphate buffer), pH 5.5 (sodium citrate buffer), and pH 4.3 (sodium citrate buffer) and ending with pH 2.3 (glycine) may provide an eluted fraction that still remains active.[9]

11.3.1.2 Antigen Antibody

Introduction: This section covers binding purified antigen to a support matrix (e.g., activated Sepharose®, magnetic beads) to be used in column chromatography for antibody purification.[10] This method requires milligram quantities of the purified antigen. One of the advantages of this method is that purification will eliminate any other immunoglobulins that do not recognize the antigen, further increasing the specificity of the purified product. This is particularly useful for improving the specificity of polyclonal antisera or ascites fluid. Because the antibody is eluted by changing the pH of the elution buffer this method is considered harsh and may lead to loss of antibody activity. Additionally, the antigen must be able to withstand the harsh elution conditions and have the ability to renature after equilibration so that you can reuse the immunoaffinity matrix. This method can be used for monoclonal antibody purification, but antibodies with low affinity to the antigen may wash off with the rest of the unbound proteins before the elution step.

Materials and solutions:

> Commercial activated resin (select from list below)*
>> Sepharose® 4B, cyanogen bromide activated (Pharmacia)
>> Affi-gel®-10 or Affi-gel®-15 (Biorad)
>
> Purified antigen
>> (approximately 2 mg of purified antigen/ml of activated resin)
>
> Binding buffer, pH 7.0
>> 0.01 *M* sodium phosphate, dibasic
>> 0.15 *M* NaCl
>> 0.01 *M* EDTA
>
> Elution buffers (Options A or B)
>> (A) 0.1 *M* glycine with 150 m*M* NaCl, pH 2.4 (adjust pH with ammonium hydroxide)
>> (B) 0.05 *M* diethylamine (pH 11.5)
>
> Neutralizing buffer (Option A or B)
>> (A) 1.0 *M* Tris-base, pH 9.0
>> (B) 1.0 *M* phosphate buffer (pH 6.8)
>
> Storage buffer
>> 100 ml binding buffer
>> 0.05% w/v sodium azide

---

* Other commercial sources may exist in addition to those listed here. The author does not recommend any one vendor.

Equipment:

Kontes Flex-column (1.5 cm × 10 cm, 18 ml bed volume)
   (Fisher Scientific, Chicago, IL)
3-way stopcock (Fisher Scientific)
Column support system, input and outlet tubing, buffer reservoir
Peristaltic pump (optional)
Fraction collector (optional)
UV spectrophotometer with UV cuvettes

Procedure:

1. Follow manufacturer's directions for binding antigen to column resin (see Reference 10 for procedure). Typically the resin will conjugate approximately 80% of the applied protein. It is important not to overload the resin. Load to a final protein concentration of 2 mg/ml bed volume.
2. Prepare a small column (4 ml). Dilute the clarified and filtered antibody solution 1:1 in binding buffer. Assume a 1:1 stoichiometry in the column's antibody binding capacity. Load an equivalent concentration of the antibody solution onto the column, in this case, approximately 8 mg of antibody.
3. Collect the column sample run through and reapply to the column two more times to optimize loading, or load at a controlled flow rate of 2 ml/h.
4. Wash the column with binding buffer (five bed volumes).
5. Elute the antibody with two column bed volumes of either 0.1 M glycine (pH 2.4) or 0.05 M diethylamine (pH 11.5). Some proteins elute better at low vs. high pH. Other elution buffers may provide better results (see Reference 12).
6. Neutralize in 1 M Tris-base (pH 9) 1/3 volume of the fraction collected for the 0.1 M glycine eluant. Neutralize in 1 M phosphate buffer (pH 6.8) at a volume of 1/20 of the fraction collected for the diethylamine eluant.

Results: It has been observed that under harsh elution conditions the yield and purity of the antibody will be good, but the antibody activity may be reduced. Under more mild elution conditions the yield may be reduced with good purity and retained antibody activity. It may be necessary to try a variety of elution conditions to optimize yield and activity for each new antibody source to be purified using the antigen-based immunoaffinity method.[11,12]

Problems: It is especially important to measure the antibody reactivity of the purified product to determine if any loss in activity has occurred during the purification. Do not overload the antigen when performing the conjugation step to the chromatography matrix. Too much antigen can result in cross-linking of the antibody to the column matrix, making it more difficult to elute the bound antibody fraction. This method does not work well for purifying monoclonal antibodies of high affinity because of the difficulty of eluting the antibody fraction. Conversely, low-affinity antibodies may not bind well to the column. Also be aware that the antigen may leach from the column as a result of the harsh elution conditions and contaminate the purified product. This could possibly be observed by SDS-PAGE of the purified product.

11.3.1.3 Thiophilic Chromatography

Introduction: Thiophilic absorbent is a modified sulfur containing silica bead that has a high affinity to all IgG subclasses in a high-salt environment (e.g., 0.5 M K_2SO_4). This method provides a fast enrichment of both monoclonal (IgG) and polyclonal antibodies (IgG and IgY — chicken), but has poor IgM binding capacity.[13–16] Purification can be completed in one step and with a high yield and good purity (20 mg goat, pig, cow IgG/ml resin, 10 mg mouse IgG/ml resin). Antibody binding occurs through sulfone and bisthioether groups on the column with phenylalanine-phenylalanine and tryptophan/tryptophan groups on the protein. The antibody is eluted in a concentrated form in low salt without the adverse effects of low pH on antibody activity that sometimes occurs during immunoaffinity chromatography elution. This method is inexpensive (e.g., Pierce, $6.50/ml resin). This column resin can also withstand pressures necessary to make it useful in HPLC columns, and the rapid binding kinetics allow for faster flow rates.[17]

Materials and solutions:

> T-gel® (Pierce, Rockford, IL) or Fractogel® EMD AFTA 650S
>   (E. Merck, Gibbstown, NJ)
> Ammonium sulfate
> Binding buffer (50 mM sodium phosphate, 0.8 M ammonium sulfate, pH 8)
> Eluting buffer (50 mM sodium phosphate, pH 8)
> Regeneration buffer (8 M guanidine HCL or 95% ethanol)
> Storage buffer (100 mM Tris-HCl, 0.05% sodium azide, pH 7.0)

Equipment:

> Kontes Flex-column (1.5 × 10 cm, 18-ml bed volume)
>   (Fisher Scientific, Chicago, IL)
> Three-way stopcock (Fisher Scientific)
> Column support system, input and outlet tubing, buffer reservoir
> UV spectrophotometer with UV cuvettes
> Fraction collector

Procedure:

1. Pour a column with one of the preceding commercial gels. The gel-bed size will depend upon the amount of antibody included in the fraction to be purified. Capacities of commercial resins range from 10 to 30 mg of IgG/ml, depending upon the species.
2. The clarified and filtered antibody fluid is adjusted to a final concentration of 0.8 M ammonium sulfate (ascites, serum, bioreactor culture fluid) or 1.2 M ammonium sulfate (static culture media) and 50 mM sodium phosphate at pH 8. This mixture is further centrifuged ($10,000 \times g$) and filtered before applying to the column.

3. Equilibrate the column in binding buffer (three column bed volumes). Load the sample onto the column at a flow rate of 1 ml/min.
4. Wash the column with the binding buffer (three column bed volumes) and then elute the bound IgG with the two column volumes of eluting buffer. Collect 20 fractions (1 ml) and monitor the IgG peak with $A_{280.}$ Calculate the protein concentration and then determine purity using SDS-PAGE.

Results: The method provides yields greater than 85% with purities comparable to immunoaffinity chromatography.[17]

Problems: The only problem foreseen with this methodology is that it does not remove the nonspecific host immunoglobulin fraction in sera and ascites fluid or the nonspecific serum immunoglobulin fraction in tissue culture media-derived antibody. The use of serum-free media would circumvent this problem with culture-derived antibodies. The use of antigen affinity columns would be an option to consider if the host immunoglobulins cause problems with nonspecific binding in ascites or polyclonal-derived antibody preparations.

11.3.2 TWO-STEP METHODS

11.3.2.1 Caprylic Acid

Introduction: Caprylic or octanoic acid, is a weak acidic buffer, and with the addition of short-chain fatty acids will precipitate most serum proteins except IgG. This method is inexpensive (e.g., Sigma, $8.00/10 ml) and a crude first step for IgG purification from serum or ascites. It is useful as an initial step in purifying IgG1, 2a, and 2b from mouse ascites, and not for IgM, Ig3 and IgA.[18–21] Additional techniques such as ammonium sulfate precipitation or anion exchange chromatography are needed to further purify the antibody fraction.

Materials and solutions:

Caprylic acid (Sigma)
60 m*M* sodium acetate (pH 4.0)
1 *M* Tris

Equipment:

Centrifuge

Procedures:

1. Add two volumes of 60 m*M* sodium acetate (pH 4) to one volume of clarified and filtered antibody fluid. Adjust the final pH of the mixture to pH 4.4 (ascites) and pH 4.8 (serum or culture fluid) with 1 *M* Tris.
2. Place the antibody fluid in a beaker with stir bar/stirring and slowly add the caprylic acid to the solution. Add 0.75 ml (caprylic acid) to 10 ml of

rabbit sera. Add 0.4 ml (caprylic acid) to 10 ml of ascites fluid and add 0.7 ml (caprylic acid) to 10 ml of goat sera.
3. Stir 2 h at room temperature.
4. Centrifuge for 15,000 × g for 30 min. Collect the supernatant and proceed to a secondary method of purification, such as ammonium sulfate precipitation or anion exchange chromatography.

Results: This method will provide yields of >80% with a purity level of immunoglobulin at approximately 50%. This method takes approximately 3 h to perform.

Problems: Other high molecular weight proteins such as albumin will contaminate the final product including the host immunoglobulins that are not specific to your antigen. This nonspecific host fraction can make up approximately 90 to 99% of the immunoglobulin purified. Antigen-affinity chromatography can be performed to remove this nonspecific fraction, if background binding remains high in the assay of choice after purification.

11.3.2.2 Ammonium Sulfate Precipitation

Introduction: This method is useful as a second step following caprylic acid precipitation negative selection method or as a first step prior to anion exchange chromatography for purifying antibody from serum and ascites fluid.[1,2,12] The high-salt concentration (i.e., small and highly ionic molecules) used in this method removes water molecules that interact with antibodies, thus decreasing the solubility of the proteins and leading to protein precipitation. Various concentrations of ammonium salt precipitate out different proteins depending upon their size and charge (as well as species of origin, fluid type, pH, temperature, and the number and position of polar groups on the protein). Typically the clarified antibody solution is mixed with a saturated ammonium sulfate solution to a 45% volume/volume ratio. Precipitation occurs for over a period of 2 h in the cold. The precipitate is resuspended in PBS and desalted via gel filtration, dialysis against PBS, or filter centrifugation. The antibody solution is then concentrated. This is an inexpensive method to perform (Sigma, $32.25/500 g).

Materials and solutions: Saturated ammonium sulfate solution: Mix 385 g of ultra-high pure ammonium sulfate with 500 ml of water. Heat to just below 100°C and let stir for 30 min with the heat off. Cool and store the solution at 4°C, using the clear solution on top as needed.

Centrifuge tubes (Corex®)
Ice
Clarified delipidized ascites, serum, or culture supernatant
Dialysis tubing (MWCO 12-14,000 Spectra/Por®, Los Angeles, CA)
Centricon® Plus 20 (Millipore Corp., Beverly, MA)

Equipment:

High-speed centrifuge (Sorval)
Stir plate

Procedures:

1. Pool the clarified and filtered antibody solutions and measure the final volume.
2. Place the fluid in a beaker and with stirring add dropwise a volume of saturated ammonium sulfate solution equivalent to a final volume of 40% saturated solution for rabbit and 45% saturated solution for other species. The saturated solution should be at 4°C and pH adjusted to 7.4 with ammonium hydroxide.
3. Transfer solution to high-speed centrifuge tubes, taking care to balance the tubes and set on ice for 2 h.
4. Centrifuge at $10,000 \times g$ (30 min) at 4°C.
5. Resuspend the pellets in 1/4 the original volume of the pooled antibody fluids in 5 mM sodium phosphate (pH 6.5).
6. Remove the residual ammonium sulfate salts using a Centricon® Plus 20 filter (19 ml capacity) with a molecular weight cutoff of 100,000. Place the solution in the filter unit above the test tube and centrifuge at $3000 \times g$ for 30 to 60 min in a swinging bucket rotor. Add the appropriate diluent for buffer exchange for the next step in the purification process.
7. Alternative methods for desalting include dialysis (three buffer changes with at least 4 h between changes against 1 L of 5 mM sodium phosphate, pH 6.5) or gel filtration chromatography.[9] These alternative methods also require a filter concentration step that will add another day to the time required to complete this method.

Results: This method will provide yields of >80% with a purity level of immuno-globulin at approximately 50%. This method takes 8 h for precipitation, desalting and concentration (via Centricon filter centrifugation).

Problems: Other high molecular weight proteins will contaminate the final product including the host immunoglobulins that are not specific to your antigen. This nonspecific host fraction can make up approximately 90 to 99% of the immunoglo-bulin purified. Antigen-affinity chromatography can be performed to remove this nonspecific fraction, if background binding remains high in the assay of choice after purification. This method doesn't work well in serum-free culture media because of the low level of protein.

11.3.2.3 Anion Exchange Chromatography

Introduction: This method is meant to be used as a secondary step in the purification process. Anion exchange chromatography separates proteins on the basis of surface charge. Proteins electrostatically bind onto a matrix bearing the opposite charge.

Typically, these bound proteins are eluted by a change in the pH or an increase the concentration of the buffered salt. Anion exchange resin [e.g., DEAE (dimethylaminoethyl) cellulose/Sepharose®)] can be used for positive (column chromatography) or negative (batch chromatography) selection of antibody.[1]

Antibodies have basic isoelectric points when compared to most of the proteins in serum. During the batch method, lowering the pH will prevent the antibodies from binding the resin, providing a negative selection for antibodies in batch quantities. An increase of the pH of the antibody solution will facilitate antibody binding to the column (positive column selection method). Initially, the antibody is purified using caprylic acid precipitation or ammonium sulfate precipitation (for IgG, see Section 11.3.2.1 or 11.3.2.2). This method is inexpensive (e.g., Sigma, $44.25/50 ml) and approximately 2 ml of resin is required for 1 ml of serum. Conditions for negative selection are 70 mM sodium phosphate buffer (pH 6.3) for rabbit, 20 mM sodium phosphate buffer (pH 8) for human, and 20 mM sodium phosphate buffer (pH 7.5) for goat.[2,12] Positive selection conditions for mouse and rat IgG binding occur at pH 8 and are then eluted in a linear gradient of 0 to 300 mM NaCl.

Batch method: A batch method for negative selection of antibodies is outlined by Harlow and Lane.[1] In brief, the anion exchange Sepharose® is equilibrated to pH 6.3 (for rabbit serum purification) and pH 7.5 (for serum purification) in sodium phosphate buffer and mixed with antibody solution (dialyzed to an equivalent pH). The mixture incubates on a rocker for 1 h and the slurry is filtered, collecting the antibody in the flow through. This method has a lower yield but a fast processing time.

Column method (DEAE anion exchange): Used in combination with ammonium sulfate precipitation (Section 11.3.2.2), this method will yield a relatively pure antibody preparation at a moderate cost. The antibody solution is adjusted to pH 9 and loaded onto a DEAE column. The antibody is eluted with a high salt (less than 0.5 M NaCl) and the fractions are collected and monitored for protein measuring the absorbance at 280 nm (OD = 1 is roughly 0.8 mg/ml). This method is useful for eliminating albumins from the antibody preparation.

Materials and solutions:

    HiTrap™ Q columns, 5 ml capacity (Pharmacia Biotech)
    Start buffer (20 mM Tris, pH 9)
    Regeneration buffer (20 mM Tris, 1 M NaCl, pH 9)
    Elution buffer (20 mM Tris, 0.2 M NaCl, pH 9)

Equipment:

    Fraction collector
    Peristaltic pump (optional)
    FPLC (optional)
    Gradient-making unit (optional)
    UV spectrophotometer

Procedure:

1. Fill a 50-ml syringe with start buffer. Remove the stopper and make the connection between the column and the syringe (Luer-lock adapter) such that no air is introduced into the column.
2. Remove the twist-off end on the column.
3. Wash the column with five column bed volumes of start buffer at a flow rate of no more than 5 ml/min for the 5-ml column to avoid compacting the column.
4. Wash the column with five column bed volumes of regeneration buffer.
5. Equilibrate the column with five column volumes of start buffer.
6. Sample should be dialyzed (three buffer changes) or filter centrifuged (Centricon®) to exchange the buffer to the start buffer prior to loading onto the column. Load the sample onto the column (capacity 25 mg/ml of column bed volume). Use a slow flow rate of 2 ml/min during the loading process. Multiple columns can be linked together for an antibody capacity of greater than 125 mg (one-column capacity).
7. Wash the column with 10 column bed volumes of start buffer.
8. Elute the antibody sample with five column bed volumes of elution buffer. The eluted fractions are collected in separate tubes, and a protein assay (UV absorbance or colorimetric assay) is performed on each fraction to determine the fractions that contain protein.
9. Adjust the pH of the pooled antibody fractions to 7.0 using 1 N HCl. Concentrate if necessary (1 to 10 mg/ml optimal concentration) and aliquot the purified antibody into usable quantities, label, and freeze. Store antibody at $-70°C$.
10. Regenerate the column for reuse by washing the column with five column bed volumes of regeneration buffer followed by five column bed volumes of start buffer. The columns are stored in 20% ethanol at 4°C after equilibration. Seal the stopper and the dome nut.

Results: Purity of the antibody, when using this method as a secondary purification step, should approach greater than 95%. These columns may be connected to a peristaltic pump or FPLC system for controlled and faster flow rates.

Anion exchange resins are available from many commercial sources and columns can be poured in-house. If you choose this route, it is important to know the binding capacity of the purchased resins to optimize the loading conditions of the column.

Problems: It may be necessary to optimize the pH for binding and the salt concentration for elution. Optimal binding can be monitored by looking for nonbound antibody during the sample loading (sample flow through) fraction on an SDS-PAGE. In the column method, a high pH is used during the loading process and a high salt concentration is used to perform a single elution step. A stepwise elution or gradient elution will allow for more control in the separation of antibody from proteins with similar isoelectric charges. Be aware that endotoxins and DNA phosphate residues can bind to DEAE anion exchange columns leading to contamination of the eluted antibody fractions in a positive selection. During a negative selection batch process, these components can be removed from the antibody fraction.

This method is not recommended for IgM purification, as the antibody may form precipitates on the column and generate an unpredictable column runoff pattern. There is also evidence that anion exchange chromatography can significantly reduce the antibody reactivity of murine IgM.[22]

11.4 PURIFICATION OF IgM

11.4.1 ONE-STEP METHOD USING AFFINITY CHROMATOGRAPHY

11.4.1.1 Protein L or Mannan Binding

Protein L binds equally well to the light chain of IgM and can be useful as a one-step method for purifying this mouse isotype. Follow the procedure outlined in Section 11.3.1.1.[5]

Mannan-binding protein (MBP) is a lectin specific to mannose and N-acetylglucosamine in mammalian sera. These binding characteristics have made it useful as a ligand in chromatography for mouse IgM purification[23,24] and purities of at least 95% have been observed following this method. This method has been outlined by Andrew et al.[25] including the appropriate buffer recipes. The immobilized MBP (Cat. No. 22212) can be purchased from Pierce, Rockford, IL at a 1999 catalog price of $695 for 10 ml of resin. The cost of this resin may make this method impractical for some researchers. However, the method provides a fast one-step method with excellent final purity and yield.

11.4.1.2 Anti-Antibody

Anti-IgM (mouse) covalently linked to agarose is available commercially for use in affinity chromatography of mouse IgM. Typically, an immunoaffinity column of this type will have 5 to 10 mg of IgG covalently attached to 1 ml of resin. The IgM binding capacity is then approximately 10% or 0.5 to 1 mg/ml of resin. Keep these values in mind should you decide to prepare your own affinity matrix using a purified anti-IgM antibody source and cyanogen bromide-activated Sepharose® (Pharmacia). Follow the manufacturer's recommendation for attaching the antibody to the resin, or see Reference 10.

Materials:

Commercial anti-IgM resins or in-house prepared resins.*
Goat anti-mouse IgM-Agarose (Sigma No. A-4540)
Buffers

---

* Other commercial sources may exist in addition to those listed here. The author does not recommend any one vendor.

Binding buffer, pH 7.2
   0.01 M sodium phosphate, dibasic
   0.5 M NaCl
Elution buffer, pH 2.4 (adjust pH with ammonium hydroxide)
   0.5 M acetic acid (14.37 ml glacial acetic acid + 485.63 ml H_2O) with 150
      mM NaCl
   or
   0.1 M glycine with 150 mM NaCl
Neutralizing buffer, pH 9.0
   1.0 M Tris
Storage buffer
   100 ml binding buffer
   0.01% v/v thimerosal

Procedure:

1. Prepare a 2-ml column bed volume and equilibrate the column by washing with four column volumes of binding buffer. Dilute the clarified and filtered antibody solution 1:1 in binding buffer and apply to the column.
2. Collect the column sample run through and reapply to the column two more times to optimize loading or load at a controlled flow rate of 2 ml/h.
3. Wash the column with binding buffer (five bed volumes).
4. Elute the antibody with two column volumes of either 0.1 M glycine (pH 2.4) or 0.5 M acetic acid solution.
5. Neutralize in 1 M Tris-base (pH 9) 1/3 volume of the fraction collected for the acidic eluant.
6. Collect the eluted fractions in separate tubes and perform a protein assay (UV absorbance or colorimetric assay) on each fraction to determine the fractions that contain protein.
7. Pool the antibody fractions and concentrate if necessary (1 to 10 mg/ml optimal concentration). Aliquot the purified antibody into usable quantities, label, and freeze. Store antibody at $-70°C$.
8. Regenerate the column for reuse by washing the column with ten column volumes of elution buffer followed by five column volumes of binding buffer. Replace the binding buffer with storage buffer and place at 4°C.

Results: It has been observed that under harsh elution conditions, the yield and purity of the antibody will be good, but the antibody activity may be reduced. Under more mild elution conditions, the yield may be reduced with good purity and retained antibody activity. It may be necessary to try a variety of elution conditions to optimize yield and activity for each new antibody source to be purified using the antigen-based immunoaffinity method.[11,12,26]

Problems: It is especially important to measure the antibody reactivity of the purified product to determine if any loss in activity has occurred during the purification.

11.4.2 TWO-STEP METHODS

11.4.2.1 Ammonium Sulfate Precipitation

This method is a common first step in IgM purification. Follow the procedure outlined in Section 11.3.2.2. Yield (>80%) and purity (<50%) are similar to that observed with IgG purification.

11.4.2.2 Gel Exclusion Chromatography

Introduction: Gel exclusion chromatography separates proteins on the basis of molecular size using porous beads of cross-linked dextran or agarose. A molecular sieve of a defined pore size sifts for the molecular weight range of interest. This method may be considered as a secondary step in a two-step purification of IgM with ammonium sulfate precipitation or ultracentrifugation as the primary first step.[27] Keep in mind the column capacity will be low, resulting in a final product that is dilute. Because a neutral wash buffer is used to elute the antibody, there are no deleterious effects on the antibody activity. This method is inexpensive (Sigma, Sephadex G-200, $33.50/10 g; bed volume 20 to 30 ml/g), but time consuming.

Materials and solutions:

> Sepharose® 6B or Sephacryl® S-300 (Pharmacia)
> Binding buffer, pH 7.2
> 0.01 *M* sodium phosphate, dibasic
> 0.5 *M* NaCl

Equipment:

> Konte Flex-column (2.5 cm × 20 cm approximate 100 ml bed volume)
> Column support system, input and outlet tubing, buffer reservoir
> UV spectrophotometer with cuvettes
> Fraction collector
> Peristaltic pump (optional)

Procedures:

1. Prepare column according to manufacturer's directions. For a good reference on column preparation, also see *Current Protocols in Immunology* (Appendix A.3I.1).[25] Column size must be poured to accommodate a sample volume that is not more than 5% of the total column volume. Keep flow rates within the range recommended for the gel (e.g., Sepharose® is a soft gel used with gravity flow; Sephacryl® is a more rigid gel that can be used with a peristaltic pump).
2. Wash the column in binding buffer and remove the liquid to the top of the gel bed. Load the clarified sample (<5 ml) onto the top of the column bed and establish column flow (1 ml/min).

3. Collect 100 (1 ml) fractions and measure the A_{280} nm ($A \times 0.84 = X$ mg/ml IgM). IgM will be the first peak to elute from the column. Verify the fractions that contain IgM using SDS-gel electrophoresis or antibody titer assay and then pool those fractions. Light chain will migrate to 25 kDa and the heavy chain will migrate to 78 kDa on SDS-PAGE.
4. Concentrate using centrifugation and the Centricon® Plus 20 filters MWCO 100,000 ($3000 \times g$, 30 min).

Results: When this method is used as a secondary purification step, it provides a good yield of IgM (>80%), good purity (>95%) with nominal effects on antibody activity.

Problems: Precipitation of IgM during gel filtration will result in retention of the IgM fraction on the column. If this occurs, it may be necessary to add 10 mM CHAPS or 100 mM imidazole to the binding buffer to enhance the solubility of the antibody.[27] The product that is collected from the column will be in a dilute form and requires concentration prior to storage.

11.5 PURIFICATION OF IgY (CHICKEN YOLK)

Introduction: Eggs from immunized chickens can be stored at 4°C for up to a year without loss of antibody and provide an economical means for making polyclonal antibody. Ammonium sulfate precipitation has been found to be the most useful primary step in the purification of antibody from yolks collected from an immunized chicken in terms of yield, purity, and activity when compared to precipitation methods that utilize polyethylene glycol 6000 or caprylic acid.[28,29] This method can be followed with secondary methods of purification, if necessary, including thiophilic chromatography, Protein L, or antigen affinity chromatography as outlined in the previous sections. This method has been adapted from Reference 29.

Materials and solutions:

Ammonium sulfate
3 mM HCl (cold)
Centrifuge tubes (Corex® or polycarbonate)
Egg yolks separated from the whites and washed with distilled water
Ice
Dialysis tubing (MWCO 12 to 14,000 Spectra/Por®, Los Angeles)
Centricon® Plus 20 100,000 MWCO (Millipore, Beverly, MA)

Equipment:

High-speed centrifuge
Stir plate

Procedures:

1. Disrupt the yolk sac and collect the yolk fluid in a graduated cylinder to measure the volume.
2. Dilute the yolk with 10 volumes of 3 mM Hcl (cold) and adjust the final pH to 5 (with 10% acetic acid). Incubate this solution for 6 h or longer at 4°C. This ensures the antibody fraction will be found in the aqueous portion of the yolk.
3. Centrifuge the yolk solution (14,000 × g for 20 min at 4°C), collecting the supernatant.
4. Place the fluid in a beaker, add solid ammonium sulfate to a final molarity of 1.75 M and stir at 4°C for 1 h.
5. Transfer this solution to high-speed centrifuge tubes, taking care to balance the tubes and centrifuge at 14000 × g (20 min) at 4°C. The pellet is then washed once with 1.75 M ammonium sulfate solution.
6. Resuspend the pellets in 50 mM sodium phosphate (pH 7.5) to a volume equivalent to the original egg yolk volume.
7a. Remove the residual ammonium sulfate salts by using the Centricon® Plus 20 filters and centrifugation at (3000 × g for 30 min). Proceed with affinity chromatography as required (see Section 11.3.1.1–2).
7b. Adjust the ammonium sulfate concentration to 0.8 M and proceed with thiophilic chromatography (see Section 11.3.1.3) if additional purification is required.[29]

Results: This method will provide yields of >80% with a purity level of immunoglobulin at approximately 50%. This method takes one full day (10 h) for precipitation, desalting, and concentration. The antigen-specific IgY fraction makes up approximately 1% of the total IgY.[29]

Problems: Other high molecular weight proteins will contaminate the final product, including the host immunoglobulins that are not specific to your antigen. This nonspecific host fraction can make up approximately 90 to 99% of the immunoglobulin purified. Antigen-affinity chromatography can be performed to remove this nonspecific fraction if background binding remains high in the assay of choice after purification.

11.6 OTHER METHODS

11.6.1 HYDROPHOBIC INTERACTION CHROMATOGRAPHY

Hydrophobic interaction chromatography (HIC) is similar to the approach of reverse phase chromatography utilizing aqueous rather than organic solvents. The antibody solution is placed in a high-salt buffer (20% saturated ammonium sulfate) to facilitate binding of hydrophobic domains in the protein structure to the column matrix of derivatized hydrocarbons. The salt concentration is reduced with a gradient to elute the antibody. An advantage to this method is minimal disruption of the antibody structure and function. This method removes endotoxins, viral particles, and nucleic acids and is invaluable in antibody production. However, since HIC does not separate albumin from immunoglobulins a preliminary ammonium sulfate precipitation may be needed. HIC's disadvantage is the variable interaction between monoclonal antibodies and the matrices. If the antibody binding to the column is too strong, the elution conditions may cause a loss of antibody activity. Thus, the optimal column derivatization for the isolation of a specific monoclonal antibody must be determined empirically. (HIC materials can be obtained from Parmacia [e.g., Source TM 15ETH and other derivatives; phenyl Sepharose® high performance HiTrap™].) If albumin is present, this method does not work well to separate albumin from the immunoglobulin fraction. Ammonium sulfate precipitation works well as a preliminary step prior to using the method. Sources of HIC materials include Pharmacia (SourceTM 15ETH and other derivatives), also available as Phenyl Sepharose® High Performance HiTrap™ columns from Pharmacia, and invaluable from a production standpoint for antibody use as bioagents because of the removal of endotoxins, virus particles, and nucleic acids. Disadvantages of this method include the variable interaction with the matrices between monoclonal. Antibody binding can be too strong and a loss of antibody activity may be observed upon elution. One must try a variety of column derivatizations to find the right affinity for each monoclonal.[2,12]

11.6.2 Liquid Polymer Precipitation

Methods have been documented in the literature which demonstrate polymer specific precipitation of antibody fractions from a variety of samples.[30] For example, PEG 6000, at a volume/volume percent of 4 to 6% can be used to precipitate murine IgM from delipidized ascites fluid (>90% pure, >80% yield). This method requires a second step of purification (e.g., ion exchange) if you are using the antibodies for ELISA to remove interfering polymers. There also tends to be variability in the purity and yield documented with this method.[2]

11.6.3 Hydroxylapatite Chromatography

This method has been used to process bulk amounts of antibody into a concentrated form in buffers that do not require post-purification dialysis. Antibodies are eluted with increasing concentrations of salt in wash buffer (120 to 300 mM PBS, pH 6.8). This method has been shown to provide a good yield and purity from ascites and sera, but has not been useful for tissue culture because of the contaminating sera immunoglobulin components.[2] As with the other column chromatography methods, this procedure is time consuming but inexpensive (Sigma, $29.10/100 ml). Typically, purification of 5.0 ml of sera will require the use of 100 ml of hydroxyapatite.

11.6.4 Continuous Flow Centrifugation and Tangential Flow Filtration

Very large-scale production of antibodies from cell culture media utilizes continuous flow centrifugation (>100 L/h capacity) to remove cells and debris. A secondary step involves the use of cross flow or tangential flow filtration devices (see Pall Corp. at http://www.pall.com) to concentrate large volume of cell culture product with reduced fouling of the membrane filter surface.[2] Pall's Mini-Ultrasette™ device can filter 100 ml to 1 L volumes with variable molecular weight cutoff pore sizes available. Flow rates can approach 5 to 8 ml/min for immunoglobulin concentration.

11.7 FINAL PRODUCT

11.7.1 YIELD AND PURITY

The use of gel electrophoresis will allow determination of non-immunoglobulin contamination of the final product. However, be aware that polyclonal sera and mouse ascites fluid will also include nonspecific immunoglobulins unless antigen-specific affinity purification was performed. In these cases, these can represent anywhere from 10 to 50% of the purified fraction. Also, tissue culture supernatant and bioreactor products can be contaminated with serum supplement immunoglobulins unless serum-free media are utilized.

11.7.1.1 SDS-PAGE

This gel electrophoresis method is useful for determining the purity of the antibody product with IgG providing 2 bands (25 and 55 kDa) and IgM (25 and 78 kDa). This method is adapted from Reference 31 and the Bio-Rad MiniPROTEAN® II instruction manual.

Materials and solutions:

MiniPROTEAN® II ready gel (12% acrylamide, Tris-HCl, Bio-Rad)
SDS-PAGE molecular weight standards (Bio-Rad)
Sample Buffer

Deionized water	3.8 ml
0.5 *M* Tris-HCl, pH 6.8	1.0 ml
Glycerol	0.8 ml
10% (w/v) SDS	1.6 ml
1% (w/v) bromophenol blue	0.4 ml
Total	7.6 ml

5× run buffer, pH 8.3

Tris base	15.1 g
Glycine	94.0 g
SDS	5.0 g

Bring to 1000 ml with water and store at 4°C.

1× run buffer
Dilute 80 mL of 5X with 320 ml of deionized water.

Coomassie blue:
    0.1% Coomassie blue-R-250
    40% methanol
    10% acetic acid
Destain
    40% methanol
    10% acetic acid

Equipment:

MiniPROTEAN® gel electrophoresis system (Bio-Rad)
Power Supply

Procedure:

1. Assemble the mini gel system and fill the upper chamber with 1× run buffer (115 ml).
2. Pour about 250 ml of the run buffer into the lower chamber to cover the bottom of the gel by at least 1 cm. Remove air bubbles that may have become trapped at the base of the gel by swirling a pipet along the bottom of the gel.
3. Prepare the protein samples, including the standards by diluting 1:4 in sample buffer and heating at 100°C for 3 min. Add 1/20th volume of 2-mercaptoethanol to the sample buffer prior to mixing with the samples.
4. Remove the comb from the gel and load the samples into individual wells. Loading 1 µg/well of the purified protein and 1 µg for each band of the standards will yield a readily visible band after staining. The load volume is kept at 5 µl/well. Leave the outer lanes open for loading the protein standards.
5. Place the lid on the electrophoresis system and attach the positive and negative electrodes from the power supply (matching red to red and black to black).
6. Turn on the power supply using 200 volts constant voltage setting. Run the gel for approximately 45 min or until the blue dye front has traveled to the bottom portion of the gel. The current should drop as the change in buffer ions in the gel causes increased resistance in the gel.
7. Remove the gel from the apparatus and carefully remove the two plastic plates that sandwich the gel, notching the corner to allow orientation of the gel front and back faces. Stain for 1 h in Coomassie blue and destain with several changes to allow visualization of the blue protein bands (approximately 1 to 3 h).

11.7.1.2 Quantitative ELISA (Mouse IgG)

Materials and solutions:

96-well Immulon®-3 plate (Dynatech)
P-200 micropipettor with tips

Vacuum aspirator
Paper towels
Timer, vortex mixer, etc.
12 × 75 mm polypropylene test tubes
Solutions
    PBS with 0.1% Tween (in 1-L wash bottle)
    PBS with 0.5% BSA
Coating
    Goat anti-mouse Fc (5 µg/ml) in bicarbonate buffer, pH 9.5 (Sigma)
    Mouse IgG (400 ng/ml) in PBS-BSA (ICN Biochemical, Costa Mesa, CA)
    Pre- and post-purification antibody IgG sample in PBS-BSA (serial dilutions from 1:10 to 1:1,000,000)
Enzyme conjugates
    Rat anti-mouse kappa-HRP (1:4000) in PBS with 0.5% BSA (Southern Biotech/Fisher)

ABTS substrate:	0.1 M citric acid (2 ml)
	0.2 M sodium phosphate (2 ml)
	Distilled water (4 ml)
	30% hydrogen peroxide (3 µl)
	ABTS 1 tab; prepare just before use
	Total (8 ml)

Unknown samples (1:10 serial dilution):
1. For each unknown set, up 6 tubes labeled 1:10, 1:100, 1:1000, 1:10,000, 1:100,000, and 1:1,000,000.
2. Add 180 µl of PBS–BSA to each tube.
3. Transfer 20 µl of each unknown to the tube labeled 1:10.
4. Mix and transfer 20 µl to the next tube.
5. Repeat step 4 for the remaining tubes.

IgG Standard (preparation):
1. Dissolve the 1 mg of purified IgG in PBS–BSA. Aliquot in 10 µl volumes and freeze (–70°C) remaining stock for future assays.
2. Dilute 4 µl of IgG stock into 10 ml of PBS–BSA (400 ng/ml).
3. Set up 6 tubes labeled 200, 100, 50, 25, 12.5, and 6.25.
4. Add 200 µl of PBS–BSA to each tube.
5. Transfer 200 µl of 400 ng/ml IgG to the tube labeled 200.
6. Mix and transfer 200 µl to the next tube.
7. Repeat step 5 for the remaining tubes.

Procedure:

1. Add 50 µl of anti-Fc (5 µg/ml) to each well and incubate for 1 h at room temperature. The use of bicarbonate buffer at pH 9.5 promotes binding of capture antibody to the plate.
2. Use phosphate-buffered saline at pH 7.4 with 0.1% Tween-20 (PBST) to remove unbound protein.
   (a) Aspirate the fluid from each well of the plate.

(b) Flood all the wells with PBST and wait 15 s.

(c) Shake out the wash fluid and pat the plate dry on paper towels.
Repeat steps (b) and (c) two more times.

3. Add 200 μl PBS-BSA to all the wells and incubate 10 min. PBS with 0.5% bovine serum albumin (BSA) blocks nonspecific protein binding sites remaining in the wells.

4. Prepare the serial dilutions for step 6.

5. Aspirate the blocking solution from the wells.

6. Following the map outlined below, add 50 μl of the appropriate solution to the appropriate well and incubate for 1 h at room temperature.

Standard	Pre-purification	Post-purification
Well no. 1, 2	3, 4	5, 6
PBS–BSA	Undiluted	Undiluted
6.25 ng/ml	1:10	1:10
12.5 ng/ml	1:100	1:100
25.0 ng/ml	1:1000	1:1000
50.0 ng/ml	1:10,000	1:10,000
100 ng/ml	1:100,000	1:100,000
200 ng/ml	1:1,000,000	1:1,000,000
400 ng/ml	PBS–BSA	PBS–BSA

7. Repeat the washing steps in 2.

8. Add 50 μl anti-mouse Kappa-HRP (1:4000) to each well and incubate for 1 h at room temperature.

9. Repeat the washing steps in 2.

10. Add 50 μl substrate solution to each well and incubate for 30 min at room temperature or until visible blue color can be observed. Measure the absorbance at 405 nm. See Figure 11.1 for represented data from an assay standard curve.

The following equations can be useful for comparing antibody yield based upon the antibody concentration using this capture ELISA method between the original and purified product.

Original Volume (ml) × Antibody Concentration = Total Antibody Concentration
[Example: 10 ml Bioreactor fluid × 1 mg/ml = 10 mg mouse IgG total]

Final Volume (ml) × Antibody Concentration = Final Antibody Concentration
[Example: 1 ml solution × 9 mg/ml = 9 mg mouse IgG total (loss in yield = 10%)]

11.7.2 SPECIFIC ACTIVITY (ELISA ASSAY/TITRATION)

Antibody titer is defined as the highest dilution that still allows observation of an antigen detection signal in the assay. A titration assay using ELISA with purified antigen as the coating layer is a common method for determining the level of enrichment in the antibody solution after purification. Samples of pre- and post-purification antibody are used in a serial dilution on replicate wells coated with

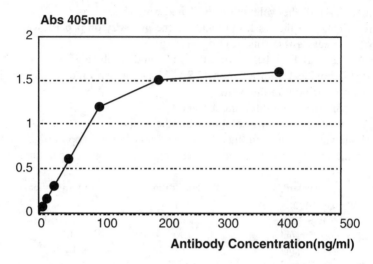

FIGURE 11.1 Mouse IgG ELISA (Standard Curve).

antigen to determine the antibody titer before and after purification. Alternatively, antibody titer can be evaluated using a dot-blot analysis, immunofluorescence assay (IFA), antibody neutralization of virus, or other methods that provide relevant information on the antibody's ability to bind antigen.

11.7.3 STORAGE

For long-term storage of purified antibody, the best scenario is in the freezer at –20°C or at –70°C (further reduces protease activity). Store the antibody at a neutral pH and at a concentration of 1 to 10 mg/ml. Use a rapid dry-ice methanol bath to freeze, and this will reduce the formation of antibody precipitation. Freeze-drying can cause aggregate formation and should be avoided. Avoid repeated freezing and thawing, as the antibody molecule, especially IgM, will denature and/or aggregate. You can add 0.05 to 0.1% sodium azide as a bactericidal agent and store at 4°C for long periods, assuming no protease activity exists. Be aware that sodium azide can have detrimental effects on alkaline phosphatase activity. Thimerosal can be used in place of azide as a bactericide. The additional precaution of filtering through a 0.2-μm membrane will also reduce microorganism growth. IgM antibodies may precipitate out in solution and can be re-dissolved with the addition of more salt to the diluent (i.e., NaCl, if PBS is used). Antibodies that have been conjugated can be stored at –20°C in a 50% glycerol solution.

REFERENCES

1. Harlow, E. and Lane, D., 1988, *Antibodies: A Laboratory Manual*, Cold Spring Harbor Laboratory, Cold Spring Harbor, NY.
2. Mohr, P., Holtzhauer, M., and Kaiser, M., 1992, Separation and purification of antibody, hapten and antigen, *Immunosorption Techniques: Fundamentals and Applications*, Akademie Verlag, Berlin, 66–101.

3. Boyle, M.D.P., Ed., *Bacterial Immunoglobulin-binding Proteins*, Vol. 1, 1990, and Vol. 2, 1991.

4. Bjorck, L. and Kronvall, G., 1984, Purification and some properties of streptococcal protein G, a novel IgG binding reagent, *J. Immunol. Meth.*, 133, 969–974.

5. Nilson, B.H.K., Logdberg, L., Kastern, W., Bjorck, L., and Akerstrom, B., 1993, Purification of antibodies using protein L-binding framework structures in the light chain variable domain, *J. Immunol. Meth.*, 164, 33–40.

6. Bjorck, L., 1988, Protein L, a novel bacterial cell wall protein with affinity for Ig L chains, *J. Immunol.*, 140, 1194–1197.

7. Akerstom, B. and Bjorck, L., 1989, Protein L: a light chain-binding bacterial protein, *J. Biol. Chem.*, 264, 19740–19746.

8. Godfrey, M.A.J., Kwasowski, P., Cliff, R., and Marks, V., 1992, A sensitive enzyme linked immunoassay (ELISA) for the detection of staphylococcal protein A (SpA) present as a trace contaminant of murine immunoglobulins purified on immobilized protein A, *J. Immunol. Meth.*, 149, 21–27.

9. Andrew, S.M. and Titus, J.A., 1997, Purification of immunoglobulin G, in *Current Protocols in Immunology*, Coligan, J.E., Kruisbeek, A.M., Margulies, D.H., Shevach, E.M., and Strober, W., Eds., John Wiley & Sons, New York, 2.7.1–2.7.12.

10. Delves, P.J., 1995, Affinity chromatography, in *Antibody Applications*, John Wiley & Sons, West Essex, U.K., 87–93.

11. Tsang, V.C.W. and Wilkins, P.P., 1991, Optimum dissociation condition for immunoaffinity and preferential isolation of antibodies with high specific activity, *J. Immunol. Meth.*, 138, 291–299.

12. Kerr, M.A. and Thorpe, R., 1994, Purification of immunoglobulins, in *Immunochemistry LABFAX*, Academic Press, New York, 83–114.

13. Belew, M., Juntti, N., Larsson, A., and Porath, J., 1987, A one-step purification method for monoclonal antibodies based on salt-promoted adsorption chromatography on a 'thiophilic' adsorbent, *J. Immnol. Meth.*, 102, 173–182.

14. Oscarsson, S., Chaga, G., and Porath, J., 1991, Thiophilic adsorbents for RIA and ELISA procedures, *J. Immnol. Meth.*, 143, 143–149.

15. Bog-Hansen, T.C., 1995, Separation of monoclonal antibody from cell culture supernatants and ascites fluid using thiophilic agarose, in *Monoclonal Antibody Protocols*, Vol. 45, Davis, W.C., Ed., Methods in Molecular Biology, Humana Press, Totowa, NJ.

16. Lihme, A. and Heegaard, P.M.H., 1991, Thiophilic adsorption chromatography: the separation of serum proteins, *J. Immunol. Meth.*, 192, 64–69.

17. Nopper, B., Kohen, F., and Wilchek, M., 1989, A thiophilic adsorbent for the one-step high performance liquid chromatography purification of monoclonal antibody, *Anal. Biochem.*

18. Russo, C., Callegaro, L., Lanza, E., and Ferrone, S., 1983, Purification of IgG monoclonal antibody by caprylic acid precipitation, *J. Immunol. Meth.*, 65, 269.

19. Temponi, M., Kekish, U., and Ferrone, S., 1988, Immunoreactivity and affinity of murine IgG monoclonal antibodies purified by caprylic acid precipitation, *J. Immunol. Meth.*, 115, 151–152.

20. Ogden, J.R. and Leung, K., 1988, Purification of murine monoclonal antibodies by caprylic acid, *J. Immunol. Meth.*, 111, 283–284.

21. Temponi, M., Kagenshita, T., Persosa, F., Ono, R., Okada, H., and Ferrone, S., 1989, Purification of murine IgG monoclonal antibodies by precipitation with caprylic acid: comparison with other methods of purification, *Hybridoma*, 8, 85–95.

22. Knutson, V.P., Buck, R.A., and Moreno, R.M., 1991, Purification of murine monoclonal antibody of the IgM class, *J. Immunol. Meth.*, 136, 151–157.

23. Nevens, J.R., Mallia, A.K., Wendt, M.W., and Smith, P.K., 1992, Affinity chromatographic purification of immunoglobulin M antibodies utilizing immobilized mannan binding protein, *J. Chromatogr.*, 597, 247–256.

24. Ohta, M., Okada, M., Yamashina, I., and Kawaski, T., 1990, The mechanism of carbohydrate-mediated complement activation of mannan-binding protein, *J. Biol. Chem.*, 265, 1980–1984.

25. Andrew, S.M., Titus, J.A., Coico, R., and Amin, A., 1997, Purification of immunoglobulin M and immunoglobulin D, in *Current Protocols in Immunology*, Coligan, J.E., Kruisbeek, A.M., Margulies, D.H., Shevach, E.M., and Strober, W., Eds., John Wiley & Sons, New York, 2.9.3–2.9.4.

26. Quitadamo, I.J. and Schelling, M.E., 1998, Efficient purification of mouse anti-FCF receptor IgM monoclonal antibody by magnetic beads.

27. Roggenbuck, D., Marx, U., Kiessig, S.T., Schoenherr, G., Jahn, S., and Porstmann, T., 1994, Purification and immunochemical characterization of a natural human polyreactive monoclonal IgM antibody, *J. Immunol. Meth.*, 167, 207–218.

28. Svendsen, L., Crowley, A., Ostergaard, L.H., Stodulski, G., and Hau, J., 1995, Development and comparison of purification strategies for chicken antibodies from egg yolk, *Lab. Anim. Sci.,* 45, 89–93.

29. Hansen, P., Scoble, J.A., Hanson, B., and Hoogenraad, N.J., 1998, Isolation and purification of immunoglobulins from chicken eggs using thiophilic interaction chromatography, *J. Immunol. Meth.*, 215, 1–7.

30. Neoh, S.H., Gordon, C., Potter, A., and Zola, H., 1986, The purification of mouse monoclonal antibodies from ascitic fluid, *J. Immunol. Meth.*, 91, 231–236.

31. Sambrook, J., Fritsch, E.F., and Maniatis, T., 1989, Detection and analysis of proteins expressed from cloned genes, in *Molecular Cloning: A Laboratory Manual*, Cold Spring Harbor Laboratory Press, Cold Spring Harbor, NY, 18.1–18.88.

32. Vilaseca, J.C., Pupo, M., Bernal, M., Matamoros, L., Gordillo, S., Rodriguez, H., Caballero, Y., and Otero, A., 1997, Quantitative ELISA for mouse monoclonal antibody determination in culture supernatants and in human serum, *Hybridoma,* 16, 557–562.

12 Molecular Characterization of Immunoglobulin Genes

Warren Ladiges and Gamal E. Osman

CONTENTS

12.1 INTRODUCTION

One of the fascinating properties of immunoglobulin (Ig) genes is the diversity of proteins (antibodies) they encode. It has been estimated that any mammalian immune system is capable of generating more than 10^8 antibodies with different specificities. Understanding this unique biological phenomenon has been a challenge to many of us. For this reason, different aspects of Ig genes such as the structure, organization, regulation, rearrangement, and expression have been the focus of very intense studies for the past several decades. In this chapter, we are going to describe different contemporary PCR methods of cloning and sequencing Ig genes. We also provide the reader with an updated reference of all mouse Ig V gene families with regard to their numbers, sequence alignments, and sequence similarities.

12.1.1 ORGANIZATION OF IG GENES

An Ig molecule consists of two identical heavy chains and two identical light chains which are covalently bonded. Each Ig chain consists of a variable region and a constant region. Threbe clusters of gene segments encode the heavy chain variable regions: variable gene segments (V_H), diversity gene segments (D_H), and joining gene segments (J_H). A complete heavy chain variable region gene (V_H-D_H-J_H) is assembled by somatic rearrangements during B cell ontogeny; a D_H to J_H rearrangement occurs first on both chromosomes followed by a V_H to D_H-J_H rearrangement. Allelic exclusion ensures that one B lymphocyte expresses Igs of only one specificity (reviewed in Alt et al. 1987). Unlike the heavy chains, there are two types of light chains: kappa (κ) light chains and lambda (λ) light chains. The light chain variable regions are encoded by only two clusters of gene segments: variable gene segments (V_L: κ or λ) and joining gene segments (J_L: κ or λ). The V_L gene segment rearranges with the J_L gene segment by a process similar to that for heavy chains.[46] However, the lambda chain in the mouse constitutes only 5% of the total murine Igs and has three V gene segments (reviewed in Eisen and Reilly 1985). The total number of murine V_H gene segments has been estimated to be 100 to 1000,[5,28,32] whereas the total number of murine Vκ gene segments has been estimated to be 90 to 200.[10,28] To simplify the study of Ig V-genes, they are organized into gene families or groups based on their sequence similarity at the nucleic acid level[5] and at the amino acid level.[14,26,39] The members of the same gene family have more than 80% nucleotide sequence similarity while members of different gene families have less than 75% sequence similarity level.[6] Accordingly, the V_H gene segments have been grouped into 15 V_H gene families (Figure 12.1), while the Vκ gene segments have been organized into 19 Vκ gene families (Figure 12.2). The largest of these families is V_H1 (J558), which is estimated to contain 60 to 1000 members.[6,32] Thus, all the V gene segments together constitute an extremely diverse pool of Ig genes for generating antibodies.

12.1.2 CLONING OF IG GENES

Classically, the rearranged Ig genes were cloned from cDNA libraries.[6,41,48,62] However, this technique is tedious, laborious, and time consuming. The advent of the PCR technique[43,61] has revolutionized the way molecular biology is performed today and has resulted in a number of rapid cloning techniques. However, cloning and sequencing members of the diverse Ig gene family have been challenging tasks. This is primarily due to the very diverse nature of the 5′ ends of the Igs, i.e., the variable regions. PCR involves the design of 5′ and 3′ primers that specifically amplify the DNA region between the two PCR primers. The 5′ ends of the Igs are encoded by the V gene segments, which are highly variable and polymorphic. In addition, not all V gene segments have been cloned. The Kabat database has been utilized[26] to design 5′ V primers to clone the Ig V-genes from humans, mice,[7–9,16,18,25,27,30,37,38,63] and rats.[29] Often, the 3′ IgH primers have been made from the constant regions of the Igs. However, in most cases the 5′ IgH primers have been designed from regions 5′ of the Ig variable gene segments and are degenerate. Furthermore, these techniques

IgVH Families	201				250	251				300
J558(V_H1)	AGTTCAAGGG	CAAGGCCACA	TTGACTGTAG	ACAAATCCTC	CAGCACAGCC	TACATGCAGC	TCAACAGCCT	GACATCTGAG	GACTCTGCAG	TCTATTACTG
Q52(V_H2)	CTTTCATGTC	CAGACTGAGC	ATCACCAAGG	ACAACTCCAA	GAGCCAAGTT	TTCTTTAAGA	TGAACAGTCT	GCAAGCTGAT	GACACTGCCA	TATACTACTG
36-30(V_H3)	CTCTAAAAG	TCGAATCTCC	ATCACTCGAG	ACACATCCAA	GAACCAGTAC	TACCTGCAGT	TGAATTCTGT	GACTACTGAG	GACACACCCA	CATATTACTG
X-24(V_H4)	CTCTAAAGGA	TAAATTCATC	ATCTCCAGAG	ACAACGCCAA	AAATACGCTG	TACCTGCAAA	TGAGCAAAGT	GAGATCTGAG	GACACAGCGC	TTTATTACTG
7183(V_H5)	CAGTGAAGGG	CCGATTCACC	ATCTCAAGAG	ACAATCCCAA	GAACACCCTG	TTCCTGCAAA	TGACCAGTCT	AAGGTCTGAG	GACACGGCCA	TGTATTACTG
J606(V_H6)	CTGTGAAAGG	GAGGTTCACC	ATATCAAGAG	ATGATTCCAA	AAGTAGTGTC	TACCTGCAAA	TGAACAACTT	AAGGGCTGAA	GACACTGAA	TTTATTACTG
S107(V_H7)	CTGTGAAGGG	TCGGTTCATC	GTCTCCAGAG	ACACTTCCCA	AAGCATCCTC	TACCTTCAGA	TGAATGCCCT	GAGAGCTGAG	GACACTGCCA	TTTATTACTG
3609(V_H8)	CCCTGAAGAG	CCAGCTCACA	ATCTCCAAGG	ATCCTCCAG	AAACCAGGTC	TTCCTCAAGA	TCACCAGTGT	GGACACTCGA	GATACTGCCA	CTTACTACTG
VGAM3.8(V_H9)	ACTTCAAGGG	ACGGTTTGCC	TTCTCTTGG	AAACCTCTGC	CATCACTGCC	TATTTGCAGA	TCAACAACCT	CAAAAATGAG	GACATGGCTA	CATATTTCTG
V_H10(DNA-4)	CAGTGAAAGA	CAGGTTCACC	ATCTCCAGAG	ATGATTCACA	AAGCATGCTC	TATCTGCAAA	TGAACAACTT	GAAAACTGAG	GACACAGCCA	TGTATTTCTG
V_H11(CP3)	CCATAAAGGA	TCGATTCACT	ATCTTCAGAG	ACAATGACAA	GAGCACCCTG	TACCTGCAGA	TGAGCAATGT	GCGATCGGAG	GACACAGCCA	CGTATTTCTG
V_H12(CH27)	CTCTCCAGAG	CCCCATCTCC	ATTACTAGAG	AAACGTCAAA	GAACCAGTTC	TTCCTCCAAT	TGAACTCTGT	GACCACAGAG	GACACAGCCA	TGTATTACTG
3609N(V_H13)	CTGTGAAAGG	CAGATTCGCC	ATTTCAAGAG	ATGATTCAAA	AAGCAGTGTC	TACCTGCAGA	TGGACAGATT	AAGAGAGGAA	GACACTGCGA	CTTATTATTG
SM7(V_H14)	AGTTCCAGGA	CAAGGCCACT	ATGATCACAG	ACACATCCTC	CAATATAGCC	TACCTGCAGT	CCAGCAGCCT	GACATCTGAG	GACACTGCCG	TCTATTACTG
VH15	AGTTTGAGGA	CAAAGCCACA	CTGGATGCAG	ACACAGTGTC	CAACACAGCC	TACTTGGAGC	TCAACAGTCT	GACATCTGAG	GACTCTGCTA	TCTACTACTG

FIGURE 12.1 Alignment of nucleotide and amino acid sequences of all mouse Ig V_H gene family prototypes. (A) The 5' mouse Ig universal primer, UmIgV_H, was designed from the framework region 1 (FR1: 1–91)[26] and its nucleotide sequence is shown above the aligned sequences. (B) Alignment of amino acid sequence of all mouse Ig V_H gene families. References for the representative sequences for the fifteen Ig V_H gene families are (1) Akolkar et al. 1987, (2) Matsuda et al. 1989, (3) Gefter et al. 1984, (4) Hartman et al. 1984, (5) Bothwell et al. 1981, (6) Ferguson et al. 1989, (7) Winter et al. 1985, (8) Meek et al. 1990, (9) Pennell et al. 1989, (10) Tutter et al. 1991, and (11) Brodeur et al., 1988. Dot (.) represents a gap in the nucleotide sequence alignment.

VH Family	1				50	51				105	Ref.
J558(V_H1)	EVQLQQSGPE	LVKPGASVKI	SCKASGYT.F	.TDYYMKWVK	QSHSKSLEWI	GDINPNNGG.	.TSYNQKFKG	KATLTCDKSS	STAYMQLNSL	TSEDSAVYYC	1
Q52(V_H2)	QVQLKQSGPS	LVQPSQSLSI	TCTVSDFSL.	.TNFGVIHWVR	QSPGKGLEWL	SVIWRGGN..	.TDYNAAFMS	RLSITKDNSK	SQVFFKMNSL	QADDTAIYYC	2
36-30(V_H3)	EVQLQESGPS	LVKPSQTLSL	TCSVTGDSL	TSG.YWNWIR	KFPGNKLEYM	GYISYSGS..	.TYYNPSLKS	RISITRDTSK	NQYYLQLNSV	TTEDTPTYYC	3
X-24(V_H4)	XVKLLESGGG	LVQPGGSLNL	SCAASGFD.F	.SRYWMSWAR	QAPGKGQEWI	GEI.NPGSS	TINYTPSLKD	KFIISRDNAK	NTLYLQMSKV	RSEDTALYYC	4
7183(V_H5)	DVQLVESGGG	LVQPGGSRKL	SCAASGFT.F	.SSFGMHWVR	QAPEKGLEWV	AYL.SSGSS	TLHYADTVKG	RFTISRDNPK	NTLFLQMSTSL	RSEDTAMYYC	5
J606(V_H6)	XVKLEESGGG	LVQPGGSMKL	SCVASGFT.F	.SNYWMSWVR	QSPEKGLEWV	AQIRLKSDNY	ATHYAESVKG	RFTISRDDSK	SSVYLQMNNL	RAEDTGIYYC	4
S107(V_H7)	EVKLVESGGG	LVQPGGSLRL	SCATSGFT.F	.SDFYMEWVR	QPPGKRLEWI	AASRNKANDY	TTEYSASVKG	RFVSRDTSQ	SILYLQMNAL	RAEDTAIYYC	6
3609(V_H8)	QVTLKESGPG	ILKPSQTLSL	TCSFSGFSLS	ASGMGVGWIR	QPSGEGLEWL	AHIWWDDD..	KYYNPSLKS	QLTSIKDTSR	NQVFLKITSV	DTRDTATYYC	7
VGAM3.8(V_H9)	QIQLVQSGPE	LKKPGETVKI	SCKASGYT.F	.TNYGLNWVK	QAPGKGLKWM	GWINTYTGK.	.STYADDFKG	RFAFSLETSA	ITAYLQINNL	KNEDMAITYFC	7
V_H10(DNA-4)	EVQLVETGGG	LVQPKGSLKL	SCPASGFS.F	.NTNAMNWVR	QAPGKGLEWV	ARIRSKSNNY	ATYYADSVKD	RFTISRDDSQ	SMLYLQMNNL	KTEDTAMYYC	8
V_H11(CP3)	EVQLLETGGG	LUXPGGSRXL	SCEGSGXT.F	.SGFWMSWVR	QTPGKTLEWI	GDX..NDDGS	AINYAPSIKD	RFTIFRDNDK	STLYLQMSNV	RSEDTATYFC	8
V_H12(CH27)	QMQLQESGPG	LVKPSQSLFL	TCSITGFPI.	TSGYYWIWIR	QSPGKPLEWM	GYITHSGE..	.TFYNPSLQS	PISITRETSK	NQFFLQLNSV	TTEDTAMYYC	9
3609N(V_H13)	QCQLVETGGG	LVRPGNSLKL	SCVTSGFT.F	.SNYRMHWLR	QPPGKRLEWI	AVITVKSDNY	GANYAESVKG	RFAISRDDSK	SSVYLQMDRL	REEDTATYYC	10
SM7(V_H14)	EVQLQQSGAE	VV.PGASVKL	SCTASGFN.I	.KDDYMHWAK	QRPDQGLEWI	GRIDPAIDD.	.TDYAPKFQD	KATMTDTSS	NIAYLQSSSL	TSEDTAVYYC	10
VH15	QVHLQQDGSE	LRSPGSSVKL	SCKDFDSEVF	.PIAYMSWVR	QKPGHGFEWI	GDILPSIGR.	.TIYGEKFED	KATLDADTVS	NTAYLELNSL	TSEDSAIYYC	11

FIGURE 12.1 (continued)

Universal Primer / IgVH Families	TGAGGTGCAG	CTGGAGGAGT	C								Ref
	1			50	51				100		
J558(VH1)	GAGGTCCAG	CTGCAACAAT	CTGGACCTGA	GCTGGTGAAG	CCTGGGGCCT	CAGTGAAGT	ATCCTGTAAG	GCTTCTGGAT	....ACAC	ATTCACTGAC	1
Q52(VH2)	CAGGTGCAG	CTGAAGCAGT	CAGGACCTAG	CCTAGTGCAG	CCCTCACAGA	GCCTGTCCAT	AACCTGCACA	GTCTCTGATT	TCTCATTAA.	.....CTAAC	2
36-30(VH3)	GAGGTGCAG	CTTCAGGAGT	CAGGACCTAG	CCTCGTGAAA	CCTTCGCAGA	CTCTGTCCCT	CACCTGTTCT	GTCACTGGCG	ACTCCATCAC	CAGTGGT...	3
X-24(VH4)	GAGGTGAAG	CTTCTCGAGT	CTGGAGGTGG	CCTGGTGCAG	CCTGGAGGAT	CCCTGAATCT	CTCCTGTGCA	GCCTCAGGAT	.....TCGA	TTTTAGTAGA	4
7183(VH5)	TGATGTGCAG	CTGGTGGAGT	CTGGGGGAGG	CTTAGTGCAG	CCTGGAGGGT	CCCGGAAACT	CTCCTGTGTT	GCCTCTGAT	.....TCAC	TTTCAGTAGC	5
J606(VH6)	GAAGTGAAG	GTTGAGGAGT	CTGGAGGAGG	CTTGGTGCAA	CCTGGGGAT	CCATGAAACT	CTCCTGTGCA	GCCTCTGGAT	.....TCAC	TTTCAGTAAC	4
S107(VH7)	TGAGGTGAAG	CTGGTGGAAT	CTGGAGGAGG	CTTGGTACAG	CCTGGGGGTT	CTCTGAGACT	CTCCTGTGCA	ACTTCTGGGT	.....TCAC	CTTCAGTGAT	6
3609(VH8)	CAAGTTACT	CTAAAAGAGT	CTGGCCCTGG	GATATTGAAG	CCCTCACAGA	CCCTCAGTCT	GACTTGTTCT	TTCTCTGGGT	TTTCACTGAG	CGCTTCTGGT	7
VGAM3.8(VH9)	CAGATCCAG	TTGGTGCAGT	CTGGACCTGA	GCTTAAGAAG	CCTGGAGAGA	CAGTCAAGAT	CTCCTGCAAG	GCTTCTGGGT	.....ATAC	CTTCACAAAC	7
VH10(DNA-4)	TGAGGTGCAG	CTGTTGAGA	CTGGTGGAGG	ATTGGTGCAG	CCTAAAGGGT	CATTGAAACT	CTCATGTCCA	GCCTCTGGAT	.....TCAG	CTTCAATACC	8
VH11(CP3)	TGAAGTGCAG	CTGTTGGAGA	CTGGAGGAGG	CTTGGTGNNA	CCTGGGGGNT	CACGGGNNCT	CTCTTGTGAA	GGCTCAGGGN	.....TCAC	TTTTAGTGGC	8
VH12(CH27)	CAGATGCAG	CTTCAGGAGT	CAGGACCTGG	CCTGGTGAAA	CCCTCACAGT	CACTCTTCCT	TACCTGCTCT	ATTACTAGTT	TCCCCATCAC	CAGTGGTTAC	9
3609N(VH13)	CAGGTGCAG	CTTGTAGAGA	CCGGGGGAGG	CTGGTGAGG	CCTGGAAATT	CTCTGAAACT	CTCCTGTGTT	ACCTGGGAT	.....TCAC	TTTCAGTAAC	10
SM7(VH14)	GAGGTTCAG	CTGCAGCAGT	CTGGGGCTGA	GGTTGT...A	CCAGGGGCCT	CAGTCAAGTT	GTCCTGCACA	GCTTCTGGCT	.....TTAA	CATTAAAGAC	10
VH15	CAGGTTCAC	CTACAACAGT	CTGGTTCTGA	ACTGAGGAGT	CCTGGGTCTT	CAGTAAAGCT	TTCATGCAAG	GATTTTGAIT	..CAGAAGT	CTTCCCTATT	11

FIGURE 12.1 (continued)

IgVH Families	101				150	151				200
J558(V_H1)	TACTACATGA	AGTGGGTGAA	GCAGAGTCAT	GGAAAGAGCC	TTGAGTGGAT	TGGAGATATT	.....AATC	CTAACAATGG	TGGTAACTAGC	TACAACCAGA
Q52(V_H2)	TTTGGTGTAC	ACTGGGTTCG	CCAGTCTCCA	GGAAAGGGTC	TGGGAGTGGTT	GGGAGTGATA	......T	GGAGAGGTGG	AAACACAGAC	TACAATGCAG
36-30(V_H3)	TACTGGAA..	.CTGGATCCG	GAAATTCCCA	GGGAATAAAC	TTGAGTACAT	GGGGTACATA	......A	GCTACAGTGG	TAGCACTTAC	TACAATCCAT
X-24(V_H4)	TACTGGATGA	GTTGGGCTCG	GCAGGCTCCA	GGGAAAGGGC	AGGAATGGAT	TGGAGAAATT	.....AATC	CAGGAAGCAG	TACGATAAAC	TATACGCCAT
7183(V_H5)	TTTGGAATGC	ACTGGGTTCG	TCAGGCTCCA	GAGAAGGGGC	TGGAGTGGGT	CGCATACATT	.....AGTA	GTGGCAGTAG	TACCCTCCAC	TATGCAGACA
J606(V_H6)	TACTGGATGT	CCTGGGTCCG	CCAGTCTCCA	GAGAAGGGGC	TTGAGTGGGT	TGCTCAAATA	AGATTGAAAT	CTGATAATTA	TGCAACACAT	TATGCGGAGT
S107(V_H7)	TTCTACATGG	AGTGGGTCCG	CCAGCCTCCA	GGGGAGGGTC	TGGAGTGGAT	TGCTGCAAGT	AGAAACAAAG	CTAATGATTA	TACAACAGAG	TACAGTGCAT
3609(V_H8)	ATGGGTGTAG	GCTGGATTCG	TCAGCCTTCA	GGAAAGGGTT	TGGAGTGGCT	GGCACACATT	......T	GGTTGGGATGA	TGATAAGTAC	TATAACCCAT
VGAM3.8(V_H9)	TATGGACTGA	ACTGGGTGAA	GCAGGCTCCA	GGAAAGGGTT	TAAAGTGGAT	GGGCTGGATA	.....AACA	CCTACACTGG	AAAGTCAACA	TATGCTGATG
V_H10(DNA-4)	AATGCCATGA	ACTGGGTCCG	CCAGGCTCCA	GGAAAGGGTT	TGGAATGGGT	TGCTCCGCATA	AGAAGTAAAA	GTAATAATTA	TGCAACATAT	TATGCCGATT
V_H11(CP3)	TTCTGGATGA	GCTGGGTTCG	ACAGACACCT	GGGAAGACCC	TGGAGTGGAT	TGGAGACATN	.....AATT	CTGATGGCAG	TGCAATAAAC	TACGCACCAT
V_H12(CH27)	TACTGGAT.	.CTGGATCCG	TCAGTCACCT	GGGAAACCCC	TAGAATGGAT	GGGGTACATC	.....A	CTCATAGTGG	GGAAACTTTC	TACAACCCAT
3609N(V_H13)	TACCGGATGC	ACTGGCTTCG	CCAGCCTCCA	GGGAAGAGGC	TGGAGTGGAT	TGCTGTAATT	ACAGTCAAAT	CTGATAATTA	TGGAGCAAAT	TATGCAGAGT
SM7(V_H14)	GACTATATGC	ACTGGGCGAA	GCAGAGGCCT	GACCAGGGCC	TGGAGTGGAT	TGGAAGGATT	.....GATC	CTGCGATTGA	TGATACTGAT	TATGCCCGA
VH15	GCTTATATGA	GTTGGGTTAG	GCAGAAGCCT	GGGCATGGAT	TTGAATGGAT	TGGAGACATA	.....CTCC	CAAGTATTGG	TAGAACAATC	TATGGAGAGA

FIGURE 12.1 (continued)

		1				50	51				100	Ref.
Universal Primer		GACATTCTGA	TGACCCAGTC	T								
VK Family												
Vκ1		GATGTTGTGA	TGACCCAAAC	TCCACTCTCC	CTGCCTGTCA	GTCTTGGAGA	TCAAGCCTCC	ATCTCTTGCA	GATCTAGTCA	GAGCCCTTGT.	..ACACAGTA	1
Vκ2		GATGTTGTGA	TGACCCAGAC	TCCACTCACT	TTGTCGGTTA	CCATTGGACA	ACCAGCCTCC	ATCTCTTGCA	AGTCAAGTCA	GAGCTCTT.	.AGATAGTG	1
Vκ4/5		CAAATTGTTC	TCACCCAGTC	TCCAGCAATC	ATGTCTGCAT	CTCCTGGGGA	GAAGGTCACC	ATGACCTGCA	GTGCCAGATC	AAGTGT...	...AAGTT	1
Vκ8		GACATTGTGA	TGACACAGTC	TCCATCCTCC	CTGGCTATGT	CAGTAGGACA	GAAGGTCACT	ATGAGCTGCA	AGTCCAGTCA	GAGCCTTTTA	AATAGTAGCA	1
Vκ9A		GACATCCAGA	TGACCCAGTC	TCCATCCTCC	TTATCTGCCT	CTCTGGGAGA	AAGAGTCAGT	CTCACTTGTC	GGGCAAGTCA	GGACATT...	....	1
Vκ9B		GACATCAAGA	TGACCCAGTC	TCCATCTTCC	ATGTATGCAT	CTCTAGGAGA	GAGAGTCAGT	ATCACTTGCA	AGGCGAGTCA	GGACATT...	....	1
Vκ10		GATATCCAGA	TGACACAGAC	TACATCCTCC	CTGTCTGCCT	CTCTGGGAGA	CAGAGTCACC	ATCAGTTGCA	GGGCAAGTCA	GGACATT...	....	1
Vκ11		GATGTTCAAA	TGACCCAGTC	TCCATCCTCC	CTGTCTGCAT	CTTTGGGTGA	AAGAGTCTCC	CTGACCTGCC	AGGCAAGTGG	GAGCATT...	....	1
Vκ12/13		GACATCCAGA	TGACTCAGTC	TCCAGCCTCC	CTATCTCAT	CTGTGGGTGA	AACTGTCACC	ATCACATGTC	GAGCAAGTGG	GAATATT...	....	1
Vκ19/28		AGTATTGTGA	TGACCCAGAC	TCCAAAATTC	CTGCTTGTAT	CAGCAGGAGA	GAGGGTTACC	ATAACCTGCA	AGGCCAGTCA	GAG......	....	1
Vκ20		....ACTG	TGACCCAGTC	TCCAGCNTCC	CTGTCCGTGG	CTACNGGAGA	AAAAGTCACT	ATCAGATGCA	TAACCAGCAC	TGATATT...	....	2
Vκ21		AACATTGTGC	TGACCCAATC	TCCAGCTTCT	TTGGCTGTGT	CTCTAGGGCA	GAGGGCCACC	ATATCCTGA	GAGCCAGTGA	AAGTGTTGAT	AGTTATTGGCA	1
Vκ22		GACATTATGA	TGACTCAGTC	TCCAACTTTC	CTTGCTGTGA	CAGCAAGTAA	GAAGGTCACC	ATTAGTTGCA	CTGCNTCTGA	GAGCCTTTAT	TCAAGCAAAC	1
Vκ23		GACATCTTGC	TGACTCAGTC	TCCAGCCATC	CGTGTCTGTGA	GTCCAGGAGA	AAGAGTCAGT	TTCTCCTGCA	GGGCCAGTCA	GAGCATT...	....	1
Vκ24/25		GATATTGTGA	TAACCCAGGA	TGAACTCTCC	AATCCTGTCA	CTTCTGGAGA	ATCAGTTTCC	ATCTCCTGCA	GGTCTAGTAA	GAGTCTCCT.	.ATATAAGG	1
Vκ31/38C		GACATCCAGA	TGACACAGTC	TCCATCCTCA	CTGTCTGCAT	CTCTGGGAGG	CAAAGTCACC	ATCACTTGCA	AGGCAAGCCA	AGACATT...	....	1
Vκ32		GACATCCAGA	TGAACCAGTC	TCCATCCAGT	CTGTCTGCAT	CCCTTGGAGA	CACAATAACC	ATCACTTGCC	ATGCCAGTCA	GAAAAT...	....	3
Vκ33/34		GACATCCAGA	TGACACAATC	TTCATCCTCC	TTTTCTGTAT	CTCTAGGAGA	CAGAGTCACC	AITACTTGCA	AGGCAAGTGA	GGACATA...	....	4
VκRF		GATGTCCAGA	TAACCCAGTC	TCCATCTTAT	CTTGCTGCAT	CTCCTGGAGA	AACCATTACT	ATTAATTGCA	GGGCAAGTAA	GAGCATT...	....	1

FIGURE 12.2 Alignment of nucleotide and amino acid sequences of all mouse Ig V$_\kappa$ gene family prototypes. (A) The 5′ mouse Ig universal primer, UmIgV$_\kappa$, was designed from the framework region 1 (FR1: 1–69)[26] and its nucleotide sequence is shown above the aligned sequences. (B) Alignment of amino acid sequence of all mouse Ig V$_\kappa$ gene families. References for the representative sequences for the nineteen Ig V$_\kappa$ gene families are (1) Strohal et al. 1989, (2) Shefner et al. 1990, (3) D'Hoostelaere and Klinman 1990, and (4) Valiante and Caton 1990. Dot (.) represents a gap in the nucleotide sequence.

VK Family	101				150	151				200
V$_\kappa$1	ATGGAAACAC	CTATTTACAT	TGGTACCTGC	AGAAGCCAGG	CCAGT...CT	CCAAAGCTCC	TGATCTACAA	AGTTTCCAA.	CCGATTTTCT	GGGGTCCCAG
V$_\kappa$2	ATGGAAAGAC	ATATTTGAAT	TGGTTGTTAC	AGAGGCCAGG	CCAGT...CT	CCAAAGCGCC	TAATCTATCT	GGTGTCTAA.	ACTGGACTCT	GGAGTCCCTG
V$_\kappa$4/5	CC.....AG	CTACTTGTAC	TGGTACCAGC	AGAAGCCAGG	ATCCT...CC	CCCAAACTCT	GGATTTATAG	CACATCCAA.	CCTGGCTTCT	GGAGTCCCTG
V$_\kappa$8	ATCAAAAGAA	CTATTTGGCC	TGGTACCAGC	AGAAACCAGG	ACAGT..CT	CCTAAACTTC	TGGTATACTT	TGCATCCAC.	TAGGGAATCT	GGGGTCCCTG
V$_\kappa$9A	....GGTAG	TAGCTTAAAC	TGGCTTCAGC	AGGAACCAGA	TGGAA...CT	ATTAAACGCC	TGATCTACGC	CACATCCAG.	TTTAGATTCT	GGTGTGCCCA
V$_\kappa$9B	....AATAG	CTATTTAAGC	TGGTTCCAGC	AGAAACCAGG	GAAAT...CT	CCTAAGACCC	TGATCTATCG	TGCAAACAG.	ATTGGTAGAT	GGGGTCCCAT
V$_\kappa$10	....AGCAA	TTATTTAAAC	TGGTATCAGC	AGAAACCAGA	TGGAA...CT	GTTAAACTCC	TGATCTACTA	CACATCAAG.	ATTACACTCA	GGAGTCCCAT
V$_\kappa$11	....AACAA	TTTTTTAAAA	TGGTTTCAGC	AAACACTGGG	GAAAA...CT	GCTAGGCTCT	TGATCTATGG	TGCAAACAA.	ATTGGAAGAT	GGGGTCCCTT
V$_\kappa$12/13	....CACAA	TTATTTAGCA	TGGTATCAGC	AGAAACAGGG	AAAAT..CT	CCTCAGCTCC	TGGTCTATAA	TGCAAAAAC.	CTTAGCAGAT	GGTGTGCCAT
V$_\kappa$119/28	.TGTGAGTAA	TGATGTAGCT	TGGTACCAGC	AGAAGCCAGG	GCAGT..CT	CCTAAACTGC	TGATATACTA	TGCATCCAA.	TCGCTACACT	GGAGTCCCTG
V$_\kappa$20	...GATGA	TGATATGAAC	TGGTACCAGC	AGAAGCCAGG	GNNA...CCG	CCTAAGCTCC	TTATTTCAGA	AGGCAATACT	CTTCGTC.CT	GGGGTCCCTG
V$_\kappa$21	AT....AG	TTTTATGCAC	TGGTACCAGC	AGAAACCAGG	ACAGC..CA	CCCAAACTCC	TCATCTATCT	TGCATCCAA.	CCTAGAATCT	GGGGTCCCTG
V$_\kappa$22	ACAAGGTGCA	CTACTTGGCT	TGGTACCAGA	AGAAACCAGA	GCAAT..CT	CCTAAACTGC	TGATATACGG	GGCATCCAA.	CCGATACATT	GGGGTCCCTG
V$_\kappa$23	...GGCAC	AAGCATACAC	TGGTATCAGC	AAAGAACA..	..AATGGTTCT	CCAAGGCTTC	TCATAAAGTA	TGCTTCTGAG	TCTA.TCTCT	GGGGATCCTT
V$_\kappa$24/25	ATGGGAAGAC	ATACTTGAAT	TGGTTTCTGC	AGAGACCAGG	ACAAT...CT	CCTCAGCTCC	TGATCTATTT	GATGTCCAC.	CCGTGCATCA	GGAGTCTCAG
V$_\kappa$31/38C	....AACAA	GTATATAGCT	TGGGACCAAC	ACAAGCCTGG	AAAAG...GT	CCTAGGCTGC	TCATACATTA	CACATCTASC	AATAGAGCCA	GGCATCCCAT
V$_\kappa$32	....AATGT	TTGGTTAAGC	TGGTACCAGC	AGAAAAAAA ^A	AGGAAATATT	CCTAAACTAT	TGATCTATAG	GACTTCCAA.	CTTGCACACA	GGCGTCCCAT
V$_\kappa$33/34	...TATAT	CGGATTAGCC	TGGTATCAGC	AGAAACCAGG	AAATGTACCT	CCTAGATTCT	TAATATCTGG	GTCAACCAG.	TTTGAAAACT	GGGGTTCCTT
V$_\kappa$RF	....AGCAA	ATATTTAGCC	TGGTATCAAG	AGAAACCTGG	GAAAA...CT	AATAAGCTTC	TTATCTACTC	TGGATCCAC.	TTTGCAATCT	GGAATTCCAT

FIGURE 12.2 (continued)

VK Family	201				250	251				300
$V_\kappa 1$	ACAGGTTCAG	TGGCAGTGGA	TCAGGGACAG	ATTTCACACT	CAAGATCAGC	AGAGTGGAGG	CTGAGGATCT	GGGAGTTTAT	TTCTGCTCTC	AAAGTACACA
$V_\kappa 2$	ACAGGTTCAC	TGGCAGTGGA	TCAGGGACAG	ATTTCACACT	GAAAATCAGC	AGAGTGGAGG	CTGAGGATTT	GGGAGTTTAT	TATTGCTGGC	AAGGTACACA
$V_\kappa 4/5$	CTCGCTTCAG	TGGCAGTGGG	TCTGGGACCT	CTTATTCTCT	CACAATCAGC	AGCATGGAGG	CTGAAGATGC	TGCCACTTTT	TACTGCCAGC	AGTACAGTGG
$V_\kappa 8$	ATCGCTTCAT	AGGCAGTGGA	TCTGGGACAG	ATTTCACTCT	TACCATCAGC	AGTGTGCAGG	CTGAAGACCT	GGCAGAITAC	TTCTGTCAGC	AACATTATAG
$V_\kappa 9A$	AAAGGTTCAG	TGGCAGTAGG	TCTGGGTCAG	ATTATTCTCT	CACCATCAGC	AGCCTTGAGT	CTGAAGATTT	TGTAGACTAT	TACTGTCTAC	AATATGCTAG
$V_\kappa 9B$	CAAGGTTCAG	TGGCAGTGGA	TCTGGGCAAG	ATTATTCTCT	CACCATCAGC	AGCCTGGAGT	ATGAAGATAT	GGGAATTTAT	TATTGTCTAC	AGTATGATGA
$V_\kappa 10$	CAAGGTTCAG	TGGCAGTGGG	TCTGGAACAG	ATTATTCTCT	CACCATTAGC	AACCTGGAGC	AAGAAGATAT	TGCCACTTAC	TTTTGCCAAC	AGGGTAATAC
$V_\kappa 11$	CAAGGTTCAG	TGGAACTGGA	TATGGGACAG	ATTTCACTTT	CACCATCAGC	AGCCAGGAGG	AAGAAGATGT	GTCAACTTAT	TTCTGTCTAC	AGCATAGGTA
$V_\kappa 12/13$	CAAGGTTCAG	TGGCAGTGGA	TCAGGAACAC	AATATTCTCT	CAAGATCAGC	AGCCTGCAGC	CTGAAGATTT	TGGGAGTTAT	TACTGTCAAC	ATTTTTGGAG
$V_\kappa 19/28$	ATCGCTTCAC	TGGCAGTGGA	TATGGGACGG	ATTTCACTTT	CACCATCAGC	ACTGTGCAGG	CTGAAGACCT	GGCAGTTTAT	TTCTGTCAGC	AGGATTATAG
$V_\kappa 20$	CCCGATTCTC	CAGCAGTGGC	TATGTACAG	ATTTGTTTTT	TACAATTGAA	AACATGCTCT	CAGAAGATGT	TGCAGAITAC	TACTGTTTGC	AAAGTGATAA
$V_\kappa 21$	CCAGGTTCAG	TGGCAGTGGG	TCTAGGACAG	ACTTCACCCT	CACCATTGAT	CCTGTGGAGG	CTGATGATGC	TGCAACCTAT	TACTGTCAGC	AAAATAATGA
$V_\kappa 22$	ATCGCTTCAC	AGGCAGTGGA	TCTGGGACAG	ATTTCACTCT	GACCATCAGC	AGTGTACAGG	TTGAAGACCT	CACACATTAT	TACTGTGCAC	AGTTTTACAG
$V_\kappa 23$	CCAGGTTTAG	TGGCAGTGGA	TCAGGGACAG	ATTTTACTCT	TAGCATCAAC	AGTGTGGAGT	CTGAAGATAT	TGCAGATTAT	TACTGTCAAC	AAGTAATAG
$V_\kappa 24/25$	ACCGGTTTAG	TGGCAGTGGG	TCAGGAACAG	ATTTCACCCT	GGAAATCAGT	AGAGTGAAGG	CTGAGGATGT	GGGTGTGTAT	TACTGTCAAC	AACTTGTAGA
$V_\kappa 31/38C$	CAAGGTTCAG	TGGAAGTGGG	TCTGGGAGAG	ATTATTCCTT	CAGCATCAGC	AACCTGGAGC	CTGAAGATAT	TGCAACTTAT	TATTGTCTAC	AGTATGATAA
$V_\kappa 32$	CAAGGTTCAG	TGGCAGTGGA	TCAGGAACAG	GTTTCACATT	AACCATCAGC	AGCCTGCAGC	CTGAAGACAT	TGCCACTTAC	TACTGTCAAC	AGGGTCAAAA
$V_\kappa 33/34$	CAAGATTCAG	TGGCAGTGGA	TCTGGAAAGG	ATTACACTCT	CAGCATTACC	AGTCTTCAGA	CTGAAGATGT	TGCTACTTAT	TACTGTCAAC	AGTATTGGAG
$V_\kappa RF$	CAAGGTTCAG	TGGCAGTGGA	TCTGGTACAG	ATTTCACTCT	CACCATCAGT	AGCCTGGAGC	CTGAAGAITT	TGCAATGTAT	TACTGTCAAC	AGCATAATGA

FIGURE 12.2 (continued)

VK Family	1				50	51				100	Ref.
Vκ1	DVVMTQTPLS	LPVSLGDQAS	ISCRSSQSLV	H.SNGNTYLH	WYLQKPGQS	PKLLIYKVSN	RFSGVPDRFS	GSGSGTDFTL	KISRVEAEDL	GVYFCSQSTH	1
Vκ2	DVVMTQTPLT	LSVTIGQPAS	ISCKSSQSLL	D.SDGKTYLN	WLLQRPGQS	PKRLIYLVSK	LDSGVPDRFT	GSGSGTDFTL	KISRVEAEDL	GVYYCWQGT H	1
Vκ4/5	QIVLTQSPAI	MSASPGEKVT	MTCSARSSV.	.S..SYLY	WYQQKPGSS	PKLWIYSTSN	LASGVPARFS	GSGSGTSYSL	TISSMEAEDA	AITYCQQYSG	1
Vκ8	DIVMTQSPSS	LAMSVGQKVT	MSCKSSQSLL	NSSNQKNYLA	WYQQKPGQS	PKLLVFAST	RESGVPDRFI	GSGSGTDFTL	TISSVQAEDL	ADYFCQQHYS	1
Vκ9A	DIQMTQSPSS	LSASLGERVS	LTCRASQDI.	...GSSLN	WLQQEPDGTI	KR.LIYATSS	LDSGVPKRFS	GSRSGSDYSL	TISSLESEDF	VDYYCLQYAS	1
VκPB	DIKMTQSPSS	MYASLGERVT	ITCKASQDI.	...NSYLS	WFQQKPGKS	PKTLIYRANR	LVDGVPSRFS	GSGSGQDYSL	TISSLEYEDM	GIYYCLQYDE	1
Vκ10	GIQMTQTTSS	LSASLGDRVT	ISCRASQDI. ...SNYLN	WYQQKPDGTV	WFQQKPGQS	.KLLIYYTSR	LHSGVPSRFS	GSGSGTDYSL	TISNLEQEDI	AITYFCQQGNT	1
Vκ11	DVQMTQSPSS	LSASLGERVS	LTCQASQSI.	...NNFLK	WFQQ.TLGKT	ARLLIYGANK	LEDGVPSRFS	GTGYGTDFTF	TISSQEEEDV	STYFCLQHRY	1
Vκ12/13	DIQMTQSPAS	LSASVGETVT	ITCRASGNI.	..HNYLA	WYQQKQGK.S	PQLLVNAKT	LADGVPSRFS	GSGSGTQYSL	KINSLQPEDF	GSYYCQHFWS	1
Vκ19/28	SIVMTQTPKF	LLVSAGERVT	ITCKASQSVS	ND.....VA	WYQQKPGQS	PKLLIYYASN	RYTGVPDRFT	GSGYGTDFTF	TISTVQAEDL	AVYFCQQDYS	1
Vκ20	.TVTQSPAS	LSVATGEKVT	IRCITSTDID	DD......MN	WYQQKQ.GXP	PKLLISEGNT	LRPGVPSRFS	SSGYGTDFVF	TIENMLSEDV	ADYYCLQSDN	2
Vκ21	NIVLTQSPAS	LAVSLGQRAI	ISCRASESV.	.DSYGNSFMH	WYQQKPGQP	PKLLIYLASN	LESGVPARFS	GSGSRTDFTL	TIDPVEADDA	AITYCQQNNE	1
Vκ22	DIVMTQSPTF	LAVTASKKVT	ISCTXSESLY	SSKHKVHYLA	WYQKKPEQS	PKLLIYGASN	RYIGVPDRFT	GSGSGTDFTL	TISSVQVEDL	THYYCAQFYS	1
Vκ23	DILLTQSPAI	LSVSPGERVS	PSCRASQSI.	GTS....IH	WYQQRT.NGS	PRLLIKYASE	SISGIPSRFS	GSGSGTDFTL	SINSVESEDI	ADYYCQQSNS	1
Vκ24/25	DIVITQDELS	NPVTSGESVS	ISCRSSKSLL	Y.KDGKTYLN	WFLQRPGQS	PQLLYLMST	RASGVSDRFS	GSGSGTDFTL	EISRVKAEDV	GVYYCQQLVE	1
Vκ31/38C	DIQMTQSPSS	LSASLGGKVT	ITCKASQDI.	...NKYIA	WDQHKP.GKG	PRLLIHYTST	IEPGIPSRFS	GSGSGRDYSF	SISNLEPEDI	ATYYCLQYDN	1
Vκ32	DIQMNQDPSS	LSASLGDTIT	ITCHASQKI.	...NVWLS	WYQQKKKGNI	PKLLIYRTSN	LHTGVPSRFS	GSGSGTGFTL	TISSLQPEDI	ATYYCQQGQN	3
Vκ33/34	DIQMTQSSSS	FSVSLGDRVT	ITCKASEDI.	...YIGLA	WYQQKPGNVP	PRFLISGSTS	LETGVPSRFS	GSGSGKDYTL	SITSLQTEDV	ATYYCQQYWS	4
VκRF	DVQITQSPSY	LAASPGETIT	INCRASKSI.	...SKYLA	WYQEKPGKT	NKLLIYSGST	LQSGIPSRFS	GSGSGTDFTL	TISSLEPEDF	AMYYCQQHN E	1

FIGURE 12.2 (continued)

have not been shown to amplify the Ig genes from all Ig V gene families. Other variants of technique, such as inverted PCR[64] and anchored PCR (Loh et al. 1989, Ratech 1992, Heinrichs et al. 1995) have been used to clone the Ig or TCR genes. However, the inverted PCR technique needs an additional optimization step before amplification and subsequent cloning. Furthermore, the cDNA concentration needs to be titrated, in order to favor the intramolecular DNA ligation over the intermolecular ligation. The anchored PCR technique, which involves the addition of a poly(dG) tail at the 5' end of the variable region involves elaborate steps; the technique is time consuming and difficult to reproduce. Anchored PCR is also very sensitive to any primer remaining from the cDNA synthesis steps.

12.1.3 APPLICATIONS

Cloning, sequencing, and expression of Ig V genes of appropriate specificities have many applications for immunologists. They can be used to (1) characterize antibodies produced by B-cell hybridomas, (2) follow the progress of B-cell lymphomas and test their heterogeneity, (3) determine B-cell repertoires at different stages during development, (4) mutate Ig V regions to study their effects on the binding properties of a given antibody, and (5) engineer chimeric antibodies consisting of mouse variable regions and human constant regions. The advantage of these chimeras is that they do not elicit anti-mouse responses when injected into humans. Similarly, chimeric immunotoxins and heteroconjugate antibodies can be engineered.

12.1.4 METHODS OF CLONING AND SEQUENCING IG GENES

We describe here two simple, rapid, and reproducible PCR-based techniques for cloning any rearranged mouse Ig V_H and V_L genes from cDNAs. The principle of the first method is the use of 5' universal primers from a highly conserved region in the framework region (FR1) of the Ig heavy and light chain V gene sequences (Figures 12.1, 12.2, and 12.3), and the 3' primers from the joining and/or constant regions of the heavy and light (κ and λ) gene segments (Figure 12.4). However, if the researcher is planning to express the cloned Ig V gene, this method is not suitable because it introduces sequence changes at the 5' end. The second method is a practical alternative for the cloning and expression of any Ig V genes. The principle of the second method is based on the ligation of a linker with known sequence to the unknown sequence of the 5' ends of any Ig V genes (for more detail, see Figure 12.5).

12.2 CLONING IMMUNOGLOBULIN V REGIONS USING PCR WITH UNIVERSAL PRIMERS

12.2.1 DESIGN OF IG PRIMERS FOR PCR

Nearly all V gene families of Ig heavy and light chains were examined and the nucleotide sequence prototypes were obtained for each heavy and light chain V gene family from Genbank/EMBL and other published sources. The 15 sequences for the

Universal Primer	CAGGCTGTTTG	TGACTCAGGA	ATCT							
VL Family	1				50	51				100 Ref.
V$_l$1	CAGGCTGTTTG	TGACTCAGGA	AITCTGCACTC	ACCACATCAC	CTGGTGAAAC	AGTCACACTC	ACTTGTCGCT	CAAGTACT..	...GGGGCT	GTTACAACTA 1
V$_l$2	CAGGCTGTTTG	TGACTCAGGA	AITCTGCACTC	ACCACATCAC	CTGGTGAAAC	AGTCATACTC	ACTTGTCGCT	CAAGTACT..	...GGGGCT	GTTACAACTA 2
V$_l$X	CAACTTGTGC	TCACTCAGTC	AITCTTCAGCC	TCTTTCTCCC	TGGGAGCCTC	AGCAAAACTC	ACGTGCACCT	TGAGTAGTCA	GCACAGTACG	TACACCATTG 3
VL Family	101				150	151				200
V$_l$1	GTAACTATGC	CAACTGGGTC	CAAGAAAAAC	CAGATCATTT	AITCCACTGGT	CTAATAGGTG	GTACCAACAA	CCGAGCTCCA	GGTGTTCCTG	CCAGATTCTC
V$_l$2	GTAACTATGC	CAACTGGGTT	CAAGAAAAAC	CAGATCATTT	AITCCACTGGT	CTAATAGGTG	GTACCAGCAA	CCGAGCTCCA	GGTGTTCCTG	TCAGATTCTC
V$_l$X	AATGGTATCA	GCAACAGCCA	CTCAAGCCTC	CTAAGTATGT	GATGGAGCTT	AAGAAAGATG	GAAGCCACAG	CACAGGTGAT	GGGATTCCTG	ATCGCTTCTC
VL Family	201				250	251				300
V$_l$1	AGGCTCCCTG	AITTGGAGACA	AGGCTGCCCT	CACCATCACA	GGGGCACAGA	CTGAGGATGA	GGCAATATAT	TTCTGTGCTC	TATGGTACAG	CAACCATT..
V$_l$2	AGGCTCCCTG	AITTGGAGACA	AGGCTGCCCT	CACCATCACA	GGGGCACAGA	CTGAGGATGA	TGCAATGTAT	TTCTGTGCTC	TATGGTACAG	CACCCATT..
V$_l$X	TGGATCCAGC	TCTGGTGCTG	AITCGCTACCT	TAGCATTTCC	AACATCCAGC	CTGAAGATGA	AGCAATATAC	AITCTGTGGTG	TGGGTGATAC	AATTAAGGAA
VL Family	1				50	51				100 Ref.
V$_l$1	QAVVTQESAL	TTSPGETVTL	TC.RSSTGA	VTTSNYANWV	QEKPDHLFTG	LIGGTNNRAP	GVPARFSGSL	IGDKAALTTT	GAQTEDEAIY	FCALWYSNH. 1
V$_l$2	QAVVTQESAL	TTSPGGTVIL	TC.RSSTGA	VTTSNYANWV	QEKPDHLFTG	LIGGTSNRAP	GVPVRFSGSL	IGDKAALTTT	GAQTEDDAMY	FCALWYSTH. 2
V$_l$X	QLVLTQSSSA	SFSLGASAKL	TCTLSSQHST	YTIEWYQQQP	LKPPKYVMEL	KKDGSHSTGD	GIPDRFSGSS	SGADRYLSIS	NIQPEDEAIY	ICGVGDTIKE 3

FIGURE 12.3 Alignment of nucleotide and amino acid sequences of all mouse V$_l$ gene family segments. (A) The 5' mouse Ig universal primer, UmIgV$_l$, was designed from the framework region 1 (FR1: 1–66)[26] and its nucleotide sequence is shown above the aligned sequences. (B) Alignment of amino acid sequences of all mouse V$_l$ gene family segments. References for the three Ig V$_l$ sequences are (1) Bernard et al. 1978, (2) Tonegawa et al. 1978, and (3) Sanchez et al. 1990. Dot (.) represents a gap in the nucleotide sequence.

A. **UmIgJ$_H$**

			CTGGGGCCAAGGGACCACGGTCAC	
	1	17	18	41	51
J$_H$1	TACTGGTACT	TCGATGT	CTGGGGCGCAGGGACCACGGTCAC	CGTTTCCTCA
J$_H$1	......TACT	TTGACTA	CTGGGGCCAAGGCACCACTCTCAC	AGTCTCCTCA
J$_H$3	TACTATGCTA	TGGACTA	CTGGGGTCAAGGAACCTCAGTCAC	CGTCTCCTCA
J$_H$4	...GCCTGGT	TTGCTTA	CTGGGGCCAAGGGACTCTGGTCAC	TGTCTCTGCA

B. **UmIgJ$_K$**

			GGGACCAAGCTGGAAATAAAA	
	1	15	16	36	39
J$_K$1	TGGACGTTCGGTGGA	GGCACCAAGCTGGAAATCAAA	CGT
J$_K$2	TACACGTTCGGAGGG	GGGACCAAGCTGGAAATAAAA	CGT
J$_K$3	TTCACGTTCGGCTCG	GGGACAAAGTTGGAAATAAAA	CGT
J$_K$4	CTCACGTTCGGTGCT	GGGACCAAGCTGGAGCTGAAA	CGT
J$_K$5	ATCACATTCAGTGAT	GGGACCAGACTGGAAATAAAA	CCT

C. **UmIgC$_K$**

	CTGCCCAACTGTATCCATCTTCCC	
	1	7	8	31	32	50
C$_K$	GCTGATG	CTGCCCAACTGTATCCATCTTCCC	ACCATCCAGTGAGCAGTTA

D. **UmIgJ$_l$**

			GGAACCAAGGTGACTGTCCTAG	
	1	15	16	37	45
J$_l$1	TGGGTGTTCGGTGGA	GGAACCAAACTGACTGTCCTAG	...	.....
J$_l$2	TATGTTTTCGGCGGT	GGAACCAAGGTCACTGTCCTAG	...	.....
J$_l$3	TTTATTTTCGGCAGT	GGAACCAAGGTCACTGTCCTAG	...	.....
J$_l$4	...GTGTTCGGAGGT	GGAACCAGATTGACTGTCCTAG	ATG	AGTGA

E. **UmIgC$_l$**

	CAGCCC	AAGTCCACTC	CCACACTC	
	1	5	30	31	50
C$_l$1	.GGC	CAGCCC	AAGTCTTCGC	CATCAGTC	ACCCTGTTTCCA	CCTTCCTCTG
C$_l$2	.GGT	CAGCCC	AAGTCCACTC	CAACTCTC	ACCGTGTTTCCA	CCTTCCTCTG
C$_l$3	.GGT	CAGCCC	AAGTCCACTC	CAACACTC	ACCATGTTTCCA	CCTTCCCCTG
C$_l$4	AGGC	CAACCC	AAGGCTACAC	CATCAGTT	AATCTGTTCCCA	CCTTCCTCTG

FIGURE 12.4 Design of 3′ mouse Ig universal primers from the highly conserved regions of J$_H$, J$_K$, C$_K$, J$_l$ and C$_l$ gene segments. The primers are shown above the aligned sequences. (A) Alignment of the four mouse Ig J$_H$ gene segments.[44] (B) Alignment of the five mouse Ig J$_K$ gene segments.[36] (C) The mouse Ig C$_K$ gene segment.[36] (D) Alignment of the four mouse Ig J$_l$ gene segments.[60] (E) Alignment of the four mouse Ig C$_l$ gene segments.[60] Dot (.) represents a gap in the primer nucleotide sequence.

heavy chain V gene families, 19 sequences for the kappa light chain V gene families, and 3 sequences for the lambda light chain V gene families were aligned, both at the nucleotide and amino acid levels (Figure 12.1, 12.2, and 12.3), using the GCG package (Genetics Computing Group, University of Wisconsin). A comparison of sequence similarity was made, both at the nucleotide and amino acid levels (see Tables 12.1 and 12.2), between all the family members using the GCG package. A highly conserved region was found in the framework 1 (FR1) region of the Ig V gene sequences. The 5′ universal primers were designed from this region, starting at the first codon, with the 3′ end of the primer at a region with perfect sequence

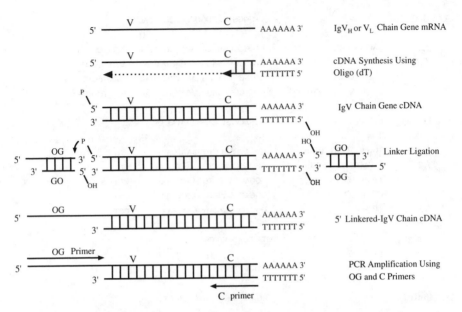

FIGURE 12.5 A schematic representation of the linkered-ligated PCR technique for amplifying any Ig V genes. The OG/GO linker is designed to have two staggered strands as shown. When the two strands of the linker are annealed, a single blunt end is formed without 5′ phosphates. This feature not only provides directionality of ligation between the linker and the Ig cDNA, but also prevents self-ligation between the linkers themselves. Only the 3′ end of the longer OG strand becomes covalently bound to the 5′ end of the Ig cDNA sense strand. During PCR amplification, the 5′ primer is the OG primer, while the 3′ primer is a primer from the constant region or the J region.

identity (Figures 12.1 and 12.2). The 3′ universal primers were designed from the joining region for the heavy chains, and joining and constant regions for the kappa and lambda light chains. The sequences were aligned as stated above and a highly conserved region was found toward the 3′ ends of the joining regions and 5′ ends of the constant regions. Hence, the 3′ universal primers were designed from these highly conserved regions (Figure 12.4).

12.2.2 PREPARATION OF cDNA

1. Total RNA extraction from B-cell hybridomas is based on the previously described method by Osman et al. (1992). Wear gloves, and be careful of RNase contamination.
2. Centrifuge 10 to 50×10^6 cells from the antibody-producing hybridoma of interest. Wash cells twice using PBS and then resuspend the cells in a total volume of 200 µl.
3. Add the cell suspension to 2.0 ml of 6 M Urea/3 M LiCl mixture and homogenize the cells for 1 min on ice at full speed using a Polytron (Kinematica, Brinkmann Instruments). Incubate at 4°C overnight.

TABLE 12.1

Sequence Similarity (Percentage) between the Representative Sequences of Different Mouse Ig V_H Gene Families

V_H Family	V_H1 J558	V_HX Q52	V_H3 36-60	V_H4 X-24	V_H5 7183	V_H6x J606	V_H7 S107	V_H8 3609	V_H9 VGAM3.8	V_H10 DNA-4	V_H11 CP3	V_H12 C_H27	V_H13 3609N	V_H14 SM7	V_H15
V_H1 (J558)	—	42	38	61	58	47	49	36	66	44	60	48	46	68	57
V_H2 (Q52)	29	—	60	45	50	39	42	52	46	42	44	44	39	40	39
V_H3 (36-60)	25	49	—	42	43	41	44	46	39	41	43	59	39	40	39
V_H4 (X-24)	45	30	26	—	74	53	49	37	54	49	77	49	52	55	46
V_H5 (7183)	45	32	25	66	—	54	51	37	58	54	74	47	52	52	44
V_H6 (J606)	33	27	23	40	42	—	73	36	45	76	51	41	80	40	33
V_H7 (S107)	32	27	24	39	38	67	—	38	42	72	52	43	72	41	35
V_H8 (3609)	14	36	36	21	22	18	19	—	35	38	37	47	37	36	41
V_H9 (VGAM3.8)	55	29	22	39	45	28	25	16	—	46	53	44	44	52	44
V_H10 (DNA-4)	30	29	26	37	41	71	66	21	28	—	48	45	72	43	35
V_H11 (CP3)	44	26	24	66	61	36	39	19	40	36	—	47	50	55	45
V_H12 (C_H27)	34	32	49	35	34	21	22	34	26	25	27	—	41	42	40
V_H13 (3609N)	31	27	24	36	37	72	65	19	28	65	36	21	—	38	35
V_H14 (SM7)	52	23	27	44	41	25	26	20	35	25	38	28	25	—	53
V_H15	44	20	25	33	28	19	20	22	26	21	28	23	16	41	—

Note: (1) Above the diagonal: comparison at the nucleic level. (2) Below the diagonal: comparison at the amino acid level.

TABLE 12.2
Sequence Similarity (Percentage) between the Representative Sequences of Different Mouse Ig V_k Gene Families

V_k family	V_k1	V_k2	$V_k4/5$	V_k8	V_k9A	V_k9B	V_k10	V_k11	$V_k12/13$	$V_k19/28$	V_k20	V_k21	V_k22	V_k23	$V_k24/25$	$V_k31/38C$	V_k32	$V_k33/34$	V_kRF
V_k1	—	81	50	54	47	52	48	49	51	56	45	56	53	49	74	39	46	38	53
V_k2	77	—	49	52	46	51	46	48	47	52	44	55	50	47	75	39	45	41	50
$V_k4/5$	43	39	—	52	52	52	54	50	52	51	46	54	48	46	50	42	48	58	52
V_k8	52	46	43	—	47	50	49	49	50	60	48	58	76	49	52	38	47	45	52
V_k9A	34	41	40	34	—	75	77	68	70	60	56	49	48	67	48	48	49	49	69
V_k9B	39	40	43	37	66	—	75	76	73	65	61	49	50	65	51	51	52	52	73
V_k10	40	38	46	42	68	64	—	72	71	64	60	48	48	66	48	52	53	49	73
V_k11	35	34	33	36	59	62	59	—	71	64	57	47	49	62	48	48	53	49	71
$V_k12/13$	35	34	39	42	56	63	59	54	—	60	59	50	47	62	51	52	53	50	69
$V_k19/28$	45	41	39	53	47	53	57	53	52	—	59	51	58	63	49	44	52	46	66
V_k20	31	33	33	35	45	49	49	49	48	48	—	48	46	59	44	44	44	42	58
V_k21	47	42	47	46	35	38	42	37	34	43	37	—	51	51	54	42	47	49	52
V_k22	45	42	39	67	34	38	39	34	39	49	34	40	—	47	50	37	48	44	49
V_k23	39	40	36	41	57	49	57	52	54	54	48	50	39	—	46	45	49	47	65
$V_k24/25$	68	71	40	45	34	37	37	33	36	39	32	40	41	38	—	36	45	41	54
$V_k31/38C$	33	32	37	34	59	66	66	58	58	51	54	35	32	54	32	—	40	48	48
V_k32	45	42	39	67	34	38	39	34	39	49	34	40	39	41	32	40	—	29	42
$V_k33/34$	25	26	42	28	34	34	34	32	34	32	29	33	29	35	27	36	29	—	49
V_kRF	40	39	47	43	57	59	64	57	61	53	48	41	42	57	38	60	25	33	—

Note: (1) Above the diagonal: comparison at the nucleic acid level. (2) Below the diagonal: comparison at the amino acid level.

4. Centrifuge the homogenate for 10 min using an Eppendorf centrifuge. Resuspend the pellet in 500 µl of 10 mM Tris.HCl, pH 7.6, 1 mM EDTA, and 0.5% SDS. Extract total RNA first with one volume of phenol:chloroform:isoamyl alcohol (25:4:1) followed by one volume of chloroform.

5. Add 50 µl of 3 M CH₃COONa and precipitate total RNA using 2.5 volumes of absolute ethanol. Carefully resuspend total RNA in RNase-free distilled H₂O and quantitate.

6. Denature RNA at 68°C and synthesize cDNA from the total RNA using any cDNA synthesis kit from a commercial source. We use the kit from Boehringer Mannheim (Indianapolis, IN).

12.2.3 PCR Amplification of Ig V Genes

7. Add 1 µl of cDNA to 19 µl PCR reaction mixture containing, 2 µl of 10X reaction buffer (100 mM Tris.Cl, pH 8.5, 500 mM KCl, and 25 mM MgCl₂), 2 µl of 10X dNTPs (2 mM of each dNTP), 1 µl each of the 5′ and 3′ universal primers (10 µM) (Table 12.3, and Figures 12.1 to 12.3), 0.2 µl of *Thermus aquaticus* (*Taq*) thermostable DNA polymerase (5 units/µl), and 12.8 µl H₂O.

8. Perform the PCR amplification reaction using a heated lid Thermo-cycler (e.g., Perkin Elmer GeneAmp 9600 PCR system). The PCR thermal cycling conditions are (a) one cycle for 2 min at 94°C; (b) 30 cycles for 15 s at 94°C; 30 s at 58°C, and 30 s at 72°C; and (c) one cycle for 3 min at 72°C.

9. Electrophorese the PCR amplified products through a 1.2% low melting point agarose gel and isolate the DNA corresponding to the predicted size (350 to 400 bp). Many thermostable DNA polymerases, such as *Taq* polymerase, leave 3′ dATP overhangs on their reaction products. These molecules can be ligated directly to a vector (T-vector) containing single T-nucleotide overhangs (e.g., pT7Blue T-vector from Novagen, Madison, WI).

10. Ligate the PCR amplified product to a T-vector and transfect into competent bacterial host suitable for the T-vector.

11. Culture positive bacterial colonies, and prepare plasmid DNA using any miniprep kit (e.g., the Wizard™ from Promega, Madison, WI).

TABLE 12.3
The Universal *Ig* Primers

Universal *Ig* Primers	Sequence
UmIgV$_H$	5′ TGAGGTGCAGCTGGAGGAGTC 3′
UmIgV$_κ$	5′ GACATTCTGATGACCCAGTCT 3′
UmIgV$_λ$	5′ CAGGCTGTTGTGACTCAGGAATCT 3′
UmIgJ$_H$	5′ GTGACCGTGGTCCCTGCGCCCCAG 3′
UmIgJ$_κ$	5′ TTTTATTTCCAGCTTGGTCCC 3′
UmIgJ$_λ$	5′ CTAGGACAGTCACCTTGGTTCC 3′
UmIgC$_κ$	5′ GGGAAGATGGATACAGTTGGGCAG 3′
UmIgC$_λ$	5′ GAGTGTGGGAGTGGACTTGGGCTG 3′

12.2.4 Sequence Analysis of Ig V Genes

12. We use the cycle sequencing technique to sequence Ig V genes. Briefly, cycle sequencing is carried out in a Thermo-cycler and uses *Taq* DNA polymerase to make multiple copies of Ig V during 25 to 30 rounds of heat denaturing, annealing, extension, and termination.
13. The cloned double-stranded Ig V genes can be sequenced directly using any cycle sequencing kit. In our lab we use the SequiTherm™ kit from Epicentre Technologies (Madison, WI).

12.3 CLONING IG V REGIONS USING LINKERED-LIGATED PCR

12.3.1 Sequence of the Linker

The linker consists of the following two strands:

OG strand: 5′ GATCGTGGTACCGAATTCGCGGCCGCGTCGACG 3′ and
GO strand: 5′ CGTCGACGCGGCCGCGAATTCGGTACC 3′

12.3.2 Preparation of cDNA and PCR Amplification of Ig V Genes

1. Mix the two oligonucleotides in equal amounts and anneal at 55°C for 30 min followed by slow cooling at room temperature to make the linker (for more detail see Dattamajumdar et. al. 1996b).
2. Prepare total RNA and then synthesize cDNA from 7 μg total RNA as described in Section 12.2.2. Resuspend the blunt-ended cDNA in 7 μl of 10 m*M* Tris, 1 m*M* EDTA, pH 8.0 (TE) buffer and ligate to 1 μg of the OG/GO linker for 10 min at room temperature. We use a rapid DNA ligation kit from BMB (Indianapolis, IN). Remove the excess linkers by washing 3 times with TE buffer using 100,000 Mr MW cut-off Ultrafree-MC filters (Millipore, Bedford, MA) and then resuspend the linkered-cDNA in 50 μl TE buffer.
3. If the researcher is planning to express the Ig gene, alternative thermo-stable DNA polymerases with efficient proofreading activity such as *pfu* (*Pyrococcus Furiossus*) should be considered. It has been estimated that during PCR amplification reaction, *pfu* polymerase exhibits eleven- to twelvefold greater replication fidelity than *Taq* polymerase (Lundberg et. al. 1991). The average error rate for *pfu* was determined to be 1.6×10^{-6}, and for *Taq* polymerase, 2.0×10^{-5}.[34] Therefore, the efficient proofreading activity of *pfu* polymerase provides a high level of replication fidelity, producing a gene sequence without any errors.
4. Optimize the PCR amplification reaction by determining the optimal Mg⁺⁺ concentration to be used with the PCR buffer (10 m*M* Tris.Cl, pH

8.5, 50 mM KCl). The optimal concentration of Mg^{++} can range from 1.5 to 3.5 mM using *Taq* DNA polymerase. We found that 2.5 mM MgCl$_2$ is optimal for amplifying the desired full length of Ig V gene using *Taq* DNA polymerase.

5. Add 1 µl of linkered-cDNA to 19 µl PCR reaction mixture containing 2 µl of 10× reaction buffer (100 mM Tris.Cl, pH 8.5, 500 mM KCl, and 25 mM MgCl$_2$), 2 µl of 10× dNTPs (2 mM of each dNTP), 1 µl of 10 µM OG primer and 1 µl of 10 µM of any 3′ primer (Figure 12.4), 0.2 µl of *Taq* DNA polymerase (5 units/µl), and 12.8 µl H$_2$O.

6. Perform the PCR amplification reaction as in Section 12.2. The PCR thermal cycling conditions are (a) one cycle for 2 min at 94°C, (b) 25 cycles for 15 s at 94°C, 30 s at 58°C, and 30 s at 72°C, and (c) one cycle for 3 min at 72°C.

7. Electrophorese the PCR product through 2% NuSieve low-melting agarose, excise the DNA fragment, and place at 68°C for 10 min.

8. Extract DNA twice with phenol, once with chloroform, and then precipitate with 2.5 volumes of absolute ethanol in the presence of 0.5 M NaCl.

9. Ligate the precipitated DNA to a T vector, as previously described in Section 2.2.2. After transformation, the appropriate plasmid can be subjected to DNA sequence analysis, as in Section 2.2.2.

12.3.3 EXPRESSION OF IG GENES

The cloned VDJ$_H$ or VJ$_L$ gene can be inserted into an appropriate Ig expression vector to study its expression, produce large quantities for therapeutic use, or generate transgenic mice. There are three essential elements that must be present in any vector in order to express any Ig genes: promoter, enhancer, and constant region (for more detail see Grosschedl et al. 1984, Storb et al. 1986, Rusconi and Kohler 1985, and Goodnow et al. 1988). The linker contains several restriction sites; *Sal* I, *Not* I, *Eco*RI, and *Kpn* I. Furthermore, the 3′ primers can be designed to contain the restriction site(s) of interest, facilitating the cloning and subsequent subcloning of Ig genes into expression vectors. The expressed Ig genes (monoclonal antibodies) can be detected using one of the appropriate methods described in Chapter 6.

REFERENCES

1. Akolkar, P. N., Sikder, S. K., Bhattacharya, S. B., Liao, J., Gruezo, F., Morrison, S. L., and Kabat, E. A., Different V-L and V-H germ-line genes are used to produce similar combining sites with specificity for alpha (1, 6) dextrans, *J. Immunol.*, 138, 4472–4479, 1987.

2. Alt, F. W., Blackwell, T. K., and Yancopoulos, G. D., Development of the primary antibody repertoire, *Science*, 238, 1079–1087, 1987.

3. Bothwell, A. L., Paskind, M., Reth, M., Imanishi-Kari, T., Rajewsky, K., and Baltimore, D., Heavy chain variable region contribution to the NP^b family of antibodies: somatic mutation evident in a gamma-2a variable region, *Cell*, 24, 625–637, 1981.

4. Bernard, O. D., Hozumi, N., and Tonegawa, S., Sequences of mouse immunoglobulin light chain genes before and after somatic changes, *Cell*, 15, 1133–1144, 1978.

5. Brodeur, P. H. and Riblet, R., The immunoglobulin heavy chain variable region (Igh-V) locus in the mouse. I. One hundred Igh-V genes comprise seven families of homologous genes, *Eur. J. Immunol.*, 14, 922–930, 1984.

6. Brodeur, P. H., Osman, G. E., Mackle, J. J., and Lalor, T. M., The organization of the mouse Igh-V locus. Dispersion, interspersion, and evolution of V_H gene family clusters, *J. Exp. Med.*, 168, 2261–2278, 1988.

7. Chaudhary, V. K., Batra, J. K., Gallo, M. G., Willingham, M. C., Fitzgerald, D. J., and Pastan, I., A rapid method of cloning functional variable-region antibody genes in *Escherichia coli* as single-chain immunoglobulin, *Proc. Natl. Acad. Sci. U.S.A.*, 87, 1066–1070, 1990.

8. Chiang, Y. L., Sheng-Dong, R., Brow, M. A., and Larrick, J. W., Direct cDNA cloning of the rearranged immunoglobulin variable region, *BioTechniques*, 7, 360–366, 1989.

9. Coloma, M. J., Larrick, J. W., Ayala, M., and Gavilondo-Cowley, J. V., Primer design for the cloning of immunoglobulin heavy-chain leader-variable regions from mouse hybridoma cells using the PCR, *BioTechniques*, 11, 152–154, 1991.

10. Cory, S., Tyler, B. M., and Adams, J. M., Sets of immunoglobulin V kappa genes homologous to ten cloned V_κ sequences: implications for the number of germline V kappa genes, *J. Mol. Appl. Genet.*, 1, 103–116, 1981.

11. Dattamajumdar, A. K., Jacobson, D. P., Ladiges, W., Hood, L. E., and Osman, G. E., Characterization of the mouse Tcra-V22 gene subfamily, *Immunogenetics*, 43, 141–151, 1996a.

12. Dattamajumdar, A. K., Li, S. W., Jacobson, D. P., Hood, L. E., and Osman, G. E., Rapid cloning of any rearranged mouse immunoglobulin variable genes, *Immunogenetics*, 44, 432–440, 1996b.

13. D'Hoostelaere, L. A. and Klinman, D., Characterization of new mouse V kappa groups, *J. Immunol.*, 145, 2706–2712, 1990.

14. Dildrop, R., A new classification of mouse V_H sequences, *Immunol. Today*, 5, 85–86, 1984.

15. Eisen, H. N. and Reilly, E. B., Lambda chains and genes in inbred mice, *Ann. Rev. Immunol.*, 3, 337–365, 1985.

16. Embleton, M. J., Gorochov, G., Jones, P.T., and Winter, G., In-cell PCR from mRNA: amplifying and linking the rearranged immunoglobulin heavy and light chain V-genes within single cells, *Nucl. Acids Res.*, 20(25), 3831–3837, 1992.

17. Ferguson, S. E., Cancro, M. P., and Osborne, B. A., Analysis of a novel V(H)S107 haplotype in CLA-1 and WSA mice. Evidence for gene conversion among IgV(H) genes in outbred populations, *J. Exp. Med.*, 170, 1811–1823, 1989.

18. Gavilondo-Cowley, J. V., Coloma, M. J., Vazquez, J., Ayala, M., Macias, A., Fry, K. E., and Larrick, J. W., Specific amplification of rearranged immunoglobulin variable region genes from mouse hybridoma cells, *Hybridoma*, 9(5), 407–417, 1990.

19. Gefter, M. L., Margolies, M. N., Near, R. I., and Wysocki, L. J., Analysis of the anti-azobenzenearsonate response at the molecular level, *Ann. Inst. Pasteur Immunol.*, 135, 17–30, 1984.

20. Goodnow, C. C., Crossbie, J., Aldelstein, S., Lavoie, T. B., Smith-Gill, S., Brink, R. A., Pritchard-Briscoe, H., Wotherspoon, J. S., Loblay, R. H., Raphael, K., Trent, R. J., and Basten, A., Altered immunoglobulin expression and functional silencing of self-reactive B lymphocytes in transgenic mice, *Nature*, 334, 676–682, 1988.

21. Grosschedl, R., Weaver, D., Baltimore, D., and Costantini, F., Introduction of a μ immunoglobulin gene into the mouse germ line: specific expression in lymphoid cells and synthesis of functional antibody, *Cell*, 38, 647–658, 1984.

22. Hartman, A. B. and Rudikoff, S., VH genes encoding the immune response to beta-(1, 6)-galactan: somatic mutation in IgM molecules, *EMBO J.*, 3(12), 3023–3030, 1984.

23. Hayashi, K., Manipulation of DNA by PCR, in *PCR: The Polymerase Chain Reaction*, K. B. Mullis, F. Ferre, and R. A. Gibbs, Eds., Birkhauser Boston, Cambridge, MA, 3–13, 1994.

24. Heinrichs, A., Milstein, C., and Gherardi, E. A., Universal cloning and direct sequencing of rearranged antibody V genes using C region primers, biotin-captured cDNA and one-sided PCR, *J. Immunol. Methods*, 178, 241–251, 1995.

25. Jones, S. T. and Bendig, M. M., Rapid PCR-cloning of full-length mouse immunoglobulin variable regions, *Bio/Technology*, 9, 88–89, 1991.

26. Kabat, E. A., Wu, T. T., Perry, H. M., Gottesman, K. S., and Foeller, C., Sequences of Proteins of Immunological Interest, U.S. Department of Health and Human Services, MD, 1991.

27. Kettleborough, C. A., Saldhana, J., Ansell, K. H., and Bendig, M. M., Optimization of primers for cloning libraries of mouse immunoglobulin genes using the polymerase chain reaction, *Eur. J. Immunol.*, 23, 206–211, 1993.

28. Kofler, R., Geley, S., Hofler, H., and Helmberg, A., Mouse variable-regions gene families: complexity, polymorphism and use in non-autoimmune responses, *Immunol. Rev.*, 128, 5–21, 1992.

29. Kutemeier, G., Harloff, C., and Mocikat, R., Rapid isolation of immunoglobulin genes from cell lysates of rat hybridomas by polymerase chain reaction, *Hybridoma*, 11(1), 23–32, 1992.

30. Larrick, J. M., Danielsson, L., Brenner, C., Abrahamson, M., Fry, K., and Borrebaeck, C.A.K., Rapid cloning of rearranged immunoglobulin genes from human hybdridoma cells using mixed primers and the polymerase chain reaction, *Biochem. Biophys. Res. Commun.*, 160, 1250–1256, 1989.

31. Larrick, J. W., Coloma, M. J., Del Valle, J., Fernandez, M. E., Fry, K. E., and Gavilondo-Cowley, J. V., Immunoglobulin V regions of a bactericidal anti-*Neisseria meningitidis* outer membrane protein monoclonal antibody, *Scand. J. Immunol.*, 32, 121–128, 1990.

32. Livant, D., Blatt, C., and Hood, L., One heavy chain variable region gene segment subfamily in BALB/c mouse contains 500–1000 or more members, *Cell*, 47, 461–470, 1986.

33. Loh, E. Y., Elliott, J. F., Cwirla, S., Lanier, L.L., and Davis, M. M., Polymerase chain reaction with single-sided specificity: analysis of T cell receptor delta chain, *Science*, 243, 217–210, 1989.

34. Lundberg, K. S., Shoemaker, D. D., Adams, M. W. W., Short, J. M., Sorge, J. A., and Mathur, E. J., High fidelity amplification using a thermostable DNA polymerase isolated from Pyrococcus Furiossus, *Gene*, 108, 1–6, 1991.

35. Matsuda, T. and Kabat, E. A., Variable region cDNA sequences and antigen binding specificity of mouse monoclonal antibodies to isomaltosyl oligosaccharides coupled to proteins: T-dependent analogues of alpha-(1–6)-dextran, *J. Immunol.*, 142, 863–870, 1989.

36. Max, E. E., Maizel, J. V., and Leder, P., The nucleotide sequence of a 5.5-kilobase DNA segment containing the mouse kappa immunoglobulin J and C region genes, *J. Biol. Chem.*, 256, 5116–5120, 1981.

37. Meek, K., Rathbun, G., Reininger, L., Jaton, J. C., Kofler, R., Tucker, P., and Capra, J. D., Organization of the murine immunoglobulin VH complex: placement of two new VH families (VH10 and VH11) and analysis of VH family clustering and interdigitation, *Mol. Immunol.*, 27, 1073–1081, 1990.

38. Orlandi, R., Gussow, D. H., Jones, P. T., and Winter, G., Cloning immunoglobulin variable domains for expression by the polymerase chain reaction, *Proc. Natl. Acad. Sci. U.S.A.*, 86, 3833–3837, 1989.

39. Osman, G. E., Brodeur, P. H., Rosenberg, N., and Wortis, H. H., The Ig V$_H$ repertoire of fetal liver-derived pre-B cells is influenced by the expression of a gene liked to X-linked immune deficiency, *J. Immunol.*, 148, 1928–1933, 1992.

40. Pennell, C. A., Mercolino, T. J., Grdina, T. A., Arnold, L. W., Houghton, G., and Clarke, S., Biased immunoglobulin variable region gene expression by Ly-1 B cells due to clonal selection, *Eur. J. Immunol.*, 19, 1289–1295, 1989.

41. Potter, M., Newell, J. B., Rudikoff, S., and Haber, E., Classification of mouse V$_κ$ groups based on the partial amino acid sequence to the first invariant tryptophan: impact of 14 new sequences from IgG myeloma proteins, *Mol. Immunol.*, 12, 1619–1630, 1982.

42. Ratech, H., Rapid cloning of rearranged immunoglobulin heavy chian genes from human B-cell lines using anchored polymerase chain reaction, *Biochem. Biophys. Res. Commun.*, 182, 1260–1263, 1992.

43. Reininger, L., Kaushik, A., Izui, S., and Jaton, J. C., A member of a new V$_H$ gene family encodes anti-bromelinized mouse red blood cell autoantibodies, *Eur. J. Immunol.*, 18, 1521–1526, 1988.

44. Rusconi, S. and Kohler, G., Transmission and expression of a specific pair of rearranged immunoglobulin μ and κ genes in a transgenic mouse line, *Nature*, 314, 330–334, 1985.

45. Saiki, R. K., Gelfand, D. H., Stoffel, S., Scharf, S. J., Higuchi, R., Horn, G. T., Mullis, K. B., and Erlich, H. A., Primer-directed enzymatic amplification of DNA with a thermostable DNA polymerase, *Science*, 239, 487–491, 1988.

46. Sakano, H., Maki, R., Kurosawa, Y., Roeder, W., and Tonegawa, S., Two types of somatic recombination are necessary for the generation of complete immunoglobulin heavy-chain genes, *Nature*, 286, 676–683, 1980.

47. Sanchez, P., Marche, P. N., Rueff-Juy, D., and Cazenave, P. A., Mouse V–lambda–X gene sequence generates no junctonal diversity and is conserved in mammalian species, *J. Immunol.*, 144, 2816–2820, 1990.

48. Shapiro, M. A. and Weigert, M., How immunoglobulin V kappa genes rearrange, *J. Immunol.*, 139, 3834–3839, 1987.

49. Shefner, R., Mayer, R., Kaushik, A., D'Eustachio, P., Bona, C., and Diamond, B., Identification of a new V kappa gene family that is highly expressed in hybridomas from an autoimmune mouse strain, *J. Immunol.*, 145, 1609–1614, 1990.

50. Siedman, J. G., Max, E. E., and Leder, P. A., A kappa-immunoglobulin gene is formed by site-specific recombination without further somatic mutation, *Nature*, 280, 370–375, 1979.

51. Songsivilai, S., Bye, J. M., Marks, J. D., and Hughes-Jones, N. C., Cloning and sequencing of human lambda immunoglobulin genes by polymerase chain reaction, *Eur. J. Immunol.*, 20, 2661–2666, 1990.

52. Storb, U., Pinkert, C., Arb, B., Engler, P., Gollahon, K., Manz, J., Brady, W., and Brinster, R., Transgenic mice with m and k genes encoding antiphosphorylcholine antibodies, *J. Exp. Med.*, 164, 627–641, 1986.

53. Strohal, R., Helmberg, A., Kroemer, G., and Kofler, R., Mouse V kappa gene classification by nucleic acid sequence similarity, *Immunogenetics*, 30, 475–493, 1989.

54. Tonegawa, S., Maxam, A. M., Tizard, R., Bernard, O. D., and Gilbert, W., Sequence of a mouse germ-line gene for a variable region of an immunoglobulin light chain, *Proc. Natl. Acad. Sci. U.S.A.*, 75, 1485–1489, 1978.

55. Tutter, A., Brodeur, P. H., Shlomchik, M., and Riblet, R., Structure, map position, and evolution of two newly diverged mouse Ig V_H gene families, *J. Immunol.*, 147, 3215–3223, 1991.

56. Valiante, N. M. and Caton, A. J., A new Igk-V kappa gene family in the mouse, *Immunogenetics*, 32, 345–350, 1990.

57. Weiss, S. and Wu, G. E., Somatic point mutations in unrearranged immunoglobulin gene segments encoding the variable region of lambda light chains, *EMBO J.*, 6, 927–932, 1987.

58. Williams, J. F., Optimization strategies for the polymerase chain reaction, *BioTechniques*, 7, 762–769, 1989.

59. Winter, E., Radbruch, A., and Krawinkel, U., Members of novel V_H gene families are found in VDJ regions of polyclonally activated B-lymphocytes, *EMBO J.*, 4, 2861–2867, 1985.

60. Zhou, H., Fisher, R. J., and Papas, T. S., Optimization of primer sequences for mouse scFv repertoire display library construction, *Nucl. Acids Res.*, 22, 888–889, 1994.

61. Zwickl, M., Zaninetta, D., McMaster, G. K., and Hardman, N., Selective cloning of B cell hybridoma-specific rearranged immunoglobulin gene loci using the polymerase chain reaction, *J. Immunol. Methods*, 130, 49–55, 1990.

13 Antibody Storage

Kathryn Elwell and Delia R. Bethell

CONTENTS

13.1 INTRODUCTION

Antibodies, a class of glycoproteins, should be handled and stored using the considerations generally applied to proteins. They are susceptible to degradation by proteases found in many of the fluids containing the antibodies and need to be protected from microbial contamination. By following a few general principles, batches of antibodies can be maintained with very little loss of activity for several years.

The most accepted method for storage of antibody material is freezing. Material should be frozen in workable aliquots in order to avoid repeated freeze-thaw cycles. The best temperature is $-70°C$; however, many laboratories do not have equipment with this temperature capability. Storage at $-20°C$ is acceptable, but only in a freezer without an automatic defrost cycle. Automatic defrost cycles have a warming phase which permits a subtle freeze-thaw cycle and frequently results in significant loss of binding activity. Some classes of antibody, notably IgM, are not known for their stability during freezing. Lower temperatures, avoiding freeze thaw, and the use of glycerol to stabilize can improve the life of IgM antibodies. If aggregation occurs following thawing, it frequently represents denatured protein. Aggregates can be removed by filtration or centrifugation. Following removal of aggregation of antibody, activity should be reevaluated. Early characterization of an antibody's stability to various storage conditions is important, since these characteristics do not generally change from batch to batch of the same antibody.

Prior to freezing, it is usually appropriate to add an antimicrobial, such as sodium azide (NaN_3). This will provide protection for the material prior to freezing, and upon thawing and short-term storage at $4°C$. Sodium azide can interfere with some immunoassay reactions and conjugations, particularly involving peroxidases. The mode of action of sodium azide is blocking of the cytochrome electron transport mechanism. It should not be added to antibodies to be used *in vivo*. Sodium azide can be removed by dialysis or gel filtration. If it is not possible to use antimicrobials, antibodies can also be filter sterilized to remove potential contaminants and handled with aseptic techniques.

In the case of purified antibodies, protein concentration, pH, and salt concentration should be taken into consideration at storage. It is best to store proteins, either frozen or at 4°C at the highest concentration possible. Even though significant dilutions must be made for use, it is best to use undiluted antibodies for storage. Very dilute antibody solutions, like other dilute protein solutions, tend to lose activity due to adsorption to the storage vessel. Because of the ready adsorption of antibodies to polystyrene, useful in many immunoassay procedures, it is best to store antibodies in glass, polypropylene, or polycarbonate. Buffer solutions at neutral pH and 150 mM salt concentrations, such as phosphate-buffered saline (PBS), should be used when freezing antibody solutions. Ammonium and tris salts and azide can interfere with some coupling reactions. If any of these salts have been used for storage, they can be dialyzed away from the antibody protein as required.

Purified antibodies, which have been conjugated to other proteins, such as enzymes or biotin, or fluorescent tags should not be frozen due to the greater sensitivity of many of the label moieties to freeze-thaw cycles. Using aseptic techniques or antimicrobials conjugated antibodies can be stored at 4°C for up to a year with little loss of activity. In some instances, conjugated antibodies can be stored frozen in the presence of 50% glycerol as a stabilizer. It is best to determine storage conditions based on the characteristics of the conjugated compound.

In addition to storage as frozen liquid, there are two convenient methods for storing antibodies in a solid state, lyophilization (freeze-dried) and ammonium sulfate precipitation. Both of these methods allow for reduction in space required for freezing and can simultaneously reduce the degradation by proteases.

13.2 STORAGE OF SERUM, ASCITES, AND TISSUE CULTURE SUPERNATANT

Serum, plasma, ascitic fluid, and tissue culture supernatant can be stored at –70°C or –20°C. Solutions should be frozen in working aliquots or in bulk with several small aliquots removed for testing. The goal is to keep the number of freeze-thaw cycles at a minimum. Repeated freezing and thawing is a potential cause of damage, especially to IgM and murine IgG3. Some monoclonal antibodies are very sensitive to low-temperature storage conditions and will precipitate; these must be stored at 4°C.

13.2.1 ADDITION OF SODIUM AZIDE (NaN$_3$)

Prepare a 2% sodium azide stock solution and store at room temperature.

> 2% NaN$_3$ is 2 g/100 ml.
> Sodium azide is added to a final concentration of 0.1 to 0.02%.
> *Note:* Sodium azide is a metabolic poison and can form explosive compounds with heavy metals, such as copper in plumbing. When disposing

down sink, follow with large amounts of water. Consult MSDS for other safety considerations.

13.2.2 REMOVAL OF PROTEASE ACTIVITY BY HEAT INACTIVATION

Serum, plasma, and ascites may contain proteases that can cause degradation of the antibody. In many instances, heat inactivation will destroy protease activity without damaging antibody activity, particularly in the case of most IgGs. Prior to treatment of an entire batch, test a small aliquot to determine the effect of heat inactivation on the antibody activity. IgMs frequently lose activity. Once the antibody is tested, it can be assumed that all batches of the antibody will react the same way.

Heat a water bath to 56°C.
Note: The temperature is important as IgG can be aggregated at 60°C.
Heat antibody for 30 min.
Cool to room temperature and aliquot for freezing.
It may be desirable to test for residual protease activity.
Note: Several vendors provide kits for the detection of residual protease activity.

13.2.3 AMMONIUM SULFATE PRECIPITATION

Tissue culture supernatant tends to be in large volumes and sometimes contains antibodies in lower concentrations. One convenient method for reducing volume prior to storage is ammonium sulfate precipitation. This method can also be used with serum and ascites. Since ammonium sulfate precipitation is frequently the first step in purification, frozen storage of the precipitated pellet saves both space and time. A 50% saturated ammonium sulfate level will efficiently precipitate both polyclonal and monoclonal antibodies. Precipitation can be done by adding grams of ammonium sulfate or by adding a volume of saturated ammonium sulfate solution.

Saturated ammonium sulfate solution:
  Saturated ammonium sulfate is 4.1 *M*.
  Add 761 g to 1 L of distilled or deionized water.
  Adjust the pH to neutral with HCl.
  Store at room temperature.

  Note: It is acceptable to see crystals in the bottom of the flask. Some investigators prefer to prepare saturated ammonium sulfate by heating the solution above 25°C and adding more than 761 g of ammonium. The solution is cooled to room temperature, resulting in crystals in the cooled solution.

Measure the volume of antibody to be precipitated.
Transfer fluid to a beaker or flask of the appropriate size.
Put in a magnetic stir bar and place on magnetic stir plate.
Slowly add an equal volume of saturated ammonium sulfate solution.

Note: This can be efficiently done by using a separation funnel with stopcock positioned in a ring stand and adjusted to slowly drip the ammonium sulfate solution.

When all the ammonium sulfate is added, move the solution to 4°C and continue to stir overnight.
Warm to room temperature.
Centrifuge the precipitate at 2500 *g* for 30 min.
Remove and discard the supernatant; tubes can be drained for thorough removal.
Store precipitated pellets at –20° or –70°C.

Note: The precipitation can also be done using powdered ammonium sulfate. Weigh 313 g of ammonium for each liter of fluid to be precipitated. Slowly add the powder to the stirring fluid. Follow the instructions as above.

13.3 STORAGE OF PURIFIED ANTIBODIES

When storing purified antibodies, several additional considerations should be observed. If possible, store the purified antibodies at an undiluted concentration, in the range of 1 mg/mL or greater. If the antibody is more sensitive to freeze-thaw, the use of 50% glycerol can allow storage at –20°C without freezing of the solution. For freezing with glycerol, mix equal portions of antibody with glycerol.

An effective method for storing purified antibodies is lyophilization or freeze-drying. Lyophilization in ammonium bicarbonate is not only an efficient method of freeze-drying and storage, it also allows reconstitution in the buffer of choice. Antibodies may also be freeze-dried in any buffer at neutral pH, with a salt concentration less than 150 m*M*. The antibody should be reconstituted using distilled or deionized water.

The amount of moisture remaining will affect the stability of the antibody. It is important to be certain the preparation is completely dry before removal. If possible, the storage vial should be capped while still under vacuum. If this is not possible, capping should be done as rapidly as possible at completion of the process.

13.3.1 METHOD

Prepare 0.1 *M* ammonium bicarbonate, enough for 2 changes of 10 to 20 times volume.
Dialyze the purified antibody 12 to 18 h against two changes at a 20× volume of 0.1 *M* ammonium bicarbonate.
Remove antibody from dialysis tubing.
Measure protein concentration if desired.
Aliquot for lyophilization.
Freeze-dry to complete dryness, cap under vacuum or immediately afterward.
Store dried antibody at –20°C.
Antibody can be reconstituted in the buffer of choice.

13.3.2 METHOD 2

Antibody may be aliquoted and lyophilized in a neutral pH buffer with less than 150 mM salt.

Use the same procedure as described above.

13.4 STORAGE OF CONJUGATED ANTIBODIES

After conjugation, most antibody solutions should be stored at 4°C or at –20°C in 50% glycerol.

Characteristics of the conjugated or coupled material will influence the final storage conditions.

14 Chemically Modifying Antibodies

Kathryn Elwell and Gary C. Howard

CONTENTS

0-8493-9445-7/00/$0.00+$.50

14.1 BASIC CONSIDERATIONS

Chemical manipulation of antibodies is often required. Modifications may be for introduction of reporter molecules (fluorescent, spectrophotometric, spin-label, or radioactive) into a protein or labeling to facilitate an isolation procedure. Some specific examples include the attachment of biotin or other ligands (e.g., avidin and streptavidin), labeling with fluorochromes, and conjugation of enzymes or other proteins.

The particular modification selected will depend upon availability of suitable attachment groups, physical characteristics of the protein and reactant, and the experience of the experimenter. Although potential sites for chemical modifications can be found on most proteins, the most accessible groups are usually the aminos at the N-terminus and on lysines, carboxy groups at the C-terminus, and on glutamic acid and aspartic acid, and carbohydrate moieties. Good quality commercial reagents and relatively simple protocols are available for each of these groups. Whatever the requirement, there are several general practical aspects to the chemical modification of amino acids. The most important is the experimental goal. Other considerations include protein sensitivity to buffer, temperature, pH, and ionic strength; potential requirements for cosolvents and their effects on the protein; reaction conditions; and methods for removal of excess labeling or modifying reagent. Since disulfide bonds are an integral part of antibody structure, reducing conditions and reagents targeting SH groups are not generally useful. Any reagent may adversely affect an antibody's conformation, binding ability, or enzymatic activity. Several conditions are briefly discussed here.

Goal. The ultimate goal of the experiment will impact the modification procedure used. For example, the number of groups bound to the antibody can be critical. Use of a similar ratio of fluorescent groups to protein to produce a fluorescent probe would be unlikely to yield a useful product. Fluorescence increases with the number of bound molecules up to a limit and then decreases due to a phenomenon called "quenching." In other cases, an excess number of protein modifications may affect the antibody's solubility or biological activity.

Buffer. The buffer used must be compatible with both the antibody to be labeled and the labeling reagent. A pH which leaves the protein group to be modified in a reactive form must be selected. Optimal pH ranges for most commonly used buffers are well known. Phosphate buffers work very well at 6.5 to 7.0. Above this, bicarbonate/carbonate buffers are the choice. Some excellent reagents are available but their reaction pH is above 10, a range destructive to many proteins. In like manner, relatively neutral pH under aqueous conditions will result in the hydrolysis of many modification reagents. Finally, the buffer must be clear of any species which may compete for binding of the reagent.

Cosolvents. Many of the modification reagents are not very soluble in aqueous solution. To attain the concentration of the reagent required for the reaction, a water-miscible cosolvent is normally used. The cosolvent must be compatible with the modification reagent and the protein. Methanol, ethanol, propanol, and dioxane meet these requirements and are often used. However, the most used are dimethyl formamide (DMF) and dimethyl sulfoxide (DMSO).

Reaction conditions. Reaction conditions include the protein concentration, reagent concentration, pH, time, ionic strength, and temperature. All of these factors must be compatible with the protein and the modification reagent. The ratio of protein to reagent is the most critical. As indicated above, the desired use of the end product will determine this ratio. Most protocols call for 1 to 2 h or overnight incubations. The reactant should be added slowly to the protein solution with moderate stirring to avoid locally high concentrations of reactant and an inconsistent product. Moderate stirring will prevent denaturation, which can occur with vigerous mixing. Most reactions are best done in the cold.

Removal of excess modification reagent. At the end of the modification reaction, the excess reagent and the protein must be separated. If the reagent is relatively water soluble, separation by gel filtration (desalting) or dialysis is ideal. These procedures are quite gentle to antibodies.

14.2 SITES FOR MODIFICATIONS

Antibodies have several groups available for modification, including α and ϵ amines, carboxyls, sulfhydrals, and carbohydrates.

14.2.1 AMINES

Amines occur as α aminos at the N-terminus of the protein and as ϵ aminos on lysines. Because only the unprotonated form is reactive, the reaction pH must be maintained so that a significant percentage of the amines is available. The ϵ aminos are good nucleophiles above pH 8.0. However, the hydrolysis rates of some modification reagents are unacceptably high at these pHs. In contrast, α amines react well at neutral pHs, and this difference with the lysine amines makes possible a selective labeling of the α amines.

Most proteins have amine groups. There are exceptions. Some proteins have no lysines and a few have α-N-acylated amines. Amine groups can normally be modified without doing harm to the protein. Antibodies, in particular, have been modified to carry various labels including biotin, fluoresceine, and rhodamine. It is important to note that modification of the amine groups may change the overall electrical charge of the protein.

N-hydroxysuccinimide (NHS) is the best example of a reactive ester. NHS has a strong preference for aliphatic amines with little reactivity for aromatic amines, alcohols, phenols, or histidines. A secondary reaction occurs with imidazoles, but the reaction product is unstable and hydrolyses rapidly. Protein concentration is a factor. At relatively high concentrations, the acylation reaction is favored. At dilute concentrations, the hydrolysis by water is favored. The optimal reaction pH for NHS is 8.0 to 9.0. The reaction product, an aliphatic amide, is very stable. Most reactions are complete in about 10 to 20 min. It should be noted that the positive charge of the amine is lost in this reaction. Many commercial modification reagents incorporate NHS including biotin, fluoresceine, rhodamine, and many heterobifunctional reagents. NHS compounds are subject to hydrolysis and must be well desiccated when stored. Many NHS compounds are not soluble in water at concentrations greater than 1 mM so an organic cosolvent must be used. The limited solubility of some NHS compounds can be improved by incorporation of sulfonate groups in the NHS moiety. These will often eliminate the requirement for cosolvents such as DMF or DMSO.

Isothiocyanates react with amines to form very stable thiourea bonds. Their optimal reaction pH is 9.0 to 9.5. They are more stable to hydrolysis than NHS esters. The leaving group is easily removed from the protein solution by dialysis or gel filtration. Fluoresceine isothiocyanate is one of the most commonly used commercial protein modification reagents.

Aldehyde reactions are commonly done by forming a Schiff base (an imine) followed by its reduction to a stable alkylamine bond by the mild reducing agent sodium cyanoborohydride.

Sulfonyl halides react with amines to form very stable sulfonamide bonds. Their one disadvantage is their instability in aqueous solutions at normal reaction pHs. The most commonly used example of this class is fluorescein DTAF. Iodoacetamide, another example of this group, reacts well at pH 9.0 to 9.5. Acid anhydrides result from the reaction of a carboxylic acid with carbitol or 2-methylpropanol chloroformate. Examples include succinic anhydride and acetic anhydride. Both can be used to eliminate the positively charged amine groups and alter the net electrical charge on the protein.

14.2.2 CARBOXYL GROUPS

Carboxyl groups occur in antibodies at the C-terminus and on the side chains of glutamic acid and aspartic acid. They are generally ionized above pH 5.0 and are extremely polar. They can be esterified, coupled with amine or other nucleophiles, and reduced to alcohols. The method most commonly employed involves the production of reactive ester by use of a water-soluble carbodiimide and then its reaction with a nucleophilic reagent like an amine or hydrazine. This reaction is one of the most useful in protein chemistry. The resulting amide bond is very stable.

14.2.3 CARBOHYDRATES

Most antibodies contain carbohydrate moieties that are available as sites for protein modification. The most commonly used is periodic acid oxidation of the carbohydrate to an aldehyde and its formation of a Schiff base with an amine or hydrazide and the subsequent reduction to an alkylamine with sodium borohydride. The great advantage of labeling or conjugating through the carbohydrate is that the antibody binding site is rarely affected.

14.3 ADDING A FLUORESCENT LABEL

The example given here will be for the binding of rhodamine isothiocynate to an antibody. Most other attachments of labels to proteins at the primary amino groups by use of the leaving group isothiocynate will behave in the same way. Some additional care must be taken with all fluorescent molecules since the binding of too many on one protein will result in a phenomenon known as quenching and a lower level of fluorescence.

Many of the fluorescent and reactive groups have problems in aqueous solution. For example, isothiocynate is labile in water and should be prepared immediately before use. The limited solubilities of rhodamine and fluoresceine in aqueous solution are improved somewhat by higher pHs (> 8.0).

14.3.1 Reagents and Supplies

Allow approximately 1 h for setup, 4 h for reaction, and 6 h for dialysis or 1 h for gel filtration. No special equipment is needed. Prepare the following reagents and other materials in advance.

RITC solution: dissolve 25 mg/ml RITC in 100 mM sodium bicarbonate or HEPES buffer, pH 8.5 (prepare just before use).
Protein solution: dissolve protein to be labeled in 100 mM sodium bicarbonate or HEPES buffer, pH 8.5, to a concentration of 2 to 10 mg/ml.
Dialysis buffer in sufficient quantity.
Dialysis tubing with an appropriate molecular weight cutoff.

14.3.2 Procedure

In advance, dissolve the protein to be labeled in the buffer or dialyze it into the bicarbonate or HEPES buffer.

1. Prepare the RITC solution immediately prior to use (the isothiocyanate groups have a fairly short half-life in aqueous solution).
2. Add the RITC solution to the protein solution in several aliquots to a final RITC concentration of 50 μg/ml.
3. Incubate at room temperature for 4 h with occasional gentle shaking.
4. Dialyze the mixture against the desired buffer for two changes of a least 3 h each.

Alternatively, pass the mixture through a Sephadex G-25 gel filtration column. The unbound RITC will be separated from the protein and the labeled protein can be collected in the column void volume.

14.3.3 Notes

    a. Fluorescent compounds (including labeled antibodies) are light sensitive. All work should be done in reduced light or darkness. Cover all containers with aluminum foil.

    b. Pilot runs may be required to determine the optimal RITC to protein ratio.

14.4 ADDING BIOTIN TO AMINO GROUPS

Biotin and avidin are among the most useful binding pairs in antibody reactions. The specificity and strength of their binding (affinity constant $>10^{15}$ M^{-1}) shorten reaction times and help to avoid nonspecific binding problems. Biotin N-hydroxy-succinimide is one of the most useful reagents for adding a biotin group to an antibody. Sulfo derivatives of this compound increase the water solubility.

14.4.1 Reagents and Supplies

Allow approximately 1 h for setup, 2 h for reaction, and 6 h for dialysis. No special equipment is needed. The following reagents and other materials should be prepared in advance:

    BNHS solution: dissolve 25 to 50 mg/ml BNHS in dimethylformamide (DMF).
    Protein solution: dissolve protein to be labeled in 100 mM sodium bicarbonate
       or HEPES buffer, pH 8.5, to a concentration of 2 to 10 mg/ml.
    Dialysis buffer in sufficient quantity.
    Dialysis tubing with an appropriate molecular weight cutoff.
    Glycine.

14.4.2 Procedure

In advance, dissolve the protein to be labeled in the buffer or dialyze it into the bicarbonate or HEPES buffer.

    1. Prepare the BNHS solution immediately prior to use. (NHS groups have a relatively short half-life in aqueous solution.)
    2. Add the BNHS solution to the protein solution so that the ratio of FNHS to protein is 1:10 (wt/wt).
    3. Incubate at room temperature for 2 h with occasional gentle shaking.
    4. After the incubation, add approximately 10 to 20 mg glycine to stop the reaction.
    5. Dialyze the mixture against the desired buffer for two changes of at lease 3 h each.
    6. Store the labeled protein in the same way the unlabeled protein is stored.

14.5 ACTIVATING CARBOXYL GROUPS WITH EDAC

EDAC (1-ethyl-3-[3-dimethylaminopropyl]-carbodiimide) is a water-soluble carbodiimide for activating carboxyl groups in antibodies and other proteins. It has many useful applications in the chemical modification of antibodies and in the joining of haptens to carrier proteins to prepare immunogens.

14.5.1 PROCEDURE

Note: EDAC can cause severe burns. Handle with appropriate care and protective clothing.

1. Prepare a 100 mg/ml EDAC solution immediately before use by dissolving the EDAC in distilled water.
2. Add the EDAC solution to the protein solution to a final EDAC concentration of 1.0 mg/ml. The ideal ratio for carboxyl groups and EDAC is 1:1. However, the exact number of carboxyls is rarely known.
3. This reaction is very rapid.
4. Add sulfo-NHS to a final concentration of 1.0 mg/ml.
5. The activated carboxyl groups are ready to bind to other reactive groups. For example, biotin hydrazide can be added to the antibody solution to a final concentration of 1.0 mg/ml and incubated overnight.
6. Remove unbound label by dialysis.

14.6 ADDING BIOTIN TO THE CARBOHYDRATE GROUP

Use of the carbohydrate groups of most antibodies involves the oxidation of the carbohydrate and its reduction by the formation of a Schiff base between a hydrazide and the oxidized sugar. The carbohydrates are not usually near the antibody binding sites and so their modification does not harm the specificity of the antibody binding. Biotin hydrazide is commercially available from a number of suppliers.

14.6.1 PROCEDURE

In advance, prepare a gel-filtration column (e.g., Sephadex G-25) in the appropriate buffer.

Dialyze the antibody against 100 m*M* sodium acetate, 150 m*M* sodium chloride, pH 5.5.

Note: The oxidation of the sugars is a light-sensitive reaction. Steps 1–6 must be done in the dark. Use aluminum foil to completely cover all reaction vessels and columns.

1. Immediately before use, prepare a solution of 100 m*M* sodium periodate in distilled water.
2. Add the periodate solution to the antibody solution in several aliquots separated by about 2 min each to a final concentration of 10 m*M*.
3. Incubate for 20 min at room temperature.

4. Separate the antibody from the unbound sodium periodate by gel-filtration chromatography in 100 mM sodium acetate, pH 5.5.
5. Add biotin hydrazide to the collected protein fraction to a final concentration of 2.0 mg/ml. Incubate 2 to 20 h at room temperature.
6. Stop the reaction by adding a small amount of solid sodium borohydride (approximately 1 mg/ml).
7. Separate the labeled antibody from the unbound label and other material by gel-filtration chromatography or dialysis.

14.7 RADIOIODINATION BY THE BOLTON-HUNTER PROCEDURE

The radioactive isotopes of iodine (^{131}I and ^{125}I) are very valuable labels for antibodies. Both are gamma emitters and require care in their use, storage, and disposal.

Bolton-Hunter reagent is a ^{125}I-labeled N-succinimidyl 3-(4-hydroxyphenylpropionate). It is commercially available with one or two iodines per molecule. The iodination method is quick and simple and also somewhat safer than the chloramine T method since the iodine is held in a less volatile form. Nevertheless, it should still be performed with appropriate care in a well-ventilated radioactive hood or glove box.

14.7.1 REAGENTS AND SUPPLIES

Well-ventilated glove box or hood and appropriate protective clothing
Appropriate radioactive disposal procedures

14.7.2 PROCEDURE

Prepare a gel-filtration column for purification of the labeled material.
Remove any azide from the antibody solution by dialysis.
1. Add dimethyl formamide to the Bolton-Hunter reagent (0.2% final concentration) if not provided by the manufacturer.
2. The antibody solution should be 0.5 to 1.0 mg/ml in 0.1 M sodium borate, pH 8.5 on ice.
3. Dry approximately 500 µCi of the Bolton-Hunter reagent in a 1.5-ml conical vial in a stream of nitrogen gas on ice.
4. Add 10 µl of the antibody solution to the vial and mix.
5. Incubate on ice for 15 min.
6. Stop the reaction by adding a solution of 0.5 M ethanolamine, 10% glycerol, 0.1 M sodium borate, pH 8.5, and incubating for 5 min at room temperature.
7. Separate the unbound reagent from the labeled antibody by gel filtration chromatography.

14.8 RADIOIODINATION BY THE CHLORAMINE T PROCEDURE

Chloramine T is an oxidant that labels antibodies and other proteins with $Na^{125}I$. Although very efficient, this method requires special procedures and training. The radioactive iodine in this method is very volatile. The procedure must be done in a contained glove box or very well-ventilated radioactive hood.

14.8.1 REAGENTS AND SUPPLIES

These are the same as those for the Bolton-Hunter procedure.

14.8.2 PROCEDURE

Prepare a gel-filtration column for the separation of the bound and unbound iodine.

Remove any azide, Tris, or reducing agents from the antibody solution by dialysis.

1. Add 10 µg of antibody in a 25 µl of 0.5 M sodium phosphate, pH 7.5, in a 1.5-ml conical vial.
2. Add 500 µCi of $Na^{125}I$ to the vial.
3. Add 25 ml of freshly made 2 mg/ml chloramine T and incubate the mixture for 1 min.
4. Stop the reaction by adding a stop solution of 2.4 mg/ml sodium metabisulfite, 10 mg/ml tyrosine, 10% glycerol, in phosphate-buffered saline.
5. Separate the unbound label from the labeled antibody by gel-filtration chromatography.

14.9 BIFUNCTIONAL REAGENTS AND CONJUGATIONS

Bifunctional reagents are those which have two reactive groups. They are used to join two other molecules together to form conjugates (e.g., antibody–enzyme, antibody–phycobiliprotein, protein–small reporter group or ligand). They can also be used to bind haptens to carrier proteins to make immunogens. Many excellent bifunctional protein cross-linking reagents are available commercially.

Separating the two reactive groups is the linker. Linkers can vary in length. The length of the linker can be useful in controlling reactions, especially in intramolecular or intracomplex reactions. Some linkers incorporate other special features, such as groups that enhance solubility in aqueous phase or, for example, disulfide groups, that allow for a "reversal" of the joining.

The reactive groups can be the same (homobifunctional reagents) or different (heterobifunctional reagents). Homobifunctional reagents are generally simpler to use.

The most common homobifunctional reagents are glutaraldehyde and formaldehyde. Their method of action is not completely understood. Others include dimethyl adipimidate (to join amines), 1, 5-diazidonaphthalene (DAN) (nonspecific, photoreactive), and dimethyl-3, 3'-dithiobispropionimidate and tartryldiazide (both cleavable). Heterobifunctional reagents require more steps and so are more complicated. For example, excess labeling reagent must be removed at each step of the reaction. However, the experimenter has greater control over the labeling and is able to target more specific groups for the cross-linking. A large number of different heterobifunctional reagents are available commercially.

14.10 CROSS-LINKING WITH GLUTARALDEHYDE

Glutaraldehyde is a commonly used and relatively efficient cross-linking reagent. The protein reactive sites are the epsilon-amino groups. Several factors favor the reaction including pH values above 7.0, higher temperatures, greater concentrations, and longer reaction times. It is important to remember that glutaraldehyde is somewhat unstable, and samples will vary in reactivity. One-step and two-step procedures for cross-linking with glutaraldehyde are indicated below. The preparations are similar for both.

14.10.1 REAGENTS AND SUPPLIES

Allow approximately 1 h for setup, 3 h for the reaction, and 2 × 3 h for dialysis. No special equipment is needed. The following reagents and other items should be prepared in advance:

> Protein A solution
> Protein B solution
> Glutaraldehyde solution: must be fresh.
> *Note:* Glutaraldehyde is toxic and can cause burns. Use with proper protection
>   (eye protection, gloves, good ventilation).
> Lysine solution: 0.5 *M* lysine in above buffer
> Dialysis buffer
> Dialysis tubing
> Gel-filtration chromatography column of appropriate separation capacity

14.10.2 ONE-STEP GLUTARALDEHYDE CROSS-LINKING METHOD

14.10.2.1 Procedure

In advance, dialyze the proteins against 100 m*M* sodium phosphate, 150 m*M* sodium chloride, pH 6.8. The dialysis ensures that the two proteins are in a buffer compatible with the cross-linking reaction, and also removes any substances that might interfere with the reaction (glycine, azide).

1. Mix the proteins in an appropriate ratio. Several pilot experiments may be necessary to determine the optimal ratio. For enzyme/antibody conjugates, ratios of 1:1 or 1:2 (antibody-enzyme) are good starting points.
2. Add the glutaraldehyde solution very slowly with stirring. The final concentration of glutaraldehyde should be 0.05% (vol/vol). Adding the glutaraldehyde too quickly may cause locally high concentrations. The resulting uneven cross-linking will yield a broad distribution of conjugate sizes. Do not stir so vigorously as to damage the proteins.
3. Incubate for 2 to 3 h.
4. Add excess lysine to stop the reaction.
5. Separate monomer proteins from complexes by gel-filtration chromatography (e.g., Sepharose S-300, Pharmacia).
6. Store complexes correctly. In general, this means in the cold with required stabilizing additives.

14.10.3 TWO-STEP GLUTARALDEHYDE METHOD

14.10.3.1 Procedure

The steps to be taken in advance are the same as those for the one-step procedure.

1. Dialyze the Protein A solution against 100 mM sodium phosphate, 150 mM sodium chloride, pH 7.0, for a minimum of two changes over 6 h.
2. Dialyze the Protein A solution once again against the same buffer with 0.2% glutaraldehyde overnight at room temperature.
3. Dialyze the Protein A solution again to remove the unreacted glutaraldehyde.
4. Mix the Protein A and Protein B solutions in the desired ratio. Incubate overnight in the cold.
5. Separate monomer proteins from complexes by gel-filtration chromatography (e.g., Sepharose S-300, Pharmacia).
6. Store the complexes correctly. In general, this means in the cold with required stabilizing additives.

14.11 PREPARING ANTIBODY-ENZYME CONJUGATES WITH SPDP

SPDP [N-succinimidyl 3-(2-pyridyldithio)propionate] is a water-insoluble solid. It must be dissolved in a water-miscible cosolvent before use. This bifunctional cross-linking reagent works by two reactions: the first attacks amines at pH 7.0 to 8.5; the second with thiols at pH 7.0 or above. An alternative cross-linking involves treatment with dithiothreitol and coupling to maleimidylated protein. SPDP has a span of approximately 7 A.

14.11.1 REAGENTS AND SUPPLIES

Allow approximately 30 min for setup, 3 h for reactions and separations, 7 h for dialysis, and 6 h for gel filtration. No special equipment is needed. The following reagents and other items should be prepared in advance:

Two G-25 columns in PBS, pH 7.4
Sepharose A-300 or other appropriate gel-filtration column in PBS

14.11.2 PROCEDURE

In advance, dialyze Protein A into PBS and Protein B into PBS at concentrations of 5 to 20 and 10 mg/ml, respectively. Prepare the columns.

1. Add an 8 M excess of SPDP dissolved in 75% ethanol to the Protein A solution and incubate for 30 min at room temperature.
2. Separate the protein from the unreacted SPDP on a Sephadex G-25 desalting column.
3. Add a 4 M excess of SPDP to the Protein B solution and incubate for 20 min at room temperature.
4. Separate the protein from the unreacted SPDP on a Sephadex G-25 desalting column.
5. Generate free thiols on the modified Protein A by incubation with 0.2 M DTT for 20 min at room temperature.
6. Separate the protein from the unreacted SPDP on a Sephadex G-25 desalting column.
7. Mix a 2 to 5 M excess of Protein B with the reduced Protein A for 60 min at room temperature.
8. Cap any remaining free thiols by reaction with iodoacetamide at a 100 M excess.
9. Dialyze at 4°C vs. several changes of PBS.
10. Separate the cross-linked protein complexes from the monomers by gel-filtration chromatography.

14.12 PREPARING ANTIBODY-ENZYME CONJUGATES WITH MBS

MBS [m-maleimidobenzoic acid N-hydroxysuccinimide ester] is a water-insoluble solid that requires the use of a water-miscible cosolvent. A water-soluble sulfosuccinimide ester is also now available. The first reaction is with amines at pH 7 to 8. The second is with thiols at pH 6.0 to 8.0. The resulting span is approximately 10 A.

14.12.1 REAGENTS AND SUPPLIES

Allow 4 h for the entire procedure. No special equipment is required.

14.12.2 Procedure

1. Add 2-iminothiolane (Traut's reagent) to Protein A if no free thiols are available.
2. Add a 5 M excess of MBS (stock solution 1 mg/ml in dimethylformamide) and incubate for 20 min at room temperature.
3. Separate the modified protein from the unreacted MBS by use of a Sephadex G-25 desalting column.
4. Mix modified Protein B with a 10 M excess of the modified Protein A for 60 min at room temperature.
5. Block any residual free thiols with N-ethylmaleimide.
6. Separate the complex from the monomers by Sepharose A-300 or other appropriate gel-filtration chromatography.

14.13 PREPARING ANTIBODY-ENZYME CONJUGATES WITH SMCC

SMCC stands for N-succinimidyl 4-(N-maleimidomethyl)-cyclohexane-1-carboxylate. SMCC is a water-insoluble reagent requiring the use of a water-miscible cosolvent. A water-soluble form is also now available. Its action is similar to that of MBS in linking between an amine and a thiol. The resulting span is approximately 12 A.

14.13.1 Reagents and Supplies

Allow 25 h for the entire procedure. No special equipment is required.

14.13.2 Procedure

1. Add a 10 M excess of SMCC (stock solution = 10 mM in dioxane) to Protein A (1 mg/ml in 100 M sodium phosphate buffer, pH 7.0, with 0.5 mM EDTA) and incubate 30 min at 30°C.
2. Separate the modified Protein A from the unreacted reagent by dialysis or by use of a desalting column.
3. Prepare Protein B to a concentration of 2 mg/ml in potassium phosphate buffer, pH 7.2, with 145 mM NaCl, 60 mM triethanolamine, and 0.1 M EDTA.
4. Degas the mixture.
5. Add 2-iminothiolane (stock solution = 0.5 M) to Protein B to a final concentration of 1 mM and incubate 90 min at 0°C.
6. Separate the unreacted 2-iminothiolane from the modified Protein B by use of a desalting column.
7. Add an equal weight of modified Protein B to modified Protein A, adjust the pH to 7.0 with triethanolamide HCl pH 8.0, and incubate at 4°C for 20 h.

8. Block any remaining free thiols by addition of 2 mM iodoacetamide for 1 h at 25°C.
9. Separate complexes from monomers by Sepharose A-300 or other appropriate gel-filtration chromatography.

14.14 PREPARING HORSERADISH PEROXIDASE-ANTIBODY CONJUGATES

Horseradish peroxidase (HRP) is a commonly used enzyme in immunohistochemistry. It contains a polysaccharide moiety that can be readily used for conjugation to antibodies. The procedure involves the oxidation of the carbohydrate with periodate, the formation of a Schiff base between the oxidized sugar and an amino group on the antibody, and the reduction of the Schiff base to form a covalent linkage.

14.14.1 REAGENTS AND SUPPLIES

The entire procedure takes approximately 3 h. Additional time is required for dialysis to remove unbound reactants.

Prepare the antibody solution to a concentration of 5 to 10 mg/ml in distilled water. Prepare HRP solution to a concentration of 5 to 10 mg/ml in 100 mM sodium bicarbonate, 100 mM sodium chloride, pH 9.5.

14.14.2 PROCEDURE

1. Immediately before use, prepare the sodium periodate by dissolving it in distilled water to 400 mM.
2. Add the periodate solution to the HRP solution in five equal aliquots at 2-min intervals to a final concentration of 40 mM.
3. Incubate for 20 min.
4. Separate the HRP from the unbound reactants by gel filtration in the same buffer. The red color of the HRP fractions makes collecting the enzyme-containing fractions easy.
5. Add the antibody solution to the pooled HRP fractions. Incubate for 3 h at room temperature.
6. Stop the reaction by adding a small amount of solid sodium borohydride to a final concentration of ~1 mg/ml.
7. Separate the monomer proteins from the conjugate by gel filtration on a Sepharose S-300 or equivalent column.

14.15 PREPARING ANTIBODY-PHYCOBILIPROTEIN CONJUGATES

Phycobiliproteins are large, somewhat stable, fluorescent proteins found in various species of algae. Several are commercially available. They offer significant advantages and some challenges. First, their fluorescence is far greater, on a molar basis, than that of most other commonly used labels. They also expand the useful excitation and emission wavelength choices.

Conjugates with antibodies, avidin, and streptavidin are very useful, especially in flow cytometry.

However, their large size limits their stability, and precipitation during conjugation is a concern. Commercial preparations are often provided as ammonium sulfate suspensions. These must be readied for conjugation by carefully dialyzing away the ammonium sulfate. The exact conditions of conjugation may have to be empirically determined.

REFERENCES

REFERENCES FOR SECTION 14.1

Anderson, G.W., Zimmerman, J.E., and Callahan, F.M., 1964, *J. Am. Chem. Soc.*, 86, 1839.
Glazer, A., Delange, R.J., and Sigman, D.S., Chemical modification of proteins, in *Laboratory Techniques in Biochemistry and Molecular Biology*, Vol. 4, Work, T.S. and Work, E., Eds., Elsevier, New York, 1976, 1–205.
Harlow, E. and Lane, D., 1988, *Antibodies. A Laboratory Manual*, Cold Spring Harbor Laboratory Press, Cold Spring Harbor, NY.
Howard, G.C., Ed., 1993, *Methods in Nonradioactive Detection*, Appleton & Lange, New York.
Means, G.E. and Freeney, R.E., *Chemical Modification of Proteins,* Holden-Day, San Francisco, CA, 1971.

REFERENCES FOR SECTION 14.3

The, T.H. and Feltkamp, T.E.W., 1970, Conjugation of fluorescein isothiocynate to antibodies. I. Experiments on the conditions of conjugation, *Immunology*, 18, 865–873.
The, T.H. and Feltkamp, T.E.W., 1970, Conjugation of fluorescein isothiocynate to antibodies. II. A reproducible method, *Immunology,* 18, 875–881.

REFERENCES FOR SECTION 14.4

Hochhaus, G., Gibson, B.W., and Sadee, W.J., 1988, *J. Biol. Chem.*, 263, 92.
Kyurkchiev, S.D. et al., 1986, *Immunology*, 57, 489.
Taki, S. et al., 1989, *J. Immunol. Methods,* 122, 33.

REFERENCES FOR SECTION 14.5

Kayser, K. et al., 1990, *Histochem. J.*, 22, 426.
Rosenberg, M.B., Hawrot, E., and Breakfield, X.O., 1986, *J. Neurochem.*, 46, 641.
Staros, J.V., Wright, R.W., and Swingle, D.M., *Anal. Biochem.*, 156, 220.

REFERENCES FOR THE USE OF CARBODIIMIDES

Hoare, D.G. and Koshland, D.E., 1967, A method for quantitative modification and estimation of carboxylic acid groups in proteins, *J. Biol. Chem.*, 242, 2447–2453.

Bauminger, S. and Wilchek, M., 1980, The use of carbodiimides in the preparation of immunizing conjugates, *Methods Enzymol.*, 70, 151–159.

Goodfriend, T.L., Levine, L., and Fasman, G.D., 1964, Antibodies to bradykinin and angiotensin: a use of carbodiimides in immunology, *Science*, 144 (Abstr.), 1344–1346.

REFERENCES FOR SECTION 14.6

Heitzman, H. and Richards, F.M., 1975, *Proc. Natl. Acad. Sci. U.S.A.*, 71, 3537.

O'Shannessy, D.J., Dobersen, M.J., and Quarles, R.H., 1984, *Immunol. Lett.*, 8, 273.

REFERENCES FOR SECTION 14.7

Bolton, A.E. and Hunter, W.M., 1973, The labeling of proteins to high specific radioactivity by conjugation to a ^{125}I-containing acylating agent, *Biochem. J.*, 133, 529–539.

Langone, J.J., 1980, Radioiodination by use of Bolton-Hunter and related reagents, *Methods Enzymol.*, 70, 221–247.

REFERENCES FOR SECTION 14.8

Greenwood, F.C., Hunter, W.M., and Glover, J.S., 1963, The preparation of ^{131}I-labeled human growth hormone of high specific radioactivity, *Biochem. J.*, 89, 114–123.

Hunter, W.M. and Greenwood, F.C., 1962, Preparation of iodine-131 labeled human growth hormone of high specific activity, *Nature*, 194, 495–496.

REFERENCE FOR SECTION 14.10.2

Avrameas, S., 1969, *Immunochemistry*, 6, 43.

REFERENCE SECTION 14.10.3

Engvall, E., 1978, *Scand. J. Immunol.*, 8 (Suppl. 7), 25.

REFERENCE FOR SECTION 14.11

O'Keefe, D.O. and Draper, R.K., 1985, Characterization of a transferrin-diphtheria toxin conjugate, *J. Biol. Chem.*, 260, 932–937.

REFERENCES FOR SECTION 14.12

Green, N., Alexander, H., Olsen, A., Alexander, S., Shinnick, T.M., Sutcliffe, J.G., and Lerner, R.A., 1982, Immunogenic structure of the influenza virus hemagglutinin, *Cell*, 28, 477–487.

Kitagawa, T. and Aikawa, T., 1976, Enzyme coupled immunoassay of insulin using a novel coupling reagent, *J. Biochem.*, 79, 233–236.

Liu, F.-T., Zinnecker, M., Hamaoka, T., and Katz, D.H., 1979, New procedures for preparation and isolation of conjugates of proteins and a synthetic copolymer of D-amino acids and immunochemical characterization of such conjugates, *Biochemistry*, 18, 690–697.

Marsh, J.W., 1988, *J. Biol. Chem.*, 263, 15993, *Proc. Natl. Acad. Sci. U.S.A.*, 77, 5483–5486.

REFERENCE FOR SECTION **14.13**

J. Biol. Chem., 260, 12035–12041, 1985.

REFERENCE FOR SECTION **14.14**

Nakane, P.K. and Kawaoi, A., 1974, Peroxidase-labeled antibody: a new method of conjugation, *J. Histochem. Cytochem.*, 22, 1084–1091.

Tijssen, P. and Kurstak, E., 1984, Highly efficient and simple methods for the preparation of peroxidase and active peroxidase-antibody conjugates for enzyme immunoassays, *Anal. Biochem.*, 136, 451–457.

REFERENCE FOR SECTION **14.15**

Festin, G., Bjorklund, B., and Totterman, T., 1987, *J. Immunol. Methods,* 101, 231.

Krokick, M.N., 1986, *J. Immunol. Methods*, 92, 1.

Oi, V., Glazer, A., and Stryer, L., 1982, *J. Cell Biol.*, 93, 981.

15 Western Blotting

Lee Bendickson and Marit Nilsen-Hamilton

CONTENTS

0-8493-9445-7/00/$0.00+$.50
© 2000 by CRC Press LLC

15.1 INTRODUCTION

Studying specific proteins in complex mixtures has been facilitated by the development of the Western blot method. This method has found wide application due to its simplicity, specificity, and sensitivity.

Western blotting is one of several methods that use the specificity of the antigen:antibody interaction to indicate the presence of particular proteins in samples. Other methods include immunoprecipitation (IP), immunohistochemistry/cytochemistry, and enzyme-linked immunosorbent assay (ELISA). Immunoprecipitation uses antibodies to preferentially precipitate the protein or protein complex of interest from a mixture of proteins. Precipitated proteins are then resolved using polyacrylamide gel electrophoresis (PAGE). If the original mixture of proteins was radiolabeled, then autoradiography is used to visualize the radioactive signal. Otherwise, proteins with modifications such as biotinylation or phosphorylation can be detected by these features, and enzymes can be detected by their enzymatic activity. Detection of biotinylated and phosphorylated proteins often involves the Western blot procedure. The two closely related methods of immunohistochemistry and immunocytochemistry detect protein *in situ* in tissue sections or intact cells, respectively, and usually employ a chromogenic substrate that leaves a stain in the region of the fixed tissue or cell where the protein of interest is located. These *in situ* methods are useful for locating the protein, but are not quantitative and do not provide further characterization of the protein such as its molecular weight. An interesting extension of these *in situ* methods is the tissue-print technique[1] in which plant tissue sections are blotted directly on nitrocellulose, leaving a surface image of the section that can be probed using specific antibodies.

The ELISA method is used when large numbers of samples are to be screened quickly. This method relies on the adsorption of protein to plastic. Adsorbed protein is detected by its binding to a specific primary antibody that, in turn, is bound by a secondary antibody that is linked to an enzyme that catalyzes the color change of a chromogenic substrate. The soluble colored product can be measured, using a spectrophotometer.

All of these methods are subject to misinterpretation if there is cross-reactivity between the antibody and proteins other than the one being studied. The Western blot procedure has the advantage that the proteins are resolved by molecular weight, and the protein of interest is usually separated from cross-reacting proteins.

Western blotting is characterized by the transfer and immobilization of complex mixtures of proteins that have been separated by electrophoresis; typically polyacrylamide gel electrophoresis (PAGE) in which sodium dodecyl sulfate is included in the gel and buffers (SDS-PAGE). The proteins are transferred to a membrane such as nitrocellulose, nylon, or PVDF. The membrane is then probed with antibodies (mono- or polyclonal) that specifically recognize the protein of interest. Conceptually, the process is similar to Southern and Northern blotting, in which DNA or RNA is separated by electrophoresis, transferred to a membrane, and then probed to detect the molecule of interest.

In large part, this chapter discusses various aspects of the Western blot procedure, its variations, benefits, and pitfalls. A step-by-step description of a typical Western blot protocol that we use successfully in our laboratory is provided at the end of the chapter.

15.2 TRANSFERRING PROTEINS

15.2.1 TRANSFER DEVICES

Following electrophoresis, protein transfer from gel to membrane can be accomplished by using an electrical field[2] or by capillary transfer.[3,4] Transfer devices employing an electrical field fall into one of two types: wet transfer or semi-dry transfer.

Wet transfer devices are typically composed of a tank that holds the transfer buffer and one or more cassettes that slightly compress the fragile polyacrylamide gel against the transfer membrane and hold it perpendicular to the electrical field generated by the unit. Platinum wire electrodes are submerged in the tank as well, and are connected to an external power supply by insulated leads, or connected directly to an integral power supply located in the lid of the unit. To dissipate heat generated during transfer, these devices usually employ some type of cooling method that may consist of (1) a buffer recirculation device connected to an external cooling coil or (2) an aluminum heat sink in the floor of the tank through which cool water is circulated. Heat can also be controlled by doing the transfer in a cold room using chilled buffer. In addition, Burnette recommends that applied voltage not exceed 10 V/cm between electrodes to avoid this heating effect.[5] We have seen buffer temperatures exceed 80°C if these precautions are not taken.

Semi-dry transfer devices are composed of two large electrode panels positioned horizontally parallel to each other and are connected to an external power supply via insulated leads. One or more gel:transfer membrane sandwiches are prepared, as for wet transfer, and placed between the two electrode panels. Buffer-saturated filter paper (e.g., Whatman 3MM chromatography paper) cut to the same size as the gel:transfer membrane sandwich separates it from the electrode panels. When properly assembled, the gel:transfer membrane sandwich completes the circuit between the electrodes resulting in protein transfer out of the gel. Because the electrodes serve as large heat sinks, heat can be dissipated rapidly and transfer can usually be completed in a short time.

A comparison of semi-dry and wet transfer of proteins to nitrocellulose has been conducted by Tovey and Baldo.[7] The semi-dry system described by Kyhse-Andersen[6] was compared to the wet transfer system using Towbin's buffer. Tovey and Baldo verified Burnette's[5] observation that low molecular-weight proteins transfer out of the gel faster than high molecular-weight (>100,000 Da) proteins, and that this is the case for both transfer systems. They also show that in both systems, 0.1 μm nitrocellulose membrane retains more protein after transfer than 0.45 μm membrane. Transfer efficiency of the two systems was comparable. The authors concluded that although the amounts of protein transferred by the two methods were similar semi-dry blotting is advantageous due to its steeper voltage gradient that results in short transfer times.

Capillary transfer is based on the DNA blotting technique developed by Southern, in which DNA fragments are drawn from the agarose resolving gel by upward capillary action and deposited onto a suitable membrane.[8] Nagy et al.[3] modified the downward capillary technique of Lichtenstein et al.,[9] applied it to protein transfer out of SDS-agarose gels and found that downward capillary transfer proceeds about twice as fast as upward transfer. Recently, Zeng et al.[4] described an upward capillary transfer method, similar to Southern blotting, that is applied to protein transfer from SDS-PAGE gels. Compared to electrotransfer, this method requires a longer blotting period, but is more efficient at retaining proteins that would otherwise pass through the membrane.

Typically, electrotransfer or capillary transfer is used to transfer protein from the resolving gel immediately after the gel run is complete. However, it has recently been shown that Coomassie Blue-stained proteins can be transferred from destained gels[10] or destained, dried gels.[11] Due to the irreversible binding of Coomassie Blue to protein, the subsequent immunodetection must be done with a nonchromogenic stain such as ^{125}I-protein A or enhanced chemiluminescent products. By contrast, proteins transferred from silver-stained gels can be detected using chromogenic methods because the proteins transfer without the stain.[10,11] Gruber showed that the transfer time required for rehydrated gels was much less than for destained wet gels, and speculated that this may be due to the removal of volatile substances during drying.[11] As discussed by Gruber, the ability to produce an acceptable protein transfer from stained and rehydrated gels allows one to gather total protein data, as well as Western blot data, from the same gel; the transfer need not be done immediately after staining the gel. Also, stained and dehydrated gels are easily stored and provide a resource for later Western blot analysis if previously unavailable antibodies become available.[11]

15.2.2 TRANSFER BUFFERS

Most Western blot electrotransfer buffers are based on the electrophoresis buffer: 25 mM Tris, 192 mM glycine, pH 8.3,[12] which Towbin later modified for transfer of protein to nitrocellulose by adding 20% methanol.[2] Since then, many different buffer compositions have been described and their effects on protein transfer and retention during Western blotting, and subsequent processing, have been studied.[13,14] These Tris/glycine/methanol buffers are contrasted with the discontinuous buffer used in semi-dry blotting described by Kyhse-Andersen in which the cathodic and anodic buffers are designed to set up an isotachophoretic system.[6] Jacobson and Karsnas[14] show that the transfer buffer most significantly affects the binding capacity of the immobilizing membrane, and that the effect of buffer composition on the transfer of protein from the gel is small. They further suggest that immobilizing transferred proteins is the most difficult problem to overcome with Western blotting. Furthermore, they and Tovey[13] conclude that the optimal electrotransfer conditions are assay dependent. That is, different buffers, membranes, and transfer times need to be tested and carefully optimized for a given assay to achieve maximum sensitivity.

15.2.3 OPTIMIZATION

To find the optimum transfer procedure, it is important to try various times of transfer and constituents of the transfer buffer. It is useful, as well, to place one or more pieces of nitrocellulose behind the piece to which the proteins are being transferred. The backup membrane(s) will catch protein that has moved through the first membrane and will help establish the maximum time for transfer before proteins move out of the membrane and into the buffer on the other side. If a large loss of protein is observed because it is not trapped by the membrane, then it is recommended to test several different membrane types. The gel from which the protein has been transferred should also be stained (Coomassie Blue, silver stain, or a combination) to determine the conditions required for the majority of the protein to be removed from the gel.

As in protein electrophoresis, protein migration during electrotransfer depends upon the protein having a net positive or negative charge; a protein at its isoelectric point will not be affected by the electrical field and will move only by diffusion. In order to ensure complete protein transfer, it may be tempting to include SDS in the transfer buffer. Although SDS works well in PAGE and encourages the transfer of protein from the gel during electrotransfer, it tends to interfere with protein binding to some transfer membranes (most notably, nylon) when included in transfer buffers.[13] Therefore, careful consideration of the advantages and disadvantages should be undertaken before deciding to include SDS in the transfer buffer.

15.2.4 Transfer Membranes

A study of the performance of nitrocellulose, mixed ester, nylon, and covalent-binding polyvinylidene difluoride (cPVDF) membranes after passive protein adsorption, and also after electrotransfer, was done using several different proteins labeled with [125]Iodine.[13] The membranes exhibited different binding capacities in passive adsorption tests with labeled bovine serum albumin (Sigma). The cPVDF showed the least binding while regenerated cellulose and nylon membranes showed the most.

In tests designed to measure protein retention, cPVDF retained the most bound protein when washed with detergents or 5% skimmed milk.[13] This result is expected due to the covalent binding properties of cPVDF. All the membranes showed virtually the same binding capacity as measured by autoradiography when tested under electrotransfer conditions using Towbin's buffer. Tovey speculated that the difference between binding performance in passive adsorption tests, in which membranes exhibited a broad range of capacities, and electrotransfer tests, in which all the membranes performed similarly, was due to: (1) active migration of protein into the membrane matrix, instead of simple diffusion, and (2) the increased hydrophobicity of Towbin's transfer buffer due to the inclusion of methanol. With SDS included in the transfer buffer, protein binding to nylon membranes was nearly completely blocked, whereas binding to cPVDF or nitrocellulose from several sources was low, variable, and dependent on the membrane source. This effect was reduced if the pH was decreased from 8.3 to 8.0 and if NaCl was added to the buffer. The reduction was presumably due to the shielding of ionized groups. Because of the observed variability in protein binding and retention by the membranes studied, Tovey concluded that assay design should include an assessment of membrane performance as it relates to a given application.

An example of the need to consider membranes as variables in assay development is provided by Chen et al.[15] In this report, cytosolic protein from bovine medulla was electrotransferred to nitrocellulose or hydrophobic polyvinylidene difluoride (PVDF) membranes and subjected to either the Western blot assay or the GTP-overlay assay. The respective blots were probed with an antibody against a portion of a GTP-binding protein or with [α-^{32}P]GTP. The results showed that GTP-binding protein was barely detectable by the GTP-overlay assay when blotted to PVDF, but clearly detected on nitrocellulose. By contrast, Western blot analysis showed the GTP-binding protein to be present on both PVDF and nitrocellulose membranes. In fact, slightly more protein was detected on PVDF. Because the same amount of protein was used in each assay and the GTP-binding protein bound to PVDF as well as, or better than, to nitrocellulose, the authors conclude that the [α-^{32}P]GTP probe used in the GTP-overlay assay did not bind to the protein even though the GTP-binding protein was present. The authors speculate that the poor performance of the PVDF in the GTP-overlay assay may have been due to an inability of protein, thus immobilized, to renature correctly. Based on these results, Chen et al.[15] recommend nitrocellulose as the membrane of choice for the GTP-overlay assay and suggest that PVDF be used for Western blots. However, nitrocellulose might be preferred for a Western blot procedure where detection requires that the transferred protein regain its native conformation after transfer, such as for a binding protein, an enzyme, or an antigenic epitope consisting of noncontiguous residues.

Materials such as nitrocellulose, PVDF, nylon, and diazo papers have been used for many years as solid phase supports for blotted protein. Recently, xerographic (photocopy) paper was reported to be an alternative to these more expensive transfer membranes.[16] Citing an inability to reliably detect bovine αS1-casein from the milk of transgenic mice by conventional transfer methods using PVDF, Yom and Bremel turned to photocopy paper and found it to be nearly 3 times as sensitive.[16] Wetting the paper in methanol prior to use was critical for protein binding as was, curiously, the exclusion of methanol from the Towbin transfer buffer. Yom and Bremel showed that log [protein] was linearly related to the signal over a range of 5 ng to 15 μg protein as measured by direct densitometry of the stained blot. Using paper instead of other blotting membranes would result in an incredible cost savings. At current prices, the cost of one nitrocellulose membrane is roughly equivalent to the cost of 600 paper membranes.

Aware that low molecular mass (<10 kDa) proteins are frequently difficult to detect using Western blot analysis, Karey and Sirbasku extended the low end of the LMW range of proteins studied by Tovey and Baldo from ~14 kDa to 5.6 kDa by studying the binding of basic fibroblast growth factor (bFGF, 15 to 17 kDa), insulin-like growth factor (IGF-1, 7.6 kDa), epidermal growth factor (EGF, 6.1 kDa), and transforming growth factor alpha (TGFα, 5.6 kDa).[17] They found that, although these proteins transferred to nylon (Zeta Probe) and nitrocellulose membranes with high efficiency using Towbin's buffer without methanol, they were not retained well on either membrane during the subsequent processing steps. Confining further study to the Zeta Probe membrane, the authors continued by treating the blot with 0.5% (v/v) glutaraldehyde after transfer and found the retention improved 1.5- to 12-fold. Concerned that the glutaraldehyde treatment may have altered the detectability of the fixed proteins, they probed the blots with specific antibodies and found that all could be detected and that less of the protein needed to be applied to the gel prior to electrophoresis in order to detect the protein after blotting. This may not be true for all antibodies because some are sensitive to fixation methods, so the effect of glutaraldehyde fixation on antibody binding should be tested with each antibody.

Extending the molecular weight range even lower, Too et al.[18] have described a method of membrane treatment in which nitrocellulose is coated with 0.5% gelatin prior to electrotransfer, followed by paraformaldehyde fixation after transfer. Using this method, neuropeptides as small as 400 Da can be detected and characterized. This method has been applied by Nishi et al.[19] to improve the sensitivity of low molecular weight EGF detection by Western blot beyond that demonstrated by Karey and Sirbasku.[17] Their results show an increase in sensitivity from a lower limit of 30 ng loaded protein using non-treated membranes to a lower limit of 0.1 to 0.3 ng using treated ones. Interestingly, the authors report that even after formaldehyde treatment, EGF transferred to PVDF is still susceptible to displacement by detergent, in this case 0.1% (w/v) Tween 20. A likely explanation is that under these conditions, the formaldehyde fixed the EGF to the larger gelatin molecules that coated the membrane, rather than to the membrane itself. Detergent treatment may have removed the gelatin-EGF complex.

15.2.5 DIRECT PROTEIN STAIN ON THE BLOT

As an indication of protein transfer quality, the transferred proteins can be visualized using stains such as Amido Black,[20] Coomassie Blue,[5] or the reversible stain Ponceau S.[21] Ponceau S has the advantage of being water soluble and can therefore be washed away prior to probing the blot, whereas Coomassie Blue and Amido Black stain protein irreversibly. Ponceau S destaining can be accelerated by washing for 1 or 2 min with 0.14 M NaCl, 2.7 mM KCl, 9.6 mM NaKPi, 0.1% Tween 20, pH 7.3. Blots stained with Amido Black or Coomassie Blue can be destained with 90% methanol and 2% acetic acid.[5,20]

In some cases, such as in 2-D gel analysis and for microsequencing, it is advantageous to produce images of specific immunodetection and total protein staining from a single blot. Several recent procedures accomplish this. Exner and Nürnberg describe a method in which the blot is first subjected to enzyme-linked immunodetection employing an enhanced chemiluminescence system, then stained for total protein using a BSA-gold conjugate.[22] In this method, the antibodies attached to the membrane bound antigens need to be removed[23] prior to gold staining. Exner et al.[22] found that gold staining of the blot was comparable to silver staining of gels in terms of sensitivity, but was incompatible with ovalbumin blocking prior to immunodetection, and incompatible with gelatin coating of the membrane prior to electrotransfer. Protein stains that do not interfere with subsequent immunode-tection obviate the need for antibody removal. Examples are India ink[24,25] and the fluorogenic dye 2-methoxy-2, 4-diphenyl-3(2H)-furanone (MDPF).[26]

15.3 ANTIGEN DETECTION

15.3.1 DETECTION

As mentioned previously, Western blotting exploits the specificity between antigen and antibody. Therefore, all the visualization techniques are indirect. The protein transferred from the gel (antigen) is detected using a complementary molecule (antibody) that presents the signal (i.e., ^{125}I - labeled IgG), is conjugated to an enzyme that catalyzes the color change of a chromogenic substrate, or acts as an intermediate to which a third signaling molecule can bind (e.g., horseradish peroxidase conjugated protein A). In each case, the presence of the antigen is implied by the signal recorded on the blot itself, a piece of film, or a phosphor storage plate.

Two parameters paramount to optimizing antigen detection are specificity and sensitivity. Specificity, is a function of the primary detection antibodies; do they recognize only the epitopes of the protein being studied or do they confound the data by recognizing other similar epitopes (cross-reactivity) or binding non-specifically to a number of unrelated sites? Specificity can be improved by blocking the membrane with one of several blocking agents such as nonfat milk or Tween 20. Blocking is intended to prevent nonspecific interactions between the detection antibodies and the membrane. Specificity can also be improved by immunoprecipitating the protein of interest prior to resolving it by PAGE.[27] In this case, specificity is increased by first allowing the antibody to react with native epitopes in solution where cross-reacting epitopes may be inaccessible. However, combining immuno-precipitation (IP) with Western blotting is potentially disadvantageous because the antibodies used to precipitate the antigen during the IP remain in the sample during gel electrophoresis and are eventually electrotransferred with the antigen. Separated into their heavy and light chain components by electrophoresis, these antibodies are likely to be detected during the Western blot and may obscure signal corresponding to the protein of interest.

A good example of this problem, coupled with a strategy for solving it, has been demonstrated by Doolittle et al.[27] They found that IgG molecules used during immunoprecipitation produced signal on the subsequent Western blot at 66 kDa, 50 kDa, and 25 kDa. Signal from these contaminating molecules (specifically the 66 kDa and 50 kDa IgG heavy chains) interfered with their study of lipoprotein lipase (LPL), a protein of about 57 kDa. Their strategy for solving the problem consists of two parts and can be generally applied to situations where the target protein is similar in size to the IgG heavy chain. First, instead of using whole immunoglobulin as the primary antibody during the IP, they used Fab fragments created by digesting the primary antibody with papain and removing the Fc fragment. Fab fragments contain the antigen-binding domains of the original antibody, but are much smaller (about 25 kDa) than the full-length heavy chain. Second, the secondary antibody used in the IP was cross-linked to killed *Staphylococcus aureus*, thus preventing its migration into the gel during electrophoresis. As a result, LPL could be studied by Western blot without interference from the IgG heavy chain.

The second parameter, sensitivity, depends on the threshold of the visualization system used and the avidity of the antibody:antigen complex.[28] Most optimized Western blot assays can detect nanogram amounts of protein. Sensitivity can be improved by increasing the proportion of the target protein in the sample — for example, by immunoprecipitating the protein of interest prior to resolving it through a gel, as discussed in the previous paragraph. Other means of selectively concentrating the protein of interest to increase sensitivity of the assay include using beads containing covalently linked ligand or a lectin that binds the carbohydrate portion of the protein. The protein, bound to the beads, is selected for by centrifugation (or magnetic attraction, if the beads are magnetic). Sensitivity can also be improved by amplifying the signal, as is the case when using the streptavidin-biotin system. This system exploits the extremely high affinity of streptavidin, a bacterial protein, for biotin. Biotinylated secondary antibodies are typically used as intermediaries between primary detection antibodies and streptavidin, which is conjugated to an enzyme capable of producing a signal. Amplification occurs when several strepta- vidin molecules bind to the biotinylated secondary antibody. Finally, Immunofiltra- tion as described by Clark et al.[29] was used to lower the detection threshold from 50 ng to 10 ng. In this method, the antibody and wash solutions were filtered through the blot instead of simply being incubated with the blot on a shaker table.

15.3.2 DETECTING ANTIBODIES ON THE BLOT

Antibodies, once bound to antigens, are typically visualized on the blot by the interaction of a secondary binding protein that is either another antibody or a bacterial protein (protein A or protein G) that specifically interacts with the Fc region of the antibody. Thus, the primary antibody is sandwiched between the antigen bound to the blot and the secondary protein. This second protein is labeled so that it can be detected visually. Labels include ^{125}I for visualization by autoradiography and enzymes for color visualization via chromogenic substrates and for fluorographic visualization via chemiluminescent substrates. The advantage of most of these sand- wich techniques is that they result in amplification of the signal. For example, each primary antibody molecule usually has more than one epitope that the secondary antibodies recognize and will bind to. Similarly, biotinylation results in multiple biotin molecules attached to a single antibody, and thus, the ratio of secondary to primary antibodies is greater than one. If enzymes are linked to the secondary antibodies, they provide another point of amplification because they catalyze the conversion of many molecules of substrate to the insoluble chromogenic or chemi- luminescent products. The sensitivity of the assay varies with the method of signal generation and depends on the extent of amplification and the sensitivity of the detection method for the signal. Many commercially available Western blot detection kits use different combinations of secondary binding proteins and means of signal generation. These are discussed by Paladichuk.[30]

Signal generation from enzyme-linked systems involves the use of an enzyme that catalyzes the conversion of a substrate to an insoluble product that is colored or chemiluminescent. The most frequently used enzymes are horseradish peroxidase and alkaline phosphatase. For example, with the alkaline phosphatase/BCIP-NBT system the signal is recorded directly on the blot as a stain in the form of a colored precipitate. However, the colored precipitates from this system create a purple stain that is often not very intense and is more difficult to capture in a photographic record of the stained blots, compared with products from procedures that use radioisotopes or chemiluminescent products.

It is important to understand the conditions under which the linked enzyme is active and when it is inactive. For example, NaN_3, a common additive used to preserve buffers from microbial contamination, inhibits the activity of horseradish peroxidase. Conditions that result in loss of enzyme activity or other problems with the assay are easily detected if a positive control is included. The positive control is a sample that contains a known amount of the protein of interest, and will give a positive signal if all of the components of the system are functional. A common source of sample for a positive control is the antigen preparation that was used to produce the primary antibody. If the primary antibody is from a commercial source, then the company can often provide a sample containing the antigen to use for a positive control. Frequently, if the protein has been cloned, expression vectors are available, and a positive control sample can be created by transiently transfecting cells such as COS cells with the expression vector.

15.3.3 QUANTITATION

Although Western blotting is often used in a qualitative way for determining the presence or absence of antigen in a particular sample, quantitation of antigens is also possible. A linear relationship between the amount of protein and its corresponding signal is desirable when attempting to quantitate an unknown. For quantitation to be valid, the unknown value must fall within this linear range. Linearity can be established by including a range of protein quantities on the same blot as the unknown. Care must be taken to use an excess of probe to preclude the possibility of exhausting the probe before fully saturating the target molecule. The quantitation method used depends on the type of signal generating molecule(s) bound to the primary antibody, as illustrated in the following examples.

^{125}I-protein A: Griswold et al.[31] quantitated blotted protein by first visualizing the signal generating molecule, ^{125}I-protein A, on X-ray film to locate the bands of interest. Corresponding regions of the blot were cut out and counted in a gamma-counter. A linear relationship was demonstrated over a range of 2.5 to 30 ng protein. Alternative to cutting the bands out and counting in a gamma-counter, a less destructive way to quantitate the signal is to expose the blot to either film or a phosphor storage plate and thereby determine the amount of radioactivity. Fang et al.[32] used this technique to detect a specific protein in serum and tissue extracts. Linearity was demonstrated between 0.5 and 15 ng of protein.

HRP-linked secondary antibody: Uhl and Newton[33] visualized the proteins of interest by staining the blot with 4-chloro-1-naphthol and H_2O_2. Peroxidase activity in the excised bands was measured spectrophotometrically by exposing them to the peroxidase chromogenic substrate o-phenylenediamine in the presence of H_2O_2. The reaction rate was linearly related to amount of protein over a range of 10 to 1000 ng.

Huang and Amero[34] used HRP-linked secondary antibody in conjunction with enhanced chemiluminescence to visualize two RNA-binding proteins found in nuclear extracts. The signal, recorded on X-ray film, was measured and plotted against total protein. In this case, the data from one of the proteins fit an asymptotic curve while the other was linear. This led the authors to conclude that "...the relationship between the amount of total protein and the antigen signal is specific and must be determined emperically." A simple explanation of an asymptotic curve is that the amount of probe is limiting relative to the amount of antigen on the blot. This example highlights the necessity for having a standard curve with reference samples that encompass the range of values derived from the unknown samples. We

have found that detection of bovine serum albumin, using an enhanced chemiluminescence signal generated by a secondary antibody linked to horseradish peroxidase,
is linear between 25 and 375 ng protein, which was the entire range tested (Bendickson and Nilsen-Hamilton, unpublished).

Fluorescent tags: Another nonradioactive means of visualizing and quantitating
proteins on Western blots is through the use of fluorescent compounds. Diamandis
et al.[35] used a streptavidin–based macromolecular complex labeled with fluorescent
europium chelate as the signal generating molecule. Quantitation was done by
scanning with a time-resolved fluorometer. The authors demonstrate a near-linear
relationship between fluorescence and protein, and also show that this method is as
sensitive as using alkaline phosphatase and BCIP-NBT to detect the protein. A more
direct method, used by Fradelizi et al.,[36] is to conjugate the fluorescent molecule,
Cy5, directly to the secondary antibody. Using this method, the authors show a linear
relationship between the signal detected by a Storm Phosphorimager and protein
over a range of 6.25 to 100 ng, and that this method is comparable to the alkaline
phosphatase:BCIP-NBT method.

15.3.4 MOLECULAR WEIGHT STANDARDS

It is often desirable to characterize the sizes of proteins on a Western blot by
estimating their apparent molecular weights. This can be accomplished by comparing
the relative electrophoretic mobility of each protein to the mobility of a set of protein
standards of known molecular weight that are included on the same gel. Because
the Western blot technique is designed to be specific for the protein(s) of interest,
the standards are typically not visualized by the same means as the antibody, and
other means of relating their positions to the antibody signal must be used. The
appropriate means used depends, of course, on the method used to visualize the
protein of interest. For example: if a chromogenic substrate is used to directly stain
the blot, a direct method such as India ink, Ponceau S, Coomassie Blue, or gold
staining would be called for. On the other hand, the protein standards can be marked
with radioactive or luminescent compounds if the signal from the protein of interest
is recorded on film or by phosphor storage media.

Prestained markers: Prestained molecular weight standards are available from
several companies and cover a wide range of molecular weights. Fluorescently
labeled standards can also be prepared in the laboratory using dansyl chloride,[37]
dabsyl chloride,[38] or fluorescamine.[39] If the blot is to be cut into several pieces after
transfer, these standards are also useful as lane indicators.[40] Multicolored prestained
standards, such as the Kaleidoscope standards from Bio-Rad Laboratories (Hercules,
CA), provide a means of estimating molecular weight with the added benefit of
unambiguous identification of each standard.

Luminescent markers: Our laboratory uses an adhesive-backed luminescent
paper (Diversified Biotech, Newton Center, MA) as a means of locating standards
on Western blot films, as well as for recording other pertinent information. After the
blot is stained with Ponceau S, the locations of the protein standards are marked
directly on the blot with a graphite pencil. Before exposure to film, a piece of
luminescent paper is cut out and applied to the blot near the standards. A mark is

then made on the paper that precisely indicates the location of the pencil mark recorded earlier and, hence, the location of the standard. This light-on-dark image will be recorded in reverse on the subsequent film exposure. We have also tried luminescent fabric paint (Ghostly Glo, #SC 350, Duncan, Fresno, CA) commonly available at craft stores. Similarly, ZnS in suspension has been suggested as an alternative marking substance.[41] Although the fabric paint and ZnS methods work well for autoradiography, we have found that they are not compatible with visualization by chemiluminescence because their required drying time (4 to 6 h with paint) does not allow exposure of the blot to film during the period of peak chemiluminescent emission.

Visualization of standards by chemiluminescence: Liu reports cross-reactivity between anti-inducible nitric oxide synthetase (anti-iNOS) and the 10 kDa ladder sold by Life Technologies.[42] The 10 kDa ladder is composed of myosin (200 kDa) and an unrelated 120 kDa protein that is partially cleaved to produce fragments from 120 kDa to 10 kDa in size. Anti-iNOS cross-reacted only with the 120 kDa protein and its cleavage fragments. Occasional chance cross-reactions such as this can be useful because the cross-reactivity makes possible the visualization of molecular weight markers and their precise locations on the same blot or film as the unknown samples.

It has been reported that molecular weight standards can be visualized by using antisera developed against them.[43] In this case, the standards can be seen using the same method for detecting the protein of interest. One disadvantage of this technique, however, is that each antiserum may contribute to nonspecific background and might cross-react with one or more other proteins in the samples. An opposite approach has been described by Lindbladh et al.[44] who, instead of making antisera against several different standards, genetically fused marker proteins to protein A and produced them in *E. coli*. The presence of the protein A moiety enables the standards to be detected at the same time as the unknowns with no additional steps, provided an antibody that binds protein A is used in the detection protocol.

15.4 ARTIFACTS AND TROUBLESHOOTING

One must be aware of potential artifacts when conducting and interpreting any assay, and Western blotting is no exception. Using protein A in concert with an enhanced chemiluminescent detection system, we periodically see spurious, amorphous signals that can usually be disregarded because they are not consistently associated with specific protein bands. These inexplicable signals can, on occasion, obscure areas of authentic signal. We speculate that these signals may be due to static discharge, the presence of air bubbles between the gel and membrane during transfer, or manufacturing defects in the membrane itself.

Another significant problem, protein band distortion, can occur if the gel is overloaded. For example, we have found that when dealing with samples containing growth medium supplemented with bovine serum, the presence of serum albumin at a final concentration greater than 1 to 2% distorts the band pattern of other proteins of similar molecular weight, making identification of these proteins difficult. If possible, it is best to avoid loading samples that contain greater than 2% serum albumin.

Kaufmann et al.[23] have observed an increase in background signal of blots blocked with bovine milk when using protein A as the secondary molecule. They attribute this effect to the weak affinity of protein A for IgG_2 found in bovine milk.[45]

Cross-reactivity, such as that noted by Liu[42] for protein standards, is another possible source of artifact and is typically a disadvantage. Although in this case, it allowed the investigators to easily visualize their standards.

When using detection molecules conjugated to enzymes, such as alkaline phosphatase or horseradish peroxidase, one needs to be concerned with the presence of endogenous activity on the blot. Indeed, Navarre et al.[46] report that peroxidase in membrane preparations from rabbit gastric mucosa is able to survive SDS-PAGE separation and produce a signal when the blot is incubated with a chemiluminescent substrate. They also note that this activity can be quenched by treating the blot with 3% H_2O_2 prior to processing. Vaitaitis et al.[47] reported that endogenous biotin-containing proteins can contribute to nonspecific signal when using the streptavidin-biotin detection system. While looking for nuclear factor kappa B (NFκB) proteins in cell extracts, they detected four bands at 72, 78, 130, and 220 kDa that were present even when the blot was incubated with streptavidin-HRP alone and developed with a chemiluminescent substrate. To solve the problem, the endogenous biotin was blocked with 0.25 μg/ml streptavidin, followed by a wash with 50 ng/ml of d-biotin (to block the bound streptavidin). Biotinylated secondary antibody was then used with streptavidin-HRP to detect only the proteins of interest.

15.5 CLINICAL APPLICATIONS

A complete review of the clinical applications of Western blotting is beyond the scope of this chapter. The following, however, will serve as a brief introduction. Immunoassays, including Western blotting, are part of the toolkit used by clinicians to diagnose infectious disease. Blood banks also use these assays to screen donors, as well as the blood supply, for the presence of antibodies against infectious agents such as human immunodeficiency virus (HIV), hepatitis C virus (HCV) and human T-cell lymphotrophic virus (HTLV).

In practice, sera are screened with an enzyme immunoassay (EIA, ELISA) that is usually confirmed, when positive, by a Western blot. Most diagnostic Western blots are essentially antibody capture assays in which the patient's serum is tested for the presence of antibodies against particular pathogens. Antigenic proteins from these pathogens are prepared and immobilized on a solid phase, such as nitrocellulose or PVDF, and sold as part of a diagnostic kit. If present, specific antibodies in sera from individuals suspected of being infected will bind to the antigen. Bound antibody is detected by applying an appropriate signal-generating molecule. The Western blot results are interpreted using criteria specifically developed for the set of antigens that were initially blotted.

The interpretation of Western blot results is sometimes rather subjective and may lead to indeterminate results, especially during early HIV infection.[48] Western blot results can also be complicated by the presence of cross-reacting proteins, as well as under-representation of certain antigenic proteins in the viral preparation.[49] Indeterminate results from assays intended to be confirmatory, such as the Western blot, present problems for clinicians regarding patient counseling, as well as for blood banks that could potentially lose donors.

These problems of interpretation have led some to suggest that, at least for HIV detection, Western blots should not be regarded as the confirmatory standard.[48,50,51] However, others have worked on making Western blots more objective by developing immunoassays that use recombinant viral proteins instead of native protein preparations. Assays based on recombinant or synthetic proteins show increased specificity, and it is hoped that they will be more objective and exhibit fewer indeterminate results.[49,52,53] The following examples show how immunoassays using native protein preparations compare to those using recombinant proteins.

15.5.1 EXAMPLE 1

Zaaijer et al.[53] compared the performance of conventional Western blot using native viral proteins to a recent immunoblot assay kit based on recombinant HIV proteins and saw an increase in specificity from 70% with the Western blot to 93% with the immunoblot. Specificity was defined as the ability of the assay in question to correctly report the HIV status of 149 noninfected blood donors whose sera are known to give false positive results in EIA screens. The authors speculate that the increase in specificity of the immunoblot assay may be due to the lack of contaminating cellular proteins in the recombinant protein preparations.

15.5.2 EXAMPLE 2

Application of the recombinant immunoassay to the diagnosis of Lyme borreliosis has been studied by Fawcett et al.[52] An immunodot assay using recombinant and purified antigens of *Borrelia burgdorferi* was compared to a conventional Western blot on which "whole *B. burgdorferi* organisms" were electrophoretically separated. The authors concluded that the immunodot assay was as sensitive as, and more specific than, the Western blot, and was easier to interpret. However, it should be noted that purified recombinant proteins were used in this immunodot assay, as they were for Example 1. When used with a mixture of proteins such as those extracted from an intact organism, the immunodot assay has the distinct disadvantage that proteins are not resolved by size, and therefore signals from contaminating proteins that also bind the antibody are superimposed on signals from the antigen–antibody interaction.

15.5.3 EXAMPLE 3

When screening for antihuman cytomegalovirus immunoglobulin type M (α-HCMV IgM), Lazzarotto et al.[54] chose to combine viral structural polypeptides with certain recombinant viral proteins that are not represented in virion preps on the same blot. The structural proteins were prepared from purified virions that had been cultured in human embryo fibroblasts. To accommodate several additional lanes of recombinant protein, the membrane was made longer than the polyacrylamide gel. After electrotransfer of the structural proteins, the recombinant proteins were spotted onto the lower portion of the membrane. The recombinant proteins were strategically chosen to help resolve potentially false-positive results. Lazzarotto et al.[54] reported that the method was more sensitive and more specific than Western blots using proteins from virion preps alone. This combination of immunoblot with purified recombinant proteins and Western blot of the complete virion is an excellent marriage of two related techniques to improve the critical analysis of clinical samples.

15.5.4 EXAMPLE 4

The recombinant viral protein p54, from African swine fever virus, was used by Alcaraz et al.[49] to improve the conventional diagnostic Western blot assay, which is based on native viral antigen. Protein p54 was chosen as the basis of the assay because of its high antigenicity. The recombinant assay was found to be as sensitive as conventional Western blot and as sensitive as an ELISA assay. Compared to the conventional Western, the p54 assay was found to be more specific, and its interpretation was less subjective.

Although it would appear that assays based on recombinant proteins will become the predominant diagnostic tools, a recent report by Hennig et al.[55] indicates that these assays are not without problems. In their report they show that in a particular hepatitis C diagnostic kit, only a portion of the HCV core protein was included (represented by a short 40 amino acid synthetic peptide). The HCV core antibodies of a recently infected blood donor were not detected until many weeks postinfection, whereas assays in which the core protein was more fully represented detected them early on. Thus, the performance of recombinant protein-based assays may be compromised by the use of truncated proteins as the antibody targets.

15.6 CONCLUSION

Western blotting is a powerful technique that has numerous variations. Its main advantage over other immunological detection techniques is the ability to show the protein of interest after it has been separated from other proteins and potential antigens. Resolution by gel electrophoresis separates the protein from potential contaminating antigens and provides independent means (other than the ability to react with the antibody) for an investigator to identify the specified protein. The protein–antibody interaction on the Western blot can be used to detect a specific protein in a mixture, such as a tissue extract, or it can be used to detect a particular group of antibodies in a mixture, such as serum. Because it includes a powerful protein separation procedure, relies on high affinity antibody–antigen interactions, and the detection systems involve amplification of the signal, the Western blot is a highly sensitive and very specific assay. In addition, with the appropriate controls and standards, the Western blot assay is linear with the amount of protein added to the system. For these reasons, the assay is widely used in research and clinical laboratories.

15.7 WESTERN BLOT PROTOCOL

This section describes the electrotransfer of protein from SDS-PAGE gel via a step-by-step procedure that is used in our laboratory. It is based on the procedure of Burnette,[5] works well for proteins of less than 80,000 Da, and results in uniform transfer of protein to the membrane. We use polyclonal primary antibodies with this method to detect proteins of interest in mammalian and bacterial cell lysates, tissue extracts, tissue fluids, and conditioned medium from cultured cells. While we have found the conditions listed to be optimal for our needs, modifications may need to be made when this procedure is used for other applications.

Many methods exist for preparing and running the SDS-PAGE gels from which proteins are to be blotted. The most popular SDS-PAGE system was described by Laemmli.[56] We prefer a system based on Ornstein[57] and Davis[12] that provides superior resolution.[58] The gels take slightly longer to run with this latter buffer system than gels using the Laemmli system (about 4.5 h vs. 3.5 h for a 10-cm-long gel).

The Western blot procedure requires transfer membrane, primary antibody, enzyme-conjugated secondary molecule, and a means to record the signal. It requires a transfer apparatus and power supply. The transfer apparatus used in our laboratory is the Hoefer TE50 electrotransfer tank. The transfer cassette requires 15 to 30 min to set up. Transfer times using this procedure range from 4 to 12 h and depend on the type of transfer device used and the thickness of the gel. For example, transfers using the very thin gels from the Phastgel system can be completed in about 20 min. With semi-dry transfer devices, transfer times can be on the order of 30 min. In our experience, the semi-dry system provides an adequate transfer, although we have occasionally observed evidence of nonuniform transfer across the gel when using a semi-dry apparatus. Once transfer is complete, subsequent antibody incubations and washes will take about 4 h. If quantitation of the results is required, a densitometer or similar device should also be available.

15.7.1 PROCEDURE

1. Cut one sheet of nitrocellulose membrane and two sheets of absorbent filter paper (Whatman 3MM) to the size of the gel.
2. Soak the gel in transfer buffer for 30 min. Wet the membrane, filter papers, and support pads in the same buffer.
3. To assemble the transfer sandwich, place the gel on a glass plate, and then place a wetted filter paper (cut to size) on top. Invert the glass plate and set it on one of the support pads. Using a spatula, gently pry the gel/filter paper off the glass. Place the membrane on top of the gel. Remove any air bubbles by gently rolling a cylinder, such as a pencil or glass rod, over the membrane. Place the second piece of filter paper on the stack and remove any air bubbles. Air bubbles left between the gel and membrane will prevent transfer in the region of the bubble.
4. Place the complete sandwich in the transfer tank with the membrane closest to the positive electrode (red) and the gel to the negative (black) electrode.
5. Fill the tank with chilled buffer and, if necessary, set up the buffer cooling system. For the Hoefer system at least 4 L of buffer are needed. The buffer can be reused at least 3 times. However, it may be necessary to add fresh buffer before reuse to counter the evaporation that occurs during transfer.

6. At 4°C, transfer at 90 V (0.6-0.8 A) for 4 h or 30 V for 12 h while stirring the buffer. Between these two extremes, other volt–hour combinations can be used as long as the volt × hour value equals 360.
7. Add the membrane to 50 ml Ponceau S staining solution and incubate for 1 to 2 min. The Ponceau S can be reused many times.
8. Wash the membrane briefly with water to remove excess stain.
9. Mark the positions of the molecular weight markers on the membrane with a pencil.
10. Photograph the stained membrane.
11. Continue washing the membrane until all the stain is gone. If stain persists where protein is abundant, wash the membrane in NaKPS + Tween 20 for 1 to 2 min, and then rinse with water for 1 to 2 min with several changes.
12. Incubate the membrane in 200 ml blocking buffer at 37°C with gentle shaking for 30 min or overnight at 4°C. After blocking, wash as follows with shaking:
    Wash procedure   (1) 100 ml NaKPS + Tween 20, one wash for 15 min
                        (2) 100 ml NaKPS, two washes for 15 min each time
13. Incubate the membrane with primary antibody incubation solution for 1.5 h at room temperature with shaking.
14. Wash as in Step 12.
15. Incubate with the HRP-conjugated protein (protein A or secondary antibody) solution for 30 min at room temperature with shaking.
16. Wash as in step 12.
17. Blot the membrane dry. Incubate with ECL substrate for 1 min. Blot excess substrate. Place membrane onto filter paper and wrap with Saran wrap. Expose to film.

15.7.2 SOLUTIONS

15.7.2.1 Transfer Buffer (4 L)

12.11 g Trizma (final = 25 mM)
57.65 g glycine (final = 190 mM)
800 ml methanol (final = 20%)
Bring to volume with distilled water.
Note: Check to make sure the pH is about 8.3. Do not adjust the pH. If it is not around 8.3, then the solution has been made incorrectly and should be remade. Degas this solution before using it.

15.7.2.2 Ponceau S Staining Solution

2 g Ponceau S (final = 0.2%) obtained from SERVA (FeinBiochemica, Heidelberg, NY)
30 g TCA (final = 3%)
Bring to 1 L with distilled water; solution can be reused at least 10 times.

15.7.2.3 Blocking Buffer

25 g nonfat dry milk (final = 5% wt/vol)
0.1 g NaN$_3$ (final = 0.02%)
500 ml TD solution
Stir the solution overnight at room temperature to completely dissolve the milk.

15.7.2.4 Primary Antibody Incubation Solution

0.2 ml antiserum (for 1/200 dilution)*
40 ml blocking buffer

15.7.2.5 HRP Conjugated Protein, Secondary Probe

40 µl of HRP secondary antibody diluted 1:100 with NaKPS (for 1/100,000
    dilution) or 4 µl of 1 mg/ml HRP protein A (for 1/10,000 dilution)**
40 ml NaKPS

15.7.2.6 4X TD (4 L)

128 g NaCl (final = 0.14 M)
6.08 g KCl (final = 5 mM)
1.60 g Na$_2$HPO$_4$ (final = 0.4 mM)
48 g Trizma (final = 25 mM)

Bring to about 3.5 L with distilled water. Add approximately 32 ml of concentrated
HCl to adjust the pH between 7.4 and 7.5 (using a pH meter). Bring volume to 4 L.
Pour into a clean 4-L bottle and store at 4°C. To make TD, dilute this stock 1:3 with
distilled water.

15.7.2.7 10X NaKPS (2 L)

160 g NaCl (final = 1.37 M)
4 g KCl (final = 27 mM)
4 g KH$_2$PO$_4$ (final = 15 mM)
142 g Na$_2$HPO$_4$ (final = 81 mM)

Dissolve in about 1500 ml of distilled water. Adjust pH to 7.3 with 10 N NaOH,
then bring to volume. For long-term storage, autoclave in aliquots of 300 to 400 ml.

---

* For most antibodies the range of appropriate dilutions is 1/100 to 1/500. The optimum dilution needs
to be determined for each antiserum. This is enough antibody solution for one gel (~13 × 10 cm by 2
mm thick) and can be reused at least four times.
** The optimum dilution needs to be determined for each application.

15.7.2.8 NaKPS (1 L)

100 ml 10X NaKPS
Bring to volume with distilled water.

15.7.2.9 NaKPS + Tween 20 (1 L)

100 ml 10X NaKPS
10 ml 10% Tween 20 (final = 0.1%)
Bring to volume with distilled water.

15.7.2.10 ECL Substrate

Mix equal parts of detection solutions #1 and #2 as per manufacturer's instructions (ECL Western blotting reagents, Amersham). The substrate can be reused for up to 48 h if kept at 4°C.

ACKNOWLEDGMENT

The authors are very grateful to Linda Lyngholm for her help in editing this chapter. Also acknowledged is journal paper no. J-18859 of the Iowa Agriculture and Home Economics Experiment Station, Ames, IA, Project No. 3096, and support by the Hatch Act and State of Iowa funds.

REFERENCES

1. Cassab, G. I., Localization of cell wall proteins using tissue-print Western blot techniques, *Methods Enzymol.*, 218, 682–688, 1993.
2. Towbin, H., Staehelin, T., and Gordon, J., Electrophoretic transfer of proteins from polyacrylamide gels to nitrocellulose sheets: procedure and some applications, *Proc. Natl. Acad. Sci. U.S.A.*, 76, 4350–4354, 1979.
3. Nagy, B., Costello, R., and Csako, G., Downward blotting of proteins in a model based on apolipoprotein(a) phenotyping, *Anal. Biochem.*, 231, 40–45, 1995.
4. Zeng, L., Tate, R., and Smith, L. D., Capillary transfer as an efficient method of transferring proteins from SDS-PAGE gels to membranes, *Biotechniques*, 26, 426–430, 1999.
5. Burnette, W. N., Western blotting: electrophoretic transfer of proteins from sodium dodecyl sulfate–polyacrylamide gels to unmodified nitrocellulose and radiographic detection with antibody and radioiodinated protein A, *Anal. Biochem.*, 112, 195–203, 1981.
6. Kyhse-Andersen, J., Electroblotting of multiple gels: a simple apparatus without buffer tank for rapid transfer of proteins from polyacrylamide to nitrocellulose, *J. Biochem. Biophys. Methods*, 10, 203–209, 1984.
7. Tovey, E. R. and Baldo, B. A., Comparison of semi-dry and conventional tank-buffer electrotransfer of proteins from polyacrylamide gels to nitrocellulose membranes, *Electrophoresis*, 8, 384–387, 1987.

8. Southern, E. M., Detection of specific sequences among DNA fragments separated by gel electrophoresis, *J. Mol. Biol.*, 98, 503–517, 1975.

9. Lichtenstein, A. V., Moiseev, V. L., and Zaboikin, M. M., A procedure for DNA and RNA transfer to membrane filters avoiding weight-induced gel flattening, *Anal. Biochem.*, 191, 187–191, 1990.

10. Ranganathan, V. and De, P. K., Western blot of proteins from Coomassie-stained polyacrylamide gels, *Anal. Biochem.*, 234, 102–104, 1996.

11. Gruber, C. and Stan-Lotter, H., Western blot of stained proteins from dried polyacrylamide gels, *Anal. Biochem.*, 253, 125–127, 1997.

12. Davis, B. J., Disc Electrophoresis. II. Method and application to human serum proteins, *Ann. N.Y. Acad. Sci.*, 404–427, 1964.

13. Tovey, E. R. and Baldo, B. A., Protein binding to nitrocellulose, nylon and PVDF membranes in immunoassays and electroblotting, *J. Biochem. Biophys. Methods*, 19, 169–183, 1989.

14. Jacobson, G. and Karsnas, P., Important parameters in semi-dry electrophoretic transfer, *Electrophoresis*, 11, 46–52, 1990.

15. Chen, L. M., Liang, Y., Tai, J. H., and Chern, Y., Comparison of nitrocellulose and PVDF membranes in GTP-overlay assay and Western blot analysis, *Biotechniques*, 16, 600–601, 1994.

16. Yom, H. C. and Bremel, R. D., Xerographic paper as a transfer medium for Western blots: quantification of bovine alpha S1-casein by Western blot, *Anal. Biochem.*, 200, 249–253, 1992.

17. Karey, K. P. and Sirbasku, D. A., Glutaraldehyde fixation increases retention of low molecular weight proteins (growth factors) transferred to nylon membranes for Western blot analysis, *Anal. Biochem.*, 178, 255–259, 1989.

18. Too, C. K., Murphy, P. R., and Croll, R. P., Western blotting of formaldehyde-fixed neuropeptides as small as 400 daltons on gelatin-coated nitrocellulose paper, *Anal. Biochem.*, 219, 341–348, 1994.

19. Nishi, N., Inui, M., Miyanaka, H., Oya, H., and Wada, F., Western blot analysis of epidermal growth factor using gelatin-coated polyvinylidene difluoride membranes, *Anal. Biochem.*, 227, 401–402, 1995.

20. Schaffner, W. and Weissmann, C., A rapid, sensitive, and specific method for the determination of protein in dilute solution, *Anal. Biochem.*, 56, 502–514, 1973.

21. Salinovich, O. and Montelaro, R. C., Reversible staining and peptide mapping of proteins transferred to nitrocellulose after separation by sodium dodecyl sulfate-polyacrylamide gel electrophoresis, *Anal. Biochem.*, 156, 341–347, 1986.

22. Exner, T. and Nurnberg, B., Immuno- and gold staining of a single Western blot, *Anal. Biochem.*, 260, 108–110, 1998.

23. Kaufmann, S. H., Ewing, C. M., and Shaper, J. H., The erasable Western blot, *Anal. Biochem.*, 161, 89–95, 1987.

24. Eynard, L. and Lauriere, M., The combination of Indian ink staining with immunochemiluminescence detection allows precise identification of antigens on blots: application to the study of glycosylated barley storage proteins, *Electrophoresis*, 19, 1394–1396, 1998.

25. Glenney, J., Antibody probing of Western blots which have been stained with india ink, *Anal. Biochem.*, 156, 315–319, 1986.

26. Alba, F. J. and Daban, J. R., Rapid fluorescent monitoring of total protein patterns on sodium dodecyl sulfate-polyacrylamide gels and Western blots before immunodetection and sequencing, *Electrophoresis*, 19, 2407–2411, 1998.

27. Doolittle, M. H., Ben-Zeev, O., and Briquet-Laugier, V., Enhanced detection of lipoprotein lipase by combining immunoprecipitation with Western blot analysis, *J. Lipid Res.*, 39, 934–942, 1998.

28. Harlow, E. and Lane, D., *Antibodies: A Laboratory Manual*, Cold Spring Harbor Laboratory, Cold Spring Harbor, NY, 1988.

29. Clark, C. R., Kresl, J. J., Hines, K. K., and Anderson, B. E., An immunofiltration apparatus for accelerating the visualization of antigen on membrane supports, *Anal. Biochem.*, 228, 232–237, 1995.

30. Paladichuk, A., How the Western was won, *Scientist*, 13, 18–21, 1999.

31. Griswold, D. E., Hillegass, L., Antell, L., Shatzman, A., and Hanna, N., Quantitative Western blot assay for measurement of the murine acute phase reactant, serum amyloid P component, *J. Immunol. Methods*, 91, 163–168, 1986.

32. Fang, Y., Lepont, M., Fassett, J., Ford, S. P., Mubaidin, A., Hamilton, R. T., and Nilsen-Hamilton, M., Signaling between the placenta and the uterus involving the mitogen-regulated protein/proliferins, *Endocrinology*, submitted.

33. Uhl, J. and Newton, R. C., Quantitation of related proteins by Western blot analysis, *J. Immunol. Methods*, 110, 79–84, 1988.

34. Huang, D. and Amero, S. A., Measurement of antigen by enhanced chemiluminescent Western blot, *Biotechniques*, 22, 454–456, 458, 1997.

35. Diamandis, E. P., Christopoulos, T. K., and Bean, C. C., Quantitative Western blot analysis and spot immunodetection using time-resolved fluorometry, *J. Immunol. Methods*, 147, 251–259, 1992.

36. Fradelizi, J., Friederich, E., Beckerle, M. C., and Golsteyn, R. M., Quantitative measurement of proteins by western blotting with Cy5™-coupled secondary antibodies, *Biotechniques*, 26, 484–494, 1999.

37. Lubit, B. W., Dansylated proteins as internal standards in two-dimensional electrophoresis and Western blot analysis, *Electrophoresis*, 5, 358–361, 1984.

38. Tzeng, M. C., A sensitive, rapid method for monitoring sodium dodecyl sulfate-polyacrylamide gel electrophoresis by chromophoric labeling, *Anal. Biochem.*, 128, 412–414, 1983.

39. Strottmann, J. M., Robinson, J. B., Jr., and Stellwagen, E., Advantages of preelectrophoretic conjugation of polypeptides with fluorescent dyes, *Anal. Biochem.*, 132, 334–337, 1983.

40. Tsang, V. C., Hancock, K., and Simons, A. R., Calibration of prestained protein molecular weight standards for use in the "Western" or enzyme-linked immunoelectrotransfer blot techniques, *Anal. Biochem.*, 143, 304–307, 1984.

41. Seto, D., Rohrbacher, C., Seto, J., and Hood, L., Phosphorescent zinc sulfide is a nonradioactive alternative for marking autoradiograms, *Anal. Biochem.*, 189, 51–53, 1990.

42. Liu, R. H., Jacob, J., and Tennant, B., Chemiluminescent detection of protein molecular weight markers in Western blot techniques, *Biotechniques*, 22, 594–595, 1997.

43. Carlone, G. M., Plikaytis, B. B., and Arko, R. J., Immune serum to protein molecular weight standards for calibrating Western blots, *Anal. Biochem.*, 155, 89–91, 1986.

44. Lindbladh, C., Mosbach, K., and Bulow, L., Standard calibration proteins for Western blotting obtained by genetically prepared protein A conjugates, *Anal. Biochem.*, 197, 187–190, 1991.

45. Lindmark, R., Thoren-Tolling, K., and Sjoquist, J., Binding of immunoglobulins to protein A and immunoglobulin levels in mammalian sera, *J. Immunol. Methods*, 62, 1–13, 1983.

46. Navarre, J., Bradford, A. J., Calhoun, B. C., and Goldenring, J. R., Quenching of endogenous peroxidase in Western blot, *Biotechniques*, 21, 990–992, 1996.

47. Vaitaitis, G. M., Sanderson, R. J., Kimble, E. J., Elkins, N. D., and Flores, S. C., Modification of enzyme-conjugated streptavidin-biotin western blot technique to avoid detection of endogenous biotin-containing proteins, *Biotechniques*, 26, 854–858, 1999.

48. Zaaijer, H. L., Exel-Oehlers, P., Kraaijeveld, T., Altena, E., and Lelie, P. N., Early detection of antibodies to HIV-1 by third-generation assays [comments], *Lancet*, 340, 770–772, 1992.

49. Alcaraz, C., Rodriguez, F., Oviedo, J. M., Eiras, A., De Diego, M., Alonso, C., and Escribano, J. M., Highly specific confirmatory Western blot test for African swine fever virus antibody detection using the recombinant virus protein p54, *J. Virol. Methods*, 52, 111–119, 1995.

50. Simon, F., Pepin, J. M., Brun-Vezinet, F., Bouchaud, O., Casalino, H., and Gerard, L., Reliability of Western blotting for the confirmation of HIV-1 seroconversion [letter], *Lancet*, 340, 1541–1542, 1992.

51. Mortimer, P. P., The fallibility of HIV Western blot, *Lancet*, 337, 286–287, 1991.

52. Fawcett, P. T., Rose, C. D., Gibney, K. M., and Doughty, R. A., Comparison of immunodot and Western blot assays for diagnosing Lyme borreliosis, *Clin. Diagn. Lab. Immunol.*, 5, 503–506, 1998.

53. Zaaijer, H. L., van Rixel, G. A., Kromosoeto, J. N., Balgobind-Ramdas, D. R., Cuypers, H. T., and Lelie, P. N., Validation of a new immunoblot assay (LiaTek HIV III) for confirmation of human immunodeficiency virus infection, *Transfusion*, 38, 776–781, 1998.

54. Lazzarotto, T., Maine, G. T., Dal Monte, P., Ripalti, A., and Landini, M. P., A novel Western blot test containing both viral and recombinant proteins for anticytomega-lovirus immunoglobulin M detection, *J. Clin. Microbiol.*, 35, 393–397, 1997.

55. Hennig, H., Kirchner, H., and Kluter, H., Failure of third-generation recombinant immunoblot assay to detect hepatitis C virus core antibodies, *Transfusion*, 39, 335–336, 1999.

56. Laemmli, U. K., Cleavage of structural proteins during the assembly of the head of bacteriophage T4, *Nature*, 227, 680–685, 1970.

57. Ornstein, L., Disc electrophoresis. I. Background and theory, *Ann. N.Y. Acad. Sci.*, 321–349, 1964.

58. Nilsen-Hamilton, M. and Hamilton, R., Detection of proteins induced by growth regulators, *Methods Enzymol.*, 147, 427–444, 1987.

16 Immunohistochemical Methods

Kendrick J. Morrell, Neil M. Hand,
and Nicholas R. Griffin

CONTENTS

16.1 INTRODUCTION

Immunohistochemistry is the application of specific antibodies for the localization of antigens in tissue sections or preparations of isolated cells. It allows the investigation of the topographical distribution of antigens within tissues, facilitating the identification of cell types expressing individual antigens. Localization of an antigen within cells is also possible, but the resolution is variable depending on the technique. Originally, immunohistochemistry was introduced in the 1940s to investigate the distribution of microbial antigens in tissues, but has since become a mainstay of investigation into fundamental aspects of cell biology and pathology. The immunohistochemical technique is thus a logical extension to traditional biochemical blotting technologies.

16.1.1 APPLICATIONS

Applications of immunohistochemistry divide into the following two basic areas:

1. Investigation of the tissue or cellular distribution of a novel antigen
2. Investigation of the tissue or cellular distribution of a known antigen to probe some aspect of cell biology

The second area has found wide application in routine diagnostic histopathology and has led to massive commercial development of applicable antibodies and associated localization technologies. Aspects of cell biology that are routinely investigated by the diagnostic pathologist include cell lineage, cell differentiation, cell degeneration, proliferation, clonality, oncogene activation, tissue invasion, and infection.

16.1.2 OVERVIEW OF METHODOLOGY

At the simplest level, antibody is applied to a tissue preparation, and sites of specific binding are revealed either by direct labelling of the antibody, or more usually, by the use of a secondary labelling method to reveal the site of antibody binding. The technique was historically developed using fluorescent labels, but this necessitates using a UV light source which prevents easy observation of tissue morphology. Alternative techniques using enzyme labels such as horseradish peroxidase or alkaline phosphatase have been developed to produce a label which can be viewed against a traditional counterstain with routine light microscopy to give excellent cytological and histological detail. While many investigations had been initially developed using frozen sections of tissue, most investigations in routine histopathology now take place on formalin-fixed, paraffin-wax embedded material. This has the considerable advantages of simple tissue preservation and storage, in addition to providing excellent morphology, but the fixation process can mask many antigens. Retrieving these antigens and rendering them detectable by immunohistochemical techniques is an aspect of technology that has rapidly advanced in recent years. Initial techniques focused on using proteolytic enzymes, but for many antigens these have been supplanted by heat-mediated antigen retrieval procedures using a microwave oven or pressure cooking.

Developments in immunohistochemistry continue apace. There is particular interest in the generation of robust primary antibodies, antigen retrieval technology, and developments in localization techniques. The emerging emphasis is on increased sensitivity leading to lower primary antibody costs, and speed of production of the final result. These concerns have recently produced innovative immunostaining techniques using dextran polymer backbones and signal amplification with tyramide. Many aspects of the immunohistochemical process can now be purchased as "off the shelf" technologies.

16.1.3 CHOICE OF ANTIBODIES IN IMMUNOHISTOCHEMISTRY

Polyclonal antibody preparations represent the products of a variety of clones reacting with different specificity to a variety of epitopes present on the immunogen. This can introduce interbatch inconsistencies in performance, as some of the antibodies present may cross-react with other antigens and the serum may contain antibodies that are unrelated to the specific immunisation procedure undertaken. This can lead to nonspecific immunohistochemical cross-reactions and false positive staining, which may need to be addressed by absorption with appropriate antigens. Alternatively, if the required antibody is present at high titer, nonspecific reactions can be removed by dilution of the antiserum. An advantage of polyclonal antisera can be their ease of use on fixed material, because one or more of the epitopes recognised by the antibody may be less prone to masking produced by fixation.

Monoclonal antibody technology has revolutionized immunohistochemistry and has led to an explosion in the number of antibodies available of precisely defined specificity and consistency. Attention needs to be paid at the screening stage of antibody production to the final applications in immunohistochemistry. Clones that recognise antigen in blotting experiments may be directed against epitopes that are sensitive to fixation, which can later lead to problems with the detection of the antigen. However, selection of clones that recognise fixation-resistant epitopes can massively increase the applicability of the final product, particularly if the vast archives of human tissues stored in pathology departments are to be utilized or if the product is likely to be of diagnostic use.

16.2 TISSUE PREPARATION

It is of paramount importance that tissue requiring immunohistochemistry must be correctly prepared if good, consistent, reliable, and meaningful staining is to be obtained. Unless this is achieved, staining may be affected and that can make accurate interpretation difficult. Two fundamental and vital stages in the preparation of the tissue which can influence staining are fixation and processing. Although there is no universal protocol for either stage or for each type of preparation, it is clear that some protocols are more suitable than others. Several types of preparations may be employed, but those discussed in this section have all been extensively used for research or diagnostic purposes and consequently are recommended for achieving high quality immunohistochemistry. Immunocytochemical methods of use at an ultrastructural level are not covered in this review.

Tissue sections may be produced either as frozen, wax, or plastic, the latter advocated when high resolution or semithin sections are required. Various procedures are suitable for examining cytological specimens. Some tissue samples can become detached from the slide during staining for various reasons, including the nature of the tissue, size of sample, or vigorous treatment (e.g., heat-mediated antigen retrieval), but an adhesive such as 3-aminopropyltriethoxysilane (APES) on the slide is suggested to reduce or prevent tissue loss.

16.2.1 PRODUCTION OF APES COATED SLIDES

1. Place the slides into racks.
2. Wash slides in acetone for 20 s.
3. Allow to drain.
4. Immerse in 2% APES (Sigma Chemicial Co.) in acetone for 20 s.

5. Quickly drain, but do not allow to dry.
6. Wash in running water.
7. Drain and allow to dry in a 37°C incubator.

APES solution must be made fresh each time, as it colorises on storage.

16.2.2 SMEARS/CYTOSPINS

1. Prepare smears/cytospins onto slides that have previously been coated with APES.
2. Air dry at room temperature for 30 min.
3. Fix in precooled, fresh acetone at 4°C for 20 min.
4. Air dry at room temperature for at least 15 min.
5. Stain smears/cytospins within 3 d.

16.2.3 FROZEN SECTIONS

1. Section unfixed frozen tissue at 4 to 7 μm.
2. Pick the sections up on slides that have previously been coated with APES.
3. Allow the sections to air dry at room temperature for 30 min.
4. Fix in precooled, fresh acetone at 4°C for 20 min.
5. Dry the sections at room temperature for at least 15 min.
6. Stain the sections within 3 d.

16.2.4 PARAFFIN WAX SECTIONS

A variety of fixatives are potentially available, but for routine purposes, tissue is usually fixed for 24 to 48 h in one of the formalin variants listed below, before being processed and embedded into paraffin wax:

10% formalin
10% formol saline
10% formol calcium
10% neutral buffered formalin

1. Section tissue at 3 to 5 μm.
2. Pick the sections up on slides that have previously been coated with APES.
3. The sections should be allowed to stand upright and drained for 30 min.
4. Place the sections on a 60°C hotplate for 15 min or in an oven at 37°C overnight prior to immunohistochemical staining.

16.2.5 CYTOBLOCK

This procedure employing a Cytospin is used for small fragments of tissue, which are too small for normal processing and embedding in paraffin wax. The reagents required to form what is called a Cytoblock (Shandon Inc.) are supplied in a commercial kit. The use of formol calcium or solutions containing phosphate ions should be avoided, as these inhibit polymerization of the gel.

1. Fix tissue in formalin for a maximum of 24 h.
2. Transfer the tissue and some fixative to one or two centifuge tubes, depending on the volume.
3. Centrifuge at 1200 rpm for 5 min.
4. Discard most of the supernatant fixative.
5. Add four drops of the blue Cytoblock fluid to the sediment.
6. Place three drops of colorless Cytoblock fluid in the well of the specialized cassette.
7. Assemble in the metal clip with specimen chamber.
8. Mix the sediment and solutions.
9. Transfer to the specimen chamber.
10. Place in the Cytospin and centifuge at 1500 rpm for 5 min.
11. Remove cassette containing Cytoblock from assembly.
12. Add one further drop of colorless Cytoblock fluid to the gel block.
13. Enclose block in the cassette and place in fixative to await processing.

Sections are cut at the standard thickness for routine paraffin blocks and prepared for subsequent immunocytochemical staining as previously described.

16.2.6 PLASTIC SECTIONS (METHYL METHACRYLATE)

Although several plastics can be employed for light microscopy immunohistochemistry, we prefer to use methyl methacrylate (MMA) which, in our experience, has produced the best and most reliable staining.

1. Fix thin slices of tissue (2 mm maximum thickness) in formalin for 24 h.
2. Dehydrate through graded ethanol (50%, 70%, 90% and 100% × 2) each for 1 h.
3. Infiltrate with 1:1 mix of MMA monomer and 100% ethanol for 1 h.
4. Infiltrate with resin mix (MMA 15 ml, dibutyl phthalate 5 ml, dried benzoyl peroxide 1 g) for 1 h.
5. Repeat step 4 at 4°C overnight.
6. Embed in a thick plastic molding tray partially immersed in water inside a glass dessicator using fresh solution of resin mix to which 125 µl of N,N dimethylaniline is added to each 10-g aliquot.
7. Polymerize in an oxygen-free atmosphere (vacuum or oxygen-free nitrogen) for approximately 3 h.
8. Cut the sections at 2 µm with a glass knife and float them on a 56°C water bath.
9. Pick up the sections on a slide coated with APES.
10. Drain and dry the sections on a hot plate for 20 min or at 37°C overnight.

16.2.7 Notes

1. Agitate specimen on a roller mixer for steps 2 through 4.
2. Benzoyl peroxide is potentially explosive when dry and care must be taken; dry samples at room temperature away from direct sunlight or heat for 24 h.
3. Handle and dispose of reagents according to local and national regulations.
4. The plastic must be removed prior to immunohistochemical staining which may easily be achieved by immersing the slides in xylene for 15 min.

16.3 ENZYME LABELS

The most commonly used enzyme labels for immunocytochemical techniques are horseradish peroxidase and to a lesser extent, calf intestine alkaline phosphatase. Other suitable but less frequently used enzymes are glucose oxidase and β-galactosidase, neither of which will be discussed in this chapter. Various chromogens of differing colors (some of which are unstable) may be employed to demonstrate the substrate.

16.3.1 Horseradish Peroxidase

Horseradish peroxidase may be bound covalently to antibodies utilizing bifunctional agents such as glutaraldehyde and 4, 4'-difluoro-3, 3'-dinitrophenyl sulfone. In the one-step procedure, because the peroxidase molecule has a paucity of reactive groups compared to the antibody molecule, more antibody molecules bind to each other than to the peroxidase. For the two-step procedure, peroxidase initially reacts with the bifunctional reagent, followed by mixing only bound peroxidase with the antibody, resulting in the prevention of unwanted polymerization.

In the peroxidase-antiperoxidase (PAP) technique, peroxidase molecules are not linked covalently to antibodies. Antibodies directed against peroxidase are used to form a soluble immune complex of two antibody and three peroxidase molecules, which results in a much higher sensitivity than those techniques that use covalently linked antibody-peroxidase complexes. A horseradish peroxidase label can be revealed with the following chromogens:

16.3.1.1 3,3'-Diaminobenzidine Tetrahydrochloride (DAB)

Electrons are donated from DAB to hydrogen peroxide via peroxidase. This results in oxidation of DAB at the site of enzyme activity and formation of an oxidative intermediate, which polymerizes rapidly to an insoluble precipitate at the site of bound antibody. The dark brown end product contrasts well if a hematoxylin counterstain is employed, and resists alcoholic dehydration and clearing in xylene.

Method:

1. Dissolve 5 mg of DAB in 10 ml 0.05 M Tris/HCl buffered saline pH 7.6.
2. Add 0.1 ml of freshly prepared 3% hydrogen peroxide. Use immediately.
3. Incubate slides for 10 min at room temperature.

Intensification of DAB end product: The DAB/peroxidase end product may be enhanced in a number of ways as follows:

1. The pH of the DAB solution may be lowered to between 5.0 and 6.0 to significantly increase the sensitivity of the substrate, but this can give rise to artefactual perinuclear staining.
2. The reaction time and/or temperature may be increased, but the technique is difficult to control, leading to increased nonspecific reactivity and less reproducibility.
3. The addition of a nitrogenous compound such as imidazole (which has been reported as one of the most popular and sensitive to detect peroxidase) to the substrate section. Imidazole increases the rate of oxidation of DAB by peroxidase, but also significantly inhibits the psuedoperoxidase activity of hemoglobin.

Method:

   a. Dissolve 5 mg of DAB in 10 ml 0.05 M Tris-HCl-buffered saline pH 7.6.
   b. Add 5 mg of imidazole and shake until dissolved.
   c. Add 60 µl of freshly prepared 1% hydrogen peroxide. Use immediately.
   d. Incubate slides for 10 min at room temperature.

4. Numerous metal salts can be added to the DAB solution or as a post-DAB step. Satisfactory results may be achieved with post-DAB solutions of 0.5 to 1.0% copper sulphate, nickel chloride, or cobalt chloride incubations. The addition of 0.9% sodium chloride to the metal salt solutions, as sometimes advocated, appears to offer no advantages. The alternative technique of adding the metal salt solution to the DAB/hydrogen peroxide substrate solution tends to result in increased levels of background reactivity, which is probably due to the ability of some metal salts to catalyse the oxidation of DAB.
5. The DAB reaction product may be intensified by incubation of the sections (which have been washed in copious amounts of water) in 1% osmium tetroxide for 5 min. This results in an intensification of the sites of DAB deposition and protects the chromogen from long-term fading due to oxidation. The major disadvantage of this procedure, however, is the significantly increased level of background staining produced.

16.3.1.2 3-Amino-9-Ethylcarbazole (AEC)

Electrons are donated from AEC to hydrogen peroxide via peroxidase, resulting in the oxidation of AEC to form an oxidative intermediate, which polymerizes rapidly to a pink/red, light-sensitive, alcohol-soluble precipitate at the site of bound antibody. The sections may be counterstained with hematoxylin, but must be mounted in an aqueous mountant.

Method:

1. Dissolve 4 mg of AEC in 1 ml of N,N-dimethylformamide (DMF).
2. Add 14 ml of 0.1 M acetate buffer (pH 5.2) and 0.15 ml of 3% hydrogen peroxide.
3. Mix and filter.
4. Incubate sections in this solution for 10 min.

16.3.1.3 4-Chloro-1-Naphthol

Electrons are donated from 4-chloro-1-naphthol to hydrogen peroxide via peroxidase resulting in the oxidation of 4-chloro-1-naphthol at the site of enzyme activity to form an oxidative intermediate, which polymerizes rapidly to a blue alcohol-soluble precipitate over the site of bound antibody. The sections are counterstained in neutral red or methyl green and mounted in acidified-buffered glycerine of pH 2.2.

Method:

1. Dissolve 40 mg of 4-chloro-1-naphthol in 0.5 ml of ethanol.
2. Add while stirring, 100 ml 50 mM Tris-HCl buffer (pH 7.6) containing 100 μl of 30% hydrogen peroxide. A white precipitate is formed.
3. Filter and incubate sections in this solution for 10 min.

16.3.2 CALF INTESTINE ALKALINE PHOSPHATASE

Calf intestine alkaline phosphatase may also be covalently bound to antibodies. However, it did not find great popularity with immunocytochemists until the unlabelled alkaline phosphatase or alkaline phosphatase-anti-alkaline phosphatase (APAAP) procedure was developed. The major advantage of the APAAP technique compared to those utilizing horseradish peroxidase, is the lack of interference from endogenous enzyme in the cells under investigation. This is an obvious advantage when studying peripheral blood and bone marrow preparations, where endogenous peroxidase activity can make horseradish peroxidase preparations uninterpretable. Furthermore, endogenous alkaline phosphatase activity, which is present in some leucocytes and tissues such as bone and kidney, may be easily and effectively inhibited by the addition of 1 mM levamisole to the substrate solution. It must be noted, however, that intestinal alkaline phosphatases are not inhibited by levamisole and, consequently, alkaline phosphatase is not recommended as an antibody label when studying tissues and cells from this region.

The rationale for these methods is based on the hydrolysis of phosphates which contain substituted naphthol groupings to produce an insoluble naphthol derivative, which then couples to a suitable diazonium salt to produce an intensely coloured, insoluble azo dye at the site of enzyme activity.

16.3.3 Naphthol AS-MX Phosphate/Fast Red TR

1. Dissolve 2 mg of naphthol-AS-MX phosphate in 0.2 ml of N,N-dimethyl-formamide (DMF).
2. Add 9.8 ml of 0.1 M Tris/HCl buffer, pH 8.2.
3. Add 2.4 mg of levamisole and 10 mg of Fast red TR salt and dissolve.
4. Filter and incubate sections in this solution for 15 min.
6. Wash sections in 0.1 M Tris/HCl buffer, pH 8.2.
7. Counterstain nuclei in an aqueous haematoxylin.
8. Mount sections in an aqueous mountant.

Results: Sites of alkaline phosphatase activity are red.

Notes:

1. Sections should be washed briefly in 0.1 M Tris/HCl buffer (pH 8.2) before incubation in the substrate solution.
2. 10 mg of Fast blue BB may be used instead of the Fast red TR, resulting in alkaline phosphatase activity staining blue. Hematoxylin is not a suitable counterstain with this chromogen, but neutral red or light green is recommended.
3. If naphthol-AS-MX phosphate sodium salt is substituted for the naphthol-AS-MX phosphate free acid, DMF can be omitted as the sodium salt is soluble in Tris/HCl buffer.

16.4 ACHIEVING SPECIFICITY

All immunohistochemistry results fall into one or more of the following categories:

1. Wanted specific reactivity
2. Unwanted specific reactivity
3. Nonspecific reactivity

The ultimate objective of the immunohistochemist is to achieve strong, well localized, wanted specific reactivity, with minimal or no unwanted or nonspecific reactivities. This section describes some techniques, which, when used as part of an immunohistochemistry method, will facilitate the achievement of this goal.

16.4.1 Wanted Specific Reactivity

This reactivity is achieved by immunological binding of the primary antibody with the protein (antigen) under investigation.

16.4.2 Unwanted Specific Reactivity

This reactivity is achieved by immunological binding of the primary antibody with a protein (antigen) other than that which is under investigation. This can occur when an impure primary antibody is used, or when the antigen under investigation shares an amino acid sequence with another protein, making it impossible for the antibody to differentiate between the two compounds.

16.4.3 NONSPECIFIC REACTIVITY

This reactivity is produced by nonimmunological reactions between the immunocytochemical reagents and tissue components. It can be eliminated, or at least reduced, by many techniques, the most common of which follow.

16.4.3.1 Dilution of Antibodies

Usually, the manufacturer of an antibody will recommend an optimal working dilution. However, while this is usually fairly accurate, it is nevertheless only a guideline, and dilutions can vary both between laboratories and depending upon the technique employed. The highest dilution that it is possible to obtain accurate results should be used, as this will usually to reduce unwanted and nonspecific binding of the antibody to tissue components. It must be remembered that the optimal dilution is influenced significantly by factors such as incubation time and temperature, and these parameters should be set and rigidly adhered to before undertaking any antibody optimizations. Using "checkerboard" titrations, the optimal dilution can be assessed, although evaluation of more than one antibody at a time should be avoided. Finally, it is vital that antibody optimization must always be undertaken on tissue sections or cell preparations that are known to contain the antigen under investigation.

16.4.3.2 Endogenous Enzyme Blocking Solutions

Some enzymes that are used as antibody labels are also present in mammalian tissues and cells, including the most commonly used labels, peroxidase and alkaline phosphatase. It is therefore necessary to remove or block this endogenous enzyme activity so that false positive results are not reported. Endogenous peroxidase is most commonly removed by incubation of the tissue sections in a methanolic or aqueous solution of hydrogen peroxide. To produce maximum blocking and minimum tissue damage when using paraffin wax sections, we prefer to use a solution consisting of one part 6% hydrogen peroxide and nine parts absolute methanol for 15 min. For frozen sections, smears, and cytospins, we use a solution consisting of one part 3% hydrogen peroxide in nine parts distilled water. Because even this weak solution can cause some tissue damage, it is only used if endogenous peroxidase makes interpretation of results difficult. For blocking of endogenous alkaline phosphatase, it is recommended that 1 mM levamisole be included in the alkaline phosphatase substrate/chromogen solution. Finally, remember that it is not always possible to remove all endogenous enzymes, and care should be taken when interpreting immunohistochemistry so that false positive results are not reported.

16.4.4 BLOCKING ELECTROSTATIC AND HYDROPHOBIC BINDING

Antibodies will readily form electrostatic and hydrophobic bonds with cells and tissue sections, resulting in poor immunocytochemical preparations. The easiest way to reduce this binding is to incubate the sections/cell preparations for 20 min in a 1:5 solution of nonimmune serum and to dilute antibodies either in a 1:20 solution of serum or use one of the commercially available antibody diluting fluids. In order to prevent any cross-reaction of the secondary antibodies used, the serum should be derived from the same species in which the secondary antibodies were raised.

16.4.5 BLOCKING ENDOGENOUS BIOTIN ACTIVITY

Some tissues, most notably gut and kidney, contain endogenous biotin. This can be particularly problematic if microwave antigen retrieval techniques have been employed. However, most commercial sources of antibodies also produce avidin/biotin blocking kits, useful for decreasing unwanted staining. These are essentially balanced solutions of avidin and biotin, in which the sections are incubated prior to the primary antibody solution.

16.5 PRETREATMENT TECHNIQUES

Tissue to be embedded in paraffin wax or plastic must be fixed to prevent putrefaction and autolysis. A variety of fixatives are available, but for routine purposes, a formalin variant is the most frequent type employed. Unfortunately, the use of certain fixatives, including formalin, causes cross-linking and changes to the protein structures, which can mask or even destroy some antigenic epitopes. In many cases, antigenicity can be unmasked by pretreating the sections prior to immunohistochemical staining with either proteolytic digestion or heat-mediated antigen retrieval, or a combination of the two. A few antigens can be unmasked by acid treatment, but there are many antigens which do not require any pretreatment. The precise way in which tissue antigens are unmasked by the various pretreatments is unclear, but it is probable that aldehyde cross-links, which form the basis of formaldehyde fixation, are broken.

Several proteolytic enzymes including trypsin, pepsin, protease, and Proteinase K (some of which are available as pre-made solutions) may be used, but for optimal staining the choice depends on the specific antigen sought. For best results and standardization, the enzyme solutions are frequently employed at 37°C. For safety and convenience, they may be quickly heated to the required temperature in a microwave oven that has a probe. The incubation times for proteolytic digestion may vary depending on the degree of fixation and, to a lesser degree, the processing schedule employed.

During the last decade, several heat-mediated antigen retrieval techniques based on treating fixed tissue sections with a high temperature solution have been introduced. These procedures have revolutionized imunohistochemistry, providing improved staining, greater standardization, increased antibody dilution, reduced influence of fixation time on staining, and the ability to demonstrate antigens which previously were only possible on frozen sections. Many antigens may be better demonstrated following these procedures rather than using proteolytic enzyme digestion, although this is not universally the case. Several solutions have been advocated, and while some may produce better results than others, the most popular is 10 m*M* citrate buffer at pH 6.0. Recently, for a selected few antigens, an EDTA solution has also been recommended. All the solutions must be heated to around boiling point, and because this may be achieved using a microwave oven, the procedure is frequently described as microwave antigen retrieval. In addition, for some antigens, superheating in a pressure cooker may produce superior immmunohistochemical staining, and more recently autoclaves and steamers have also been used. No uniformly accepted protocol exists, and laboratories must optimize the technique to their own circumstances.

It is advised that all sections required for any pretreatment are mounted on slides coated with a strong adhesive, such as APES (see tissue preparation), to reduce the possibility of the section detaching from the slide during this stage. The sections must be dewaxed or deresinated and hydrated before pretreatment is commenced.

Frozen sections that have undergone light adehyde fixation or, more usually, have been subjected to a nonadditive fixative, such as acetone, do not require pretreatment for the demonstration of antigens. This also is also the case with smear or cytospin cytological preparations which may have been fixed with methanol.

16.5.1 PROTEOLYTIC DIGESTION WITH TRYPSIN IN A MICROWAVE OVEN

Fixation:

10% formol saline 24 to 48 h

Sections:

Paraffin wax or plastic sections (2 to 5 μm) mounted on APES coated slides

Method:

1. Remove wax or plastic and hydrate.
2. Using a magnetic stirrer, mix 0.3 g trypsin and 0.3 g dihydrate calcium chloride vigorously in 300 ml 0.05 *M* Tris/HCl buffer pH 7.6 in a staining trough.
3. Adjust the pH of the solution using 1 *M* NaOH to pH 7.8.
4. Wash slides in distilled water.
5. Place the sections in a plastic rack and immerse in the trypsin solution.
6. Put the trough into the microwave oven and plug the temperature probe into the top of the oven. Ensure that the other end of the probe is immersed into the trypsin solution and shut the door.
7. Switch on the microwave oven.
8. Select the *Power* and the *Temperature* buttons for operation.
9. Touch *Start* and watch the temperature display reading rise to 37°C.

10. When the set temperature is reached, set a timer to measure the desired length of time of trypsinization. (approximately 15 to 20 min).
11. When the set time has elapsed, remove the trough and wash the slides well in running tap water before proceeding with immunohistochemical staining.

Notes:

Do not allow the sections to dry at any stage during the technique.
Enzyme solutions may cause skin irritation if splashed onto the skin.
Metal objects must never be placed inside the microwave oven.
Alternatively, trypsin tablets can be purchased and used as instructed by the manufacturer.

16.5.2 PROTEOLYTIC DIGESTION WITH PROTEINASE K

Fixation:

10% formol saline 24 to 48 h

Sections:

Paraffin wax (3 to 5 μm) mounted on APES coated slides

Method:

1. Remove wax or plastic and hydrate.
2. Wash slides in distilled water.
3. Place 2 or 3 drops of Proteinase K (Dako) onto the section for 15 min.
4. Rinse off the Proteinase K with distilled water.
5. Wash the slides well in running tap water before proceeding with immunohistochemical staining.

Note:

Alternative souces of Proteinase K are available.

16.5.3 ANTIGEN RETRIEVAL WITH 10 mM CITRATE BUFFER pH 6.0 IN A MICROWAVE OVEN

Fixation:

10% formol saline 24 to 48 h

Sections:

Paraffin wax or plastic sections (2 to 5 μm) mounted on APES coated slides

Method:

1. Remove wax or plastic and hydrate.
2. Wash the slides in distilled water.
3. Place the sections in a plastic rack into suitable (deep) plastic container containing 650 ml of 10 m*M* citrate buffer pH 6.0 solution ensuring that the slides are completely immersed.
4. Place the the lid on container so that there is a small gap for air/vapour to escape.
5. Place the container inside the microwave oven in the centre of the turn-table, and shut the oven door.
6. Select the *Power* and the *Temperature* buttons for operation
7. Key in a time of 20 min.
8. Press the *Start* button and observe. The temperature will now slowly rise and the solution should be boiling after approximately 5 to 9 min, depending on the power selected. Check the slides to ensure that the level of solution does not fall below the level of the slides.
9. After 20 min the container should be removed carefully from the microwave oven and taken to a sink to run cold tap water into the solution until it is sufficiently cool to allow removal of the slides.
10. Wash the slides well in running cold tap water for 15 min before proceeding with immunocytochemical staining.

Notes:

Do not allow the sections to dry out at any stage during the technique.
Boiling citrate buffer will cause severe scalds if splashed onto the skin. Wear heat-resistant gloves when transferring the buffer from the microwave oven to the sink.
Metal objects must never be placed inside the microwave oven.

16.5.3.1 Preparation of 10 m*M* Citrate Buffer, pH 6.0

21 g citric acid
10 L distilled water
Adjust to pH 6.0 with 1 *M* NaOH (approximately 250 ml).

16.5.4 ANTIGEN RETRIEVAL WITH 10 M*M* CITRATE BUFFER PH 6.0 IN A PRESSURE COOKER

Fixation:

10% formol saline 24 to 48 h

Sections:

Paraffin wax or plastic sections (2 to 5 μm) mounted on APES coated slides

Method:

1. Remove wax or plastic and hydrate.
2. Wash the slides in distilled water.
3. Approximately 15 min before antigen retrieval, pour 1500 ml of 10 mM citrate buffer pH 6.0 solution into the stainless-steel pressure cooker. Loosely fit the lid and place cooker on a hot plate. Switch on the hot plate and set the ring to full power. The solution will take several minutes to heat.
4. Place the sections in a clean metal rack and carefully lower into the hot solution in the pressure cooker (wear heat-resistant gloves). Fit the lid and check that the cook control is set to Manual so that after few minutes, the pintle will rise. A few minutes later the "Rise N Time" indicator will also rise, when the timer should be set for 3 min and the hot plate turned down to a low setting.
5. When the time is completed, move the cooker onto an unheated area, turn off the power of the hot plate, and carefully move the cook control to Auto. The cooker will now steam vigorously until the pintle drops and standard pressure is resumed. At this point, place the cooker in a sink one third full of water, carefully remove the lid, and allow the solution inside to cool slowly.
6. When the solution has cooled, remove the slides and wash them well in running cold tap water for 15 min.
7. The slides are now ready to continue immunostaining.

Notes:

Do not allow the sections to dry out at any stage during the technique.
Boiling citrate buffer will cause severe scalds if splashed onto the skin. Wear heat-resistant gloves.
The citrate buffer solution may be topped up to 1500 ml again and reused up to five times.

16.6 IMMUNOENZYME TECHNIQUES

The number of immunoenzyme techniques that are currently available to the immunohistochemist are many and infinitely variable. This section discusses some of the more common and less often-used techniques in a format that will enable them to be performed with confidence. If the techniques are followed exactly, an acceptable end result is likely, although it is acknowledged that some workers may want to slightly modify some of the procedures to optimize results for their own laboratories.

With few exceptions the techniques described all relate to sections of formalin-fixed, paraffin wax-embedded mammalian tissue, although similar procedures can be employed for frozen and plastic sections and cytological preparations. Obviously, frozen sections, smears, and cytospin preparations do not require procedures prior to hydration. Most of the techniques employ a horseradish peroxidase label, which is subsequently visualized with 3,3′-diaminobenzidene tetrahydrochloride (DAB) and hydrogen peroxide, but other enzyme labels and peroxidase substrates may also be substituted if required. Fundamental modifications that may be required to accommodate the substitutions are included.

16.7 THE INDIRECT PEROXIDASE TECHNIQUE

Rationale: In this technique, the unlabelled primary antibody is first applied. The sites of antigen/antibody reactivity are then localized by means of a horseradish peroxidase labeled secondary antibody, which is directed against immunoglobulins from the species and class of the primary antibody.

Method:

1. Dewax sections in xylene for 5 min.
2. Wash sections in a clean bath of xylene, followed by 2 baths of absolute alcohol.
3. Block endogenous peroxidase activity in methanolic hydrogen peroxide (1 part 6% hydrogen peroxide and 9 parts absolute methanol) for 15 min.
4. Hydrate sections in descending strengths of alcohol.
5. Wash in running tap water.
5a. Insert pretreatment procedure if required.
6. Incubate sections in 1:5 nonimmune serum (derived from the same species as the secondary antisera) for 20 min.
7. Drain and wipe off the excess serum and incubate in the appropriately diluted primary antisera for 30 min.
8. Wash off the unbound antisera in 0.05 *M* Tris/HCl buffer for 5 min.
9. Wipe off excess buffer around the section and apply appropriately diluted, peroxidase labeled secondary antisera for 30 min.
10. Wash off the unbound antisera in 0.05 *M* Tris/HCl buffer for 5 min.
11. Incubate sections in the DAB solution for 10 min.
12. Wash sections well in running tap water.
13. Counterstain in hematoxylin.
14. Dehydrate in ascending concentrations of alcohol.
15. Clear in 2 baths of xylene.
16. Mount in a synthetic mounting medium.

Results:

Sites of antigen/antibody reactivity: Brown
Nuclei: Blue

Preparation 0.05 M Tris/HCl buffer pH 7.6:

1. 8.1 g sodium chloride
2. 6 g TRIS (hydroxymethyl) aminomethane

3. 4 ml 1 *N* HCl
4. 1 L distilled water
5. Adjust to pH 7.6 with 1 *N* HCl or 1 *M* NaOH

DAB solution:

1. Dissolve 5 mg of 3,3′-diaminobenzidene tetrahydrochloride in 10 ml 0.05 *M* Tris/HCl buffered saline, pH 7.6.
2. Add 0.1 ml of freshly prepared 3% hydrogen peroxide. Use immediately.

Antibody dilutions: Prepare working dilution of antibody in a 1:20 dilution of nonimmune serum derived from the same species as the secondary antisera.

16.8 THE LABELED STREPTAVIDIN/BIOTIN (LSAB) AND THE STREPTAVIDIN BIOTIN COMPLEX (ABC) TECHNIQUES

16.8.1 LSAB Technique Rationale

This method relies upon the high affinity of avidin (a large glycoprotein found in egg white) or streptavidin (a large glycoprotein derived from *Streptomyces avidinii*) for biotin (a small glycoprotein found in egg yolk). Avidin is composed of 4 subunits which form a tertiary structure possessing 4 biotin binding hydrophobic pockets. The oligosaccharide residues present in egg white avidin, together with its charge properties, have some affinity for tissue components (particularly lectin-like proteins) resulting in nonspecific binding. Streptavidin, however, lacks oligosaccharide residues and its neutral isoelectric point offers significant advantages. The low molecular weight biotin (also known as vitamin H) can be easily conjugated to both antibodies and enzymes, with the possiblity that up to 150 biotin molecules can attach to one antibody molecule. Its strong affinity for avidin is used in complexing secondary reagents.

As a result of the high number of biotin molecules bound to a single antibody, a high tracer to antibody ratio is achieved with all of the avidin/biotin techniques. This leads to high sensitivity and allows the use of high dilutions of primary antisera that in turn can lead to reduced levels of nonspecific reactivity.

16.8.2 ABC Technique Rationale

In this technique, the required primary antibody is applied first, followed by incubation in the appropriate biotinylated secondary antibody and then a preformed complex consisting of avidin and peroxidase labeled biotin (ABC complex). Only some of the available biotin-binding sites on the avidin molecules are utilized, leaving the remaining sites free to bind to the biotinylated secondary antibody. The relatively high number of peroxidase molecules bound to sites of primary antibody/antigen reactivity provides a very high degree of sensitivity and, as with the labeled avidin technique, peroxidase labeled streptavidin may be substituted without any change in protocol.

Method:

1. Dewax sections in xylene for 5 min.
2. Wash sections in a clean bath of xylene followed by two baths of absolute alcohol.
3. Block endogenous peroxidase activity in methanolic hydrogen peroxide (one part 6% hydrogen peroxide and nine parts absolute methanol) for 15 min.
4. Hydrate sections in descending strengths of alcohol.
5. Wash in running tap water.
5a. Insert pretreatment procedure if required.
6. Incubate sections in 1:5 nonimmune serum (derived from the same species as the secondary antisera) for 20 min.
7. Drain and wipe off the excess serum and incubate in the appropriately diluted primary antisera for 30 min.
8. Wash off the unbound antisera in 0.05 M Tris/HCl buffer for 5 min.
9. Wipe off excess buffer from around the section and apply appropriately diluted, biotinylated secondary antisera for 30 min.
10. Wash off the unbound antisera in 0.05 M Tris/HCl buffer for 5 min.
11. Wipe off excess buffer from around the section and apply appropriately diluted, peroxidase labeled streptavidin or preformed streptavidin/biotinylated peroxidase Complex (ABC) for 30 min.
12. Wash off the unbound reagent in 0.05 M Tris/HCl buffer for 5 min.
13. Incubate sections in the DAB solution for 10 min.
14. Wash sections well in running tap water.
15. Counterstain in hematoxylin.
16. Dehydrate in ascending concentrations of alcohol.
17. Clear in 2 baths of xylene.
18. Mount in a synthetic mounting medium.

Results:

Sites of antigen/antibody reactivity: Brown
Nuclei: Blue

Notes: For the preparation of 0.05 M Tris/HCl buffer, DAB solution, and details relating to the diluent employed for the antibody dilutions, refer to the indirect peroxidase technique previously described. The streptavidin/biotinylated peroxidase complex should be prepared according to the manufacturer's instructions.

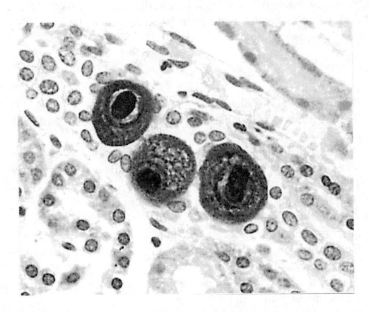

FIGURE 16.1 Paraffin section of kidney fixed in formol saline showing immunoperoxidase staining of cytomegalovirus by LSAB technique and a hematoxylin counterstain. The section was pretreated with proteinase K. Original magnification × 1250.

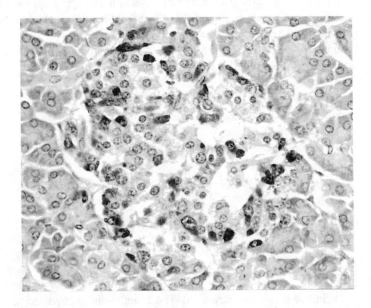

FIGURE 16.2 Paraffin section of pancreas fixed in formol saline showing immunoperoxidase staining of glucagon in an islet of Langerhans LSAB technique and a hematoxylin counterstain. No pretreatment was employed. Original magnification × 500.

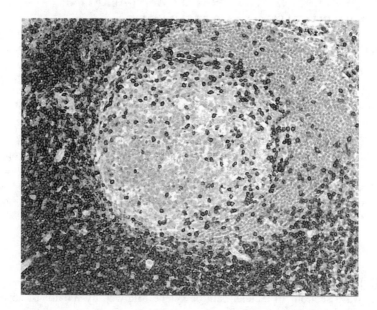

FIGURE 16.3 Paraffin section of tonsil fixed in formol saline showing immunoperoxidase staining of T lymphocytes with anti-CD3. After microwave antigen retrieval, the section was stained with an LSAB technique and a hematoxylin counterstain. Original magnification × 325.

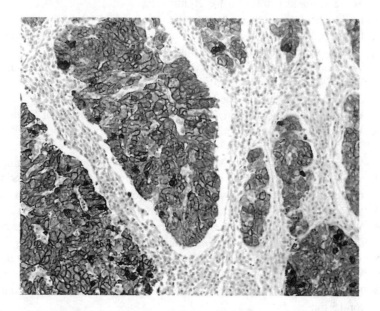

FIGURE 16.4 Paraffin section of an ovarian tumour fixed in formol saline showing immunoperoxidase staining of cytokeratin 7. After microwave antigen retrieval, the section was stained by LSAB technique and a hematoxylin counterstain. Original magnification × 325.

16.9 THE ALKALINE PHOSPHATASE ANTI-ALKALINE PHOSPHATASE (APAAP) TECHNIQUE

16.9.1 RATIONALE

The APAAP is also an unlabeled antibody enzyme complex method. It is only applicable to murine monoclonal antibodies and utilizes complexes consisting of two molecules of alkaline phosphatase and one molecule of mouse anti-alkaline phosphatase. These complexes are used as a third layer which is bound to unconjugated primary murine monoclonal antibodies via a second layer of "bridging" antibody directed against mouse immunoglobulins. The bridging antibody is applied in excess, so that one of its two identical binding sites binds to the primary antibody, and the other to the mouse immunoglobulins in the APAAP complex. In the following technique, the sensitivity is increased by repetition of the bridging antibody and APAAP incubations.

Method:

1. Dewax sections in xylene for 5 min.
2. Wash sections in a clean bath of xylene followed by 2 baths of absolute alcohol.
3. Hydrate sections in descending strengths of alcohol.
4. Wash in running tap water.
5. Incubate sections in 1:5 nonimmune serum (derived from the same species as the secondary antisera) for 20 min.
5a. Insert pretreatment procedure if required.
6. Drain and wipe off the excess serum and incubate in the appropriately diluted primary antisera for 30 min.
7. Wash off the unbound antisera in 0.05 M Tris/HCl buffer for 5 min.
8. Wipe off excess buffer from around the section and apply appropriately diluted unconjugated secondary antibody for 30 min.
9. Wash off the unbound antisera in 0.05 M Tris/HCl buffer for 5 min.
10. Wipe off excess buffer around the section and apply appropriately diluted APAAP complex for 30 min.
11. Wash off the unbound antisera in 0.05 M Tris/HCl buffer for 5 min.
12. Wipe off excess buffer from around the section and apply appropriately diluted unconjugated secondary antibody for a second time (30 min).
13. Wash off the unbound antisera in 0.05 M Tris/HCl buffer for 5 min.
14. Wipe off excess buffer from around the section and apply appropriately diluted APAAP complex for a second time (30 min).
15. Wash off the unbound antisera in 0.05 M Tris/HCl buffer for 5 min.
16. Wash sections in 0.1 M Tris/HCl buffer, pH 8.2 (see below) for 1 min.
17. Incubate sections in the naphthol AS-MX phosphate/Fast red TR solution for 15 min.
18. Wash sections well in 0.1 M Tris/HCl buffer, pH 8.2.

19. Counterstain in an aqueous hematoxylin.
20. Mount sections in an aqueous mountant.

Results

Sites of antigen/antibody reactivity: Red
Nuclei: Blue

Notes: For the preparation of 0.05 *M* Tris/HCl buffer (pH 7.6) and details relating to the diluent employed for the antibody dilutions, refer to the indirect peroxidase technique previously described.

16.9.2 PREPARATION OF NAPHTHOL AS-MX PHOSPHATE/FAST RED TR

1. Dissolve 2 mg of naphthol-AS-MX phosphate, free acid, in 0.2 ml of N,N-dimethyl formamide (DMF).
2. Add 9.8 ml of 0.1 *M* Tris/HCl buffer, pH 8.2.
3. Add 2.4 mg of levamisole and 10 mg of Fast red TR salt and dissolve.
4. Filter and use immediately.
5. Incubate sections in this solution for 15 min.
6. Wash sections in 0.1 *M* Tris/HCl buffer, pH 8.2.

16.9.3 PREPARATION OF 0.1 *M* TRIS/HCL BUFFER, PH 8.2

Solution A: 1.21 g Tris in 100 ml of distilled water
Solution B: 0.1 *N* HCl
Working solution
1. Mix 25 ml Solution A with 11 ml Solution B.
2. Add 64 ml of distilled water.
3. Adjust to pH 8.2.

Notes:

1. 10 mg of Fast blue BB may be used instead of the Fast red TR, resulting in sites of alkaline phosphatase activity stained blue. Hematoxylin is not a suitable counterstain with this chromogen, and therefore neutral red or light green is recommended.
2. Naphthol-AS-MX phosphate sodium salt may be substituted for naphthol-AS-MX phosphate-free acid. As the sodium salt is soluble in the Tris buffer, DMF can be omitted.
3. Phosphate containing buffers, such as phosphate buffered saline (PBS), should not be used, as they interfere with the reaction between the alkaline phosphatase and its substrate.

16.10 IMMUNOFLUORESCENCE TECHNIQUES

Some of the first reported immunohistochemical techniques utilized fluorescent protein conjugates, and this soon led to the production of the antibodies conjugated to fluorescent dyes. As the technique became more refined, and the quality of fluorescence microscopes improved, immunofluorescence became an attractive and readily available new tool for the biologist.

The discovery that antibodies could be labeled with enzymes without any significant loss of immunoreactivity subsequently resulted in a shift of interest away from immunofluorescence techniques toward the more versatile and stable enzyme-linked preparations. However, the use of fluorescent antibodies has not been totally superseded, and they are still widely used in a number of clinical immunology laboratories and specialized areas of immunohistochemistry, where immunofluorescence techniques are used routinely for the diagnosis of autoimmune and other immunologically related diseases.

16.10.1 FLUORESCEIN ISOTHIOCYANATE

Several new fluorochromes have become commercially available over recent years, each with its own particular advantages and disadvantages, but the isomer 1 form of fluorescein isothiocyanate (FITC) first used some 35 years ago still remains the most predominantly used fluorescent label. Proteins which have been conjugated to fluorescein show a maximum absorption of 495 nm with strong apple-green emissions. This is advantageous, in that apple-green autofluorescence is rarely expressed by mammalian tissue and the human eye is particularly sensitive to light of this wavelength.

16.10.2 RHODAMINE TETRAMETHYL ISOTHIOCYANATE

The second most commonly used fluorochrome is rhodamine. Proteins that have been conjugated to this compound show a maximum absorption of 555 nm with strong orange-red emissions. This provides a good contrast with FITC when multiple labeling studies are undertaken.

16.10.3 TEXAS RED

Proteins that have been conjugated to Texas Red show a maximum absorption of 596 nm with orange-red emissions. Texas Red is sometimes preferred to rhodamine in double labeling techniques, because it is further removed from FITC.

16.11 THE DIRECT IMMUNOFLUORESCENCE
TECHNIQUE

16.11.1 RATIONALE

In this technique the fluorescent label is linked to a secondary antibody which is directed against immunoglobulins from the species that provides the primary antibody. The indirect method is relatively quick, easy to perform, and provides greater sensitivity.

The method explained here is for fresh or fixed frozen sections or cell preparations. However, if paraffin wax sections are to be used, reference should be made to the protocol for dewaxing sections discussed in Section 16.6 on immunoenzyme techniques.

Method:

1. Wash slides in phosphate buffered saline (PBS), pH 7.2 for 5 min.
2. Drain, wipe off the excess buffer, and incubate in the appropriately diluted primary antisera for 30 min.
3. Wash off the unbound antisera in PBS for 10 min.
4. Apply appropriately diluted fluorochrome conjugated secondary antibody for 30 min.
5. Wash off unbound antisera in PBS for 20 min.
6. Mount in a suitable mounting medium.

Results: Sites of antigen/antibody reactivity express fluorescence relating to the characteristics of the fluorochrome used.

16.11.2 PREPARATION OF 0.2 *M* PHOSPHATE-BUFFERED SALINE, pH 7.2

Solution A: 31.2 g sodium dihydrogen phosphate in 1 L of distilled water
Solution B: 28.3 g disodium hydrogen phosphate in 1 L of distilled water
Working solution
1. Mix 140 ml Solution A with 360 ml Solution B.
2. Add 500 ml distilled water.
3. Add 8.1 g sodium chloride and stir to dissolve.
4. Adjust to pH 7.2 with 1 *N* HCl or 1 *M* NaOH.

16.12 SPECIALIZED TECHNIQUES

16.12.1 AMPLIFICATION OF IMMUNOCYTOCHEMICAL STAINING

In recent years, a new procedure has been introduced based on the deposition of biotinylated phenolic tyramide catalysed by peroxidase, resulting in the amplification of the number of biotin molecules that are available for binding to the subsequent reagent streptavidin peroxidase. The effect of this reaction is the development of a highly sensitive technique. At present, available are the Renaissance Tyramide Signal Amplification (TSA) kit from Dupont and the Catalysed Signal Amplification (CSA) kit from Dako. Advantages of using this procedure include the amplification of a weak signal when using certain antibodies, the possible reduction of incubation time, and the potential of a much greater dilution of primary antibody.

16.12.2 ENHANCED POLYMER ONE-STEP (EPOS™) TECHNIQUE

This is a direct method that employs a dextran polymer backbone which has attached a large number of primary antibody and enzyme peroxidase molecules. These antibodies bind to the antigens, but the technique is more sensitive than the conventional direct method due to the presence of an increased number of peroxidase molecules. Although several antibodies linked to the backbone are commercially available, the total number is not extensive, and therefore, the EPOS™ technique may not be considered to be suitable for many research uses.

16.12.3 ENVISION™

This is a further development of dextran polymer technology. A two-step indirect method is employed, in which secondary antibodies are conjugated with enzyme molecules to the polymer backbone. The commercial kits which are available for either peroxidase or alkaline phosphatase substrates (Dako) provide increased sensitivity and, of course, greater flexibility over the EPOS™ technique.

REFERENCES

Blythe, D., Hand, N.M., Jackson, P., Barrans, S.L., Bradbury, R.D., and Jack, A.S., The use of methyl methacrylate resin for embedding bone marrow trephine biopsies, *J. Clin. Pathol.*, 20, 35–38, 1997.

Elias, J.M., *Immunohistopathology: A Practical Approach to Diagnosis*, ASCP Press, Chicago, 1990.

Hand, N.M., Blythe, D., and Jackson, P., Antigen unmasking using microwave heating on formalin fixed tissue embedded in methyl methacrylate, *J. Cell Pathol.*, 1, 31–37, 1996.

Hand, N.M. and Church, R.J., Superheating using pressure cooking: its use and application in unmasking antigens embedded in methyl methacrylate, *J. Histotechnol.*, 21, 231–236, 1998.

Larsson, L.-I., Peptide immunocytochemistry, *Prog. Histochem. Cytochem.*, 13, 1981.

Miller, K., Immunocytochemical techniques, in *Theory and Practice of Histological Techniques*, J.D. Bancroft and A. Stevens, Eds., 4th ed., Churchill Livingstone, New York, 1996.

Naish, S.N., *Immunochemical Staining Methods*, DAKO Corp., 1989.

Index

MONGOLIA

op Nor

aklamakan   Sunwei   Yellow River
                         LANZHOU
                                              XI'AN

BE   CHINA

Y a
EPAL

es

                                                       South China
                                                            Sea

y of
ngal